National
Health Insurance

A Conference Sponsored by the
American Enterprise Institute for Public Policy Research

National Health Insurance

What Now, What Later, What Never?

Edited by Mark V. Pauly

American Enterprise Institute for Public Policy Research
Washington, D.C.

Library of Congress Cataloging in Publication Data

Main entry under title:

National health insurance.

    (AEI symposia ; 80C)
    Proceedings of a conference held by AEI's
Center for Health Policy Resarch in Washington, D. C.
    1.   Insurance, Health—United States—Congresses.
2.   Medical care, Cost of—United States—Congresses.
I.   Pauly, Mark V., 1941–
II.   American Enterprise Institute for Public Policy Research.
Center for Health Policy Research.
III.   Series: American Enterprise Institute for Public
Policy Research. AEI symposia ; 80C.
HD7102.U4N277   368.4′2′00973   80-22761
ISBN 0-8447-2184-0
ISBN 0-8447-2185-9 pbk.

AEI Symposia 80C

Printed in the United States of America

Contributors

Robert Glen Beck
Professor of Economics
University of Saskatchewan

Edgar K. Browning
Professor of Economics
University of Virginia

Linda A. Burns
Director, Center for Ambulatory Care
American Hospital Association

Karen Davis
Assistant Secretary for Public Health
U.S. Department of Health, Education, and Welfare

H. E. Frech III
Professor of Economics
University of California, Santa Barbara

Bernard Friedman
Professor of Economics
Northwestern University

Gilbert R. Ghez
Associate Professor of Economics
Roosevelt University

Paul B. Ginsburg
Congressional Budget Office

Thomas W. Grannemann
Mathematica Policy Research, Inc.

Michael Grossman
Director–Health Economics
National Bureau of Economic Research, Inc.
and Professor of Economics
City University of New York

Jeffrey E. Harris, M.D.
Associate Professor of Economics
Massachusetts Institute of Technology

Clark C. Havighurst
Professor of Law
Duke University

Edward F. X. Hughes, M.D.
Director, Center for Health Services
and Policy Research and Director, Program in
Hospital and Health Services Management
Northwestern University

Robert P. Inman
Associate Professor of Finance
and Economics
The Wharton School of the
University of Pennsylvania

William R. Johnson
Professor of Economics
University of Virginia

Harold S. Luft
Associate Professor of Health Economics
University of California, San Francisco

Glenn R. Markus
Congressional Research Service

Jack A. Meyer
Resident Fellow in Economics
American Enterprise Institute

Joseph P. Newhouse
The Rand Corporation

Mark V. Pauly
Professor of Economics
Northwestern University

Rudolph G. Penner
Director of Tax Policy Studies
American Enterprise Institute

Charles E. Phelps
Director, Regulatory Policies
and Institutions Program
The Rand Corporation

John B. Reiss
Director, Office of Health Regulation
Health Care Financing Administration
U.S. Department of Health, Education, and Welfare

Louis B. Russell
Senior Fellow
The Brookings Institution

Laurence S. Seidman
Professor of Economics
Swarthmore College

W. Kip Viscusi
Associate Professor of Economics
Northwestern University

Ronald J. Vogel
Director, Division of Economic Analysis
Health Care Financing Administration
U.S. Department of Health, Education, and Welfare

Contents

PART THREE
SOLVING THE PROBLEM OF OVERINSURANCE

PART FOUR
COST CONTAINMENT: LONG- AND SHORT-RUN STRATEGIES

National
Health Insurance
What Now, What Later, What Never?

Foreword

Almost a decade ago, Professor Mark Pauly, the editor of this volume, wrote an analysis for AEI of the ten major national health insurance bills then being considered.[1] He began that analysis with the statement, "The idea of national health insurance (NHI) is not new."[2] After giving a brief synopsis of the history of NHI, he pointed out that the renewed interest in the early 1970s was due to dissatisfaction with the rising cost of health care and that "those who favored greater public control over the medical care sector saw in NHI a vehicle for achieving such control. . . ."[3]

At first sight it would seem that the 1970s have contributed no fundamental change to the debate about NHI. Although several congressional hearings led to repeated predictions that passage of NHI legislation was "imminent" and "inevitable," Congress has still not passed an NHI bill. Both the prices of health services and the total private and public expenditures for them have continued to increase at very rapid rates. There is still concern that some segments of society do not receive adequate health care even though we have become a wealthier nation (real per capita disposable income has increased by 2.5 percent per year since 1970). In addition, the cost of Medicare and Medicaid has soared while at the same time significant gaps in coverage have persisted.

Even though these concerns are still with us, this volume illustrates that the character of the debate has changed since 1971. As a result of a decade of policy-related research, there now appears to be a greater willingness to question the basic concept of NHI as a grand solution to all the perceived problems in health. This skepticism is based in part on analysis of the growing cost of Medicare and Medicaid and of how these open-ended entitlement programs might affect government expenditures and hence other policy objectives. Research has increased our aware-

---

[1] Mark V. Pauly, *National Health Insurance: An Analysis* (Washington, D.C.: American Enterprise Institute, August 1971).

[2] Ibid., p. 1.

[3] Ibid., p. 2.

ness of how consumers use various kinds of insurance, especially their tendency to overuse health services when insurance pays most of the bill. Research has also begun to seek objective evidence about whether government programs, such as child health care, dental programs, and preventive health programs, actually do improve health. Research into the economic and political effects of direct government regulation has cast doubt on its ability to achieve effective cost control when conducted in a political atmosphere.

With the growth of skepticism about the ability of national health insurance to solve the real problems, health policy research has turned to the design of policies that might reduce the growth in public and private expenditures without reducing the high quality of care and the freedom of individual choice that we value in our present system. This volume brings together a group of people who have contributed important research to this debate and have the expert knowledge needed to discuss possible reforms. No one would claim that this or any other collection of experts has all the answers to the complex problems we face in health. They cannot tell us exactly what reforms should be made now, later, or never. But they can, as they have done in the last decade, lead us into a more realistic discussion of what change is needed and what changes might logically meet our objectives. In fact, in health, as in all areas of public policy addressed by this institute, AEI is dedicated to the principle that the development of good public policy requires this kind of informed debate. Although "the idea of national health insurance is not new" (as Professor Pauly reminded us in 1971), we feel that this volume will make a real contribution to the continuing debate, a debate that may now take a more meaningful direction.

We at AEI especially thank Professor Pauly for the excellent job he has done planning the conference, assembling such an outstanding group of authors and discussants, and editing the volume. We also thank Dr. Edward Hughes and the Center for Health Services and Policy Research of Northwestern University for their help with this conference and volume.

WILLIAM J. BAROODY, JR.
President
American Enterprise Institute
for Public Policy Research
August 1980

Introduction

Mark V. Pauly

Purpose and Framework for the Conference

Over the past decade, few issues have generated more public and legislative discussion, but less completed legislation, than national health insurance (NHI). One result of the lengthy debate is that issues and principles, even if once clearly stated, tend to be forgotten. Another result is that positions and programs, even if forcefully advocated, tend to be overshadowed by the sheer repetition of other arguments (though more arguments have clearly fallen by the wayside). A third and somewhat surprising characteristic of the discussion is that there are some important points that have so far been left unsaid or undeveloped. The purpose of this conference, held in Washington, D.C., in October 1979—approximately the tenth anniversary of the beginning of the NHI debate—was to address these problems.

NHI deals with both the deprivation of care and the absence of financial protection by providing more insurance than people presently have. In this sense, the present situation might be said to be characterized by "underinsurance." The conference dealt with the problem of underinsurance at considerable length, in a manner to be discussed below. But it is also important to note that there is at present an equally significant problem of "overinsurance"; many people have too much insurance of the wrong kind. The problem of overinsurance can only be exacerbated by piling more public insurance on top of presently excessive levels of private insurance. The topic of overinsurance—what it means and what its causes are—was also given serious discussion at the conference.

Whether NHI is to be general or selective, virtually all proposals involve additional outlays of public funds. With the federal budget already in serious deficit, and with the depressing influence of taxation on economic activity already a subject of much debate, it was appropriate for the the conference to investigate the budgetary and tax-incentive consequences of alternative NHI plans. Because some plans propose covering people who are not poor under mandated employer

1

benefits, it is also useful to look at this off-budget method of compulsory financing, to see whether it really avoids the deleterious effects of taxation or involves the introduction of new distortions of its own.

Finally, the support (such as it is) that many give to NHI may come not from any positive affection for an increase in taxation or public-sector activity, but rather from a feeling that there are no practical solutions to the health care crisis other than ones involving more government control and government financing. But there are "market-oriented" approaches that do provide alternatives—ones that rely on health maintenance organizations and on the greater competition and cost consciousness that accompanies increased out-of-pocket payments for easily budgeted expenses. The conference therefore gave a careful look at three practical aspects of such alternatives—income-related cost sharing, greater reliance on health maintenance organizations, and alteration of regulation to permit the emergence of competitive systems.

Main Themes Presented at the Conference

Underinsurance. Underinsurance does exist. The three papers that dealt with this subject reinforced concerns that already seem to be present in virtually all NHI legislation—that coverage needs to be improved for the poor, especially poor mothers and infants, and for persons suffering catastrophic expenses. They also point out that existing gaps in coverage are, by and large, caused not by "market failure" but rather by "government failure"—the failure of the political process to deal appropriately with the situation. The failure to pass legislation to deal with these tragic problems—virtually the only ones to have measurable health consequences—cannot be traced to opposition to NHI as such. Perhaps it has occurred because proponents of comprehensive NHI have been unwilling, for strategic reasons, to permit passage of a "partial" approach, out of fear that a good deal of the support for additional coverage would evaporate after the most pressing needs were met. In this sense, the poor and those with catastrophic illness have been held hostage for comprehensive NHI.

Although all three papers conclude that coverage should be increased, they suggest that such increases should have a scope and a method of implementation different from what is commonly suggested. First, Gilbert Ghez and Michael Grossman show that little of what is termed "preventive" care is effective, so that a general extension of insurance coverage to all preventive care is simply unwarranted on health grounds. They do show, in contrast, that care for pregnant women and infants does have measurable health benefits and that poor families could improve their levels of health if their preventive care were improved. But even here one cannot find a justification on the grounds of health for subsidizing additional insurance for children in upper income families.

Thomas Grannemann shows that the extensive cross-state variation in Medicaid eligibility criteria and maximum benefits is not the result of a failure of some states to appreciate the benefits of care for poor people or of a stubborn refusal of some states to shoulder their social burden. Rather, he shows that the present pattern is a rational response by states to incentives in the present Medicaid program. The fault, then, is in the design of the federal program, not in the states' responses. In particular, Grannemann shows that disparity in benefit levels is traceable to a suboptimal level of federal matching, while high eligibility requirements are a rational response of states to an excessive scope of services required to be covered. Readjustment of the matching rate—lowering it for low income states and raising it for high income states—plus a reduction in the scope of covered services, would reduce cross-state disparity and might induce states to bring in the poor who now are not categorically eligible for Medicaid.

Finally, Bernard Friedman examines the market for catastrophic insurance. He finds, contrary to the wisdom conventional in some circles, that catastrophic insurance coverage that would put a limit on a family's out-of-pocket expenses is easily available, cheap, and growing. The absence of coverage for some families is traceable not to a failure of markets for insurance to emerge, but rather to the existence of public catastrophic insurance—in the forms of spend-down provisions in Medicaid, public and private charity, and the willingness of hospitals to tolerate bad debts—with a deductible roughly equal to the family's wealth. If wealth is low, purchase of private catastrophic insurance only substitutes an insurance one must pay for in place of an insurance one received for free, and so such purchase could hardly be rational. Friedman, then, develops the case for mandated and income-conditioned catastrophic insurance.

Overinsurance. Overinsurance, its meaning, and its causes were the subjects of the next three papers. Unlike most other insurances, health insurance provides an incentive to the consumer to consume more of the product whose cost is being covered, because insurance reduces the out-of-pocket price for the service. Moreover, because of this price reduction, consumers are induced to buy care that is excessive in the sense of being worth less to them than its cost. Unless the community has some interest in encouraging greater use of medical care, the ideal amount of insurance for a family to have is an amount that

3

balances the risk reduction benefits of more insurance with the inducement to more excessive amounts of care.

Pauly defines insurance in excess of this amount as overinsurance. He argues that, in addition to the causes discussed in the other two papers in this session, it is possible that overinsurance is caused by a kind of spillover effect in which one person's purchase of additional insurance brings about an increase in the style, intensity, and cost of the medical care purchased by others. If this happens, then there should probably be a modest excise tax on noncatastrophic health insurance purchases by middle and upper income families.

The paper by Ronald Vogel points out that, at present, not only is health insurance tax exempt, it is in fact heavily subsidized via loopholes in the tax system. The deductibility of health insurance premiums and medical care costs in the federal personal income tax is one such loophole, but the most important tax subsidy is the exclusion of employer contributions for employee group health insurance from taxable income. For workers at most income levels, the effect of this subsidy is to make it cheaper to the worker to buy medical care, no matter how modest in amount, via insurance rather than through direct purchase. But the excessive insurance not only involves more administrative costs, it also induces excessive use of medical care. Vogel estimates the amount of the tax subsidy (from all sources) to be $10.6 billion in 1980.

Another kind of tax subsidy—this time to not-for-profit Blue Cross and Blue Shield plans—is indicated by H. E. Frech as a cause of overinsurance. Frech argues that the Blues use their tax advantages and other special concessions, such as lower rates for hospital care, to push for overly comprehensive insurance. The reason is both the ideological conviction that comprehensive coverage is somehow desirable and the historical association between the Blues and provider groups who benefit from the increased demand additional insurance causes. But the moral hazard associated with the increase in demand represents a loss in the overall welfare of society and a stimulus to the rising spiral of health care costs.

Financing of NHI. Another session at the conference dealt with the financing of any new NHI system, focusing especially on the financing of comprehensive NHI. The paper by Jack Meyer and Rudolph Penner of the American Enterprise Institute looks at the consequences of a typical expensive NHI scheme for the federal budget. They find that, even under the most favorable assumptions with regard to the success of a (now defeated) hospital cost containment bill, the cost of comprehensive NHI will add $27 billion to the federal budget. Enactment of NHI means that the tax increase that would be needed to reach the president's goal of a balanced budget by 1984 would have to be more than twice as large as it would need to be in the absence of NHI. Put another way, if NHI were not enacted and its cost were applied to the defense budget, defense spending could be increased (in real terms) by 4 percent rather than by 1.5 percent without unbalancing the president's budget.

In addition to the explicit budgetry cost, Edgar Browning and William Johnson show that there are some important implicit tax effects of a tax-financed NHI. A typical $50 billion NHI program would have two major effects. First, it would redistribute approximately $10 billion in income from the highest 20 percent of the income distribution to the lowest 20 percent. That leaves, of course, $40 billion which is returned in the form of health insurance to the same households that pay for it in taxes. But Browning and Johnson show that this transaction has costs of its own; there are substantial costs of economic distortion which accompany higher taxes. While precise estimation of this cost is not easy, Browning and Johnson show that it is far from trivial. Their best guess is that the welfare distortion cost of an extra dollar raised through taxation is about 20 cents. This implies that the replacement of private insurance and out-of-pocket spending by public tax-financed insurance would have to somehow yield additional benefits of at least 20 percent of the total expenditure. If much of NHI is just a "pass through" of funds, as even its supporters suggest, these estimates indicate that it would involve serious inefficiency.

An alternative way of financing NHI plans is through mandated employer payments. Charles Phelps shows, however, that this off-budget method of taxation has problems of its own. In particular, it will cause temporary unemployment or wage reductions. In the case of workers earning near the minimum wage, the temporary unemployment is highly likely to become permanent.

Phelps also shows that, during the 1970s, there was an "astonishing" increase in employer contributions to health insurance premiums. This means that the *additional* premium cost imposed on employers by mandated employer payments under NHI is reduced. Nevertheless, the required increases in 1980 expenditures are still substantial—$21 billion for an "intermediate" plan and $9 billion for the initial Carter administration proposal. The "tax expenditure" or reduction in federal income tax collections associated with these plans would generally amount to $3 to $7 billion. Unemployment would increase by a small but not trivial amount.

Improving Competition. The final set of papers deals with ways to improve the functioning of the competitive system in medical care, as an alternative to comprehensive public insurance and government planning. Larry Seidman shows that a system of income-conditional copayments can achieve an appropriate blend of equity and efficiency. It can contribute to the provision of adequate care for those in need, while preserving competitive influences and options for free choice for all. He contrasts this mixed competitive system with that of a fully regulated system financed by taxes, and finds the latter to be distinctly inferior. What is equally important, he shows that the federal income tax system provides a feasible and efficient way of handling the administrative problems of income-related copayments. In fact, the tax system could even be used to help people finance large medical bills by spreading out payments over time.

Harold Luft examines the potential value of the health maintenance organization (HMO) as a device for combining cost curtailment with comprehensive coverage in an NHI. He finds that the evidence that HMOs bring about a large reduction in medical care costs for their members is unconvincing and the evidence that introduction of HMOs into an area increases competition and thereby reduces expenditures is inconclusive. Although the evidence is strong that HMO members have lower costs than nonmembers and that this reduction comes about almost entirely from reductions in hospital use, Luft argues that this evidence does not prove that HMOs *cause* an expenditure reduction of the same order of magnitude. Comparisons are bedeviled by the problem of self-selection of HMO members; they voluntarily choose to join. This means that some (if not all) of the HMO "savings" could come from the self-selection of HMOs by people who are unwilling and unlikely to use hospitals in the first place—people with tastes against hospitalization. He reviews some evidence that people who join HMOs were relatively low hospital users even before they joined. He also looks at the evidence on the effect of HMOs on market-area expenditures and finds it inconclusive because of the difficulty of finding areas with significant HMO penetration outside of the West. In one of the few such areas—Minneapolis—Luft finds that significant HMO growth is not associated with an overall reduction in hospital use, providing further evidence of self-selection.

Finally, Clark Havighurst calls our attention to recent changes in federal health planning legislation which require area planners to take into account the effect of their decisions on competition and to give favorable treatment to applications that are likely to increase competition. He argues that, in at least some areas, these changes could be associated with strong encouragement to competitive systems and could be a way of bringing about coexistence between regulation and competition.

Conclusion

Several themes characterized the conference. The first, covered by virtually all the papers and many discussants, is that it is difficult to find an economic rationale for universal comprehensive first-dollar government health insurance. Such insurance would be expensive, would overload the federal budget, would increase tax burdens and tax distortions, but would be quite unnecessary. Indeed, for many Americans the problem is not too little insurance but too much. The gaps that do exist could be filled most effectively by programs, such as reforms of Medicaid and provision of catastrophic coverage, targeted particularly to those gaps.

The rising costs of medical care could be brought to a more appropriate level by increasing rather than reducing the public's opportunities to make tradeoffs between benefits and costs. Reduction or elimination of tax deductibility for individual and, especially, employer group health insurance would go a long way to reducing overinsurance. Income-conditioned public insurance, administered through the personal income tax system and probably integrated with a catastrophic insurance program, would greatly increase consumer cost-consciousness and competition.

Part
One

Initiating a
National Health Insurance Program:
Political and Economic Concerns

Impact of National Health Insurance Proposals on the Budget

Jack A. Meyer and Rudolph G. Penner

The purpose of this paper is to develop a framework for assessing the cost of national health insurance (NHI) proposals and to indicate the sort of sacrifices that would be necessitated by the introduction of such plans. Primary emphasis is placed on critically evaluating the Carter administration's cost projections for its National Health Plan, along with an assessment of the implications of implementing Phase I of this plan with regard to other goals such as balancing the federal budget, reducing the proportion of GNP accounted for by federal spending, and avoiding an increase in, or actually reducing, the burden of federal taxes.

A Framework for Analyzing Costs

Estimates of the cost of national health insurance depend not only upon the scope and coverage of alternative plans, which vary widely, but also upon the perspective on costs that is selected. Some proposals would cost more than others because they would cover more people, or cover a given population more comprehensively. But, for any given level of coverage for a stipulated universe, it is important to distinguish on-budget federal costs from total payments by individuals for health care, and to be cognizant of the difference between initial and ultimate costs of implementing a national health insurance blueprint.

Most national health insurance proposals affect health-care spending primarily by shifting the *composition* of spending or altering the *route* through which consumer outlays for health care flow. The proposals often call for new federal programs or funds, but federal outlays through these funnels typically displace some combination of federal and state spending already occurring under existing law.

In addition to affecting government outlays, most national health insurance plans would also alter federal tax revenues by changing the amount of allowable tax deductions for both households and firms. Mandated increases in employer payments for health insurance, for example, provide more tax-free income to employees as a result of the exclusion of such payments from employee income. By contrast, if

11

direct outlays by consumers are reduced as a result of greater employer or government payments on behalf of individuals, the value of the itemized deduction for medical expenses will decrease, increasing the federal taxes of households. Forgone federal income tax revenues from these two sources of health care-related deductions and exclusions are estimated to total $14.5 billion in 1980, of which $9.6 billion is accounted for by the exclusion of employer contributions.[1]

Although the focus of this discussion is on the impact of NHI plans on the federal budget, it is important to recognize that such plans typically generate substantial costs that do not appear in the federal budget. They do this by mandating costs in the private sector that appear as line-item expenses in business budgets or (in cases where mandated costs are shared by individuals) as rising direct outlays for health by households. The tendency to focus primarily on the impact of NHI proposals on the federal budget, glossing over its impact on private spending, is a specific case of a more general tendency to place exclusive emphasis on the impact of changes in the federal budget on inflation while the effect of government regulation receives insufficient attention. Our understandable urge to control what the government spends often overrides the need to scrutinize what it orders others to spend, as well as what it loans, legislates, and negotiates. This imbalance is exemplified by the contrast between the ferocious battling over President Carter's proposed $600 million reduction in Social Security benefits for fiscal year 1980 and the general acceptance of an EPA ozone standard (with questionable benefits), estimated to cost $14–19 billion per year.[2]

It is also important to distinguish what might be called "first-round" costs of NHI proposals from those costs that kick in during subsequent "phases" of a multi-year program, as well as from costs that would be induced by behavioral changes resulting from new programs and rules. Direct initial costs, which are easier to identify and estimate, include such items as insurance expenditures (by government, employers, or households) for households previously uninsured, increased expenditures for more comprehensive and expensive insurance for those previously insured (for example, covering previously uncovered services), and increased rates of reimbursement authorized for providers of health care serving particular subgroups of the population. Of course, some program features promise to *decrease* health spending, such as those that might establish reviews of the need for further treat-

[1] Congressional Budget Office, *Tax Subsidies for Medical Care: Current Policies and Possible Alternatives*, Washington, D.C., January 1980, pp. 1–3.

[2] Robert W. Crandall, "Is Government Regulation Crippling Business?" *Saturday Review* (January 20, 1979), p. 32.

ment by a group of professional "peers" or establish ceilings on physicians' fees or hospital charges. In addition, various program features may affect administrative costs. Some would create additional administrative costs (largely resulting from making new groups eligible for government assistance) while others would reduce such costs (for example, through cost savings resulting from standardizing health insurance policies).[3]

By altering the system of signals and incentives for participants in the health care system, new program features can raise or lower health costs. Moreover, changes in the rules of the game that impose little or no short-term cost may lead to significant long-run costs (or savings), while other changes may have a large, but one-time, impact on costs.

One important example of these dynamic properties of NHI proposals involves the relationship between insurance coverage and the demand for health care services. An increase in the proportion of health costs paid by insurance leads patients and their doctors to demand a greater amount (and a more expensive variety) of health services.[4] Furthermore, numerous studies have shown that the more patients pay for health care indirectly, through higher taxes, premiums and prices—rather than by direct payment of all or part of the fees and charges for diagnosis and treatment—the more health care they will demand.[5] National health insurance proposals obviously involve an extension of coverage to individuals previously uncovered, and in this respect are likely to increase the demand for health services. Similarly, most proposals entail more comprehensive coverage for various groups (for example, removing limits on hospital stays, adding drug benefits). But, proposals differ with respect to their provision for such practices as patient cost-sharing, prospective reimbursement (giving providers a fixed amount of revenue at the beginning of a period so that they have an incentive to limit the use of health services during the period), and peer reviews, which have the potential for reducing cost increases over

[3] See Gordon Trapnell, *A Comparison of the Costs of Major National Health Insurance Proposals*, U.S. Department of Commerce, National Technical Information Service, PB-259-153, Washington, D.C., September 1976, pp. 29–44.

[4] Martin Feldstein, "Quality Change and the Demand for Hospital Care," *Econometrica*, vol. 45, no. 7 (October 1977), pp. 1681–1702.

[5] See Anne A. Scitovsky and Nelda McCall, "Coinsurance and the Demand for Physician Services: Four Years Later," *Social Security Bulletin*, vol. 40, no. 5 (May 1977), pp. 19–27; Emmett B. Keeler, Daniel T. Morrow, and Joseph Newhouse, "The Demand for Supplemental Health Insurance: Do Deductibles Matter?" *Journal of Political Economy*, vol. 85, no. 4 (August 1977), pp. 789–801; and Jay Helms, Joseph Newhouse, and Charles E. Phelps, "Copayments and the Demand for Medical Care: The California Medicaid Experience," *Bell Journal of Economics*, vol. 9, no. 1 (Spring 1978), pp. 192–208.

time. In assessing the cost of NHI proposals, it is important to evaluate the merits of accompanying plans to offset or "finance" extensions of insurance coverage. Indeed, a major difference among alternative health care proposals (discussed further below) involves the type of approach each envisions for containing the added costs that would result from increased demand for medical services.

National health insurance proposals will all affect the demand for health care in the ways just described. But some proposals would also affect the supply of health services through a variety of controls or limitations on providers. Such constraints may include strengthening investment controls on hospitals, limiting physician fees and hospital charges, and influencing the number of physicians who train for various specialties. NHI proposals may also involve support for particular types of health service delivery mechanisms (for example, health maintenance organizations).

An assessment of the long-term implications of an NHI proposal on health care spending must account for the interaction of the effects on both the demand for care and the supply of care.

It is also important (and very difficult) to consider the ways in which a new health care program would interact with other health care programs and government programs in other areas, such as transfer payments for food or housing purchases. Will subsidized insurance be accounted for in these other programs in the calculation of benefit levels, and vice versa? How will reimbursement rules established by new health programs relate to limitations that might arise under incomes policy formulas?

Some uncertainty about the cost of an NHI program arises from the inability to predict the extent of utilization by the eligible population. Initial cost estimates may be predicated upon an assumption of 100 percent utilization for a particular group of eligibles, which may overestimate costs under actual program experience. But, it is also possible (as we learned with the food stamp program) that the eligible population will turn out to be larger than initially expected. The size of the group ultimately receiving benefits, of course, will affect the magnitude of the administrative costs associated with the program.

Finally, it is important to recognize that while consumers are concerned about rising health costs, they are interested in having services readily available. They are also concerned with the quality of those services. In this connection new health programs that promise both to extend demand and to limit supply may result in unwanted (and perhaps unforeseeable) side effects such as reduced access to care, longer waiting times, or a slowdown in health care advances.

14

Moreover, consumers are also concerned about general inflation, the growth of government, and the rising taxes needed to finance that growth. The tradeoff between those objectives and the objectives embodied in NHI proposals will be discussed in the final section of this paper.

The Administration's National Health Plan

The Carter administration's National Health Plan (NHP) would eventually provide health insurance coverage for all Americans.[6] In the initial phase of a five-stage plan, the program would provide the poor who are covered by Medicaid with unlimited hospital and physician services. It would also provide fully subsidized health benefits to an estimated 10.6 million people not covered by Medicaid, but whose income is less than 55 percent of the federal government's poverty standard, and another 4 million whose health expenses cause them to "spend down" to this 55 percent line. For an estimated 24 million nonpoor aged and disabled people, cost-sharing would be limited to $1,250 per person per year, the limit on fully subsidized hospital days would be removed, and physicians would be prohibited from billing patients for nonreimbursable charges. A standard package of benefits providing comprehensive protection against catastrophic costs would cover an estimated 156 million members of families with a full-time worker. Initially, the NHP would limit out-of-pocket expenses for these families to $2,500 per year. All Americans would receive complete coverage (with no cost-sharing) for prenatal, delivery, and first-year care of infants.

In subsequent phases the NHP would be converted into a universal, comprehensive plan by such measures as reducing cost-sharing, raising the 55 percent low-income standard, and extending fully subsidized infant care to the child's sixth year.

Under the NHP most employers would be directed to purchase coverage from private insurance firms with plans certified to meet federal standards. Those employers whose premiums would exceed 5 percent of payroll costs have the option of purchasing coverage, at subsidized rates, from a new government-sponsored insurance fund called Health Care, or of applying to Health Care for a comparable subsidy which could be applied to private premiums. Health Care would also cover the unemployed, the aged, the poor, and individual

---

[6] For an elaboration of the details of this plan see U.S. Department of Health, Education, and Welfare, *Fact Sheet: President Carter's National Health Plan Legislation*, Washington, D.C., June 12, 1979. Also, see the administration's proposed legislation—S.1812, 96th Congress, 1st session.

high-risk consumers. If NHP were enacted, employers would be required to pay at least 75 percent of the premiums in what is termed Phase I. The $2,500 cap on direct payments by households would be lowered as the plan developed.

The administration's hospital cost containment plan would determine reimbursement for hospital services under the NHP. Physicians who provide services to Health Care patients would be paid on the basis of a publicly set fee schedule, based initially on Medicare statewide averages and updated through a process of negotiation between the government and physicians. Private plans would be encouraged to use this fee schedule, and the names of physicians who adhere to it would be published by the government. The NHP would also attempt to decrease the number of physicians who train for specialties now considered to be in oversupply, while increasing the number of family practitioners. It would strengthen the federal government's role in health planning and controlling capital expenditures, further assist in the development of health maintenance organizations, and support preventive care and health education. The NHP would be financed through multiple sources—general tax revenues, premium payments by employers and employees, the Medicare payroll tax, and special excise taxes on alcohol and cigarettes.

Cost Estimates

In order to estimate the impact of the NHP on total spending and the federal budget, it is necessary to develop baseline estimates of the value of health spending by households and governments in the absence of any new initiatives. The Carter administration estimates total health system spending in FY 1980 at $148 billion for NHP covered services.[7] Of this projected total, $52.0 billion is accounted for by individual payments, $45.0 billion by federal spending, $42.6 billion by employer contributions, and $8.4 billion by state outlays. The administration's estimate of total health care spending under Phase I of the NHP (in FY 1980 dollars) is $166.3 billion, or an increase of $18.3 billion over the level of system-wide outlays that would occur under current law (see Table 1). This total increase is virtually identical to the projected increase in federal outlays ($18.2 billion), as the $6.1 billion increase in employer payments envisioned under Phase I is roughly offset by a decline in individual payments of $4.0 billion and a $2.0 billion drop in state payments. The bulk of the federal cost increase

---

[7] HEW, *Fact Sheet.* Actual total spending, including those services not covered by NHP, is likely to be roughly $230 billion in fiscal 1980.

TABLE 1

EXPENDITURES FOR COVERED SERVICES, CURRENT LAW AND UNDER THE NATIONAL HEALTH PLAN—PHASE I, FISCAL 1980
(in billions of dollars)

	Current Law	NHP Phase I	Change
Total spending[a]	$148.0	$166.3	+$18.3
Federal	45.0	63.2	+ 18.2
Employer	42.6	48.7	+ 6.1
Individual	52.0	48.0	− 4.0
State	8.4	6.4	− 2.0

[a] For NHP covered services.

is attributable to improved coverage for the poor ($10.7 billion) and the aged and disabled ($3.9 billion).[8]

At the present time the administration has not released cost figures beyond the first year of Phase I and is in the process of revising its Phase I figures. Phase I is scheduled to be implemented in 1983. A preliminary estimate of a $23–25 billion increase in systemwide outlays in 1983 dollars (and assuming a 1983 population) was noted in the June 1979 White House release. This range is $5–7 billion greater than the $18.3 billion estimate for the cost of Phase I in 1980 dollars. Presumably, the difference reflects the change in the population and health care inflation during the 1980–1983 period, as tempered by the anticipated impact of the proposed hospital cost containment legislation.

Assessment of Cost Estimates

The Carter administration seems unduly sanguine about the prospect of fully offsetting the cost increases emerging from its NHI proposal:

> Reductions from cost controls and system reform incentives are estimated to more than offset the expanded utilization and expenditures generated by the Phase I plan after the third year of operation. Even with the expansion to the fully implemented universal, comprehensive plan, total health

[8] Other categories of projected federal expenditures include $2.1 billion for administrative expense, $1.6 billion for subsidized care for low-wage or high-risk workers, $0.5 billion for Health Care fund coverage of those who do not fall into the employment, aged, disabled, or poverty groups and $ −0.6 billion for tax effects.

spending is expected to be lower than it would be under the current system.[9]

There are several reasons why these expectations are unlikely to be fulfilled. First, the hospital cost containment legislation, a mainstay of the administration's plan to control cost increases, has not been enacted by Congress though it has been under consideration for more than two years.

Second, the particular form of the current cost-control proposal seems to be so riddled with exclusions, exceptions, and contingencies as to make it unlikely that it would have any bite. Three triggers must go off before any hospital can possibly be in jeopardy. Labor costs, now accounting for about 50 percent of total costs for the average hospital, are, in effect, exempted from the controls. There are numerous ways in which hospitals could unbundle services or spin off functions to evade the intent of the proposal.[10] Finally, there is wide latitude for HEW to grant special adjustments or exemptions for various special circumstances.

Third, even with more bite, the proposal would seem capable of producing only short-term results, and some of these results, especially service cutbacks or quality reductions, may not be desirable.

Since the system of financial incentives and reimbursement mechanisms would essentially remain unchanged, there is little reason to believe that the legislation would spur hospitals to eliminate inefficiencies rather than redefine, relocate, or simply cut services. The legislation seems to presume (probably incorrectly) that hospital administrators, responding to an overall spending ceiling, would be able easily to recognize and isolate wasteful expenditures. Instead, this proposal might cut cost increases largely by cutting back on the quality of care in ways not desired by consumers.

CBO's estimates of the savings arising from the proposed 1979 Hospital Cost Containment Act are considerably lower than the administration's estimates. CBO's estimated reduction in annual hospital inpatient revenues in fiscal year 1980 is $1.2 billion,[11] as compared with the administration's estimated savings of $2.3 billion. The corresponding figures for FY 1984 are $11.3 and $19.2 billion.[12] The

---

[9] From HEW, *Fact Sheet*, p. 35.

[10] See Congressional Budget Office, *Controlling Rising Hospital Costs*, Budget Issue Paper for Fiscal Year 1980, September 1979, pp. 29–30.

[11] Includes small savings from fiscal 1979. Figures apply to version of the administration's bill reported by the Senate Committee on Labor and Human Resources (S.570).

[12] CBO, *Controlling Rising Hospital Costs*, pp. 29–38. The CBO estimate of $11.3 billion in 1984 savings comprises $4.1 billion and $0.62 billion in reduced

latter figure—the administration's estimate of 1984 savings from cost containment—roughly corresponds with its estimate of the NHI cost for the first year in which it would be implemented ($18.3 billion in FY 1983), explaining its contention that the two bills would offset one another from a cost viewpoint. But, the CBO figure of $11.3 billion—almost $8 billion less projected savings—suggests that this contention is overoptimistic. Moreover, the CBO report states that its own estimates may be too high because of such factors as offsets arising from increased outpatient expenditures (not accounted for in the CBO estimates), exceptions granted by HEW, and possible evasion techniques employed by hospitals, such as spinning off various hospital functions.[13]

The CBO estimate of the cumulative savings from the administration's cost containment bill over the 1980–1984 period is $24.6 billion. Its corresponding estimate for an alternative bill reported by the Senate Committee on Labor and Human Resources (S. 570) is $28.6 billion, while the comparable figure for the House version (H.R. 2626) is $20.3 billion.

Finally, even if the administration's estimate of cost containment savings is accepted for the first or second year of NHI implementation, it is highly unlikely that any ongoing savings would fully offset the swelling cost of NHI in its subsequent phases. Furthermore, to the extent that many hospitals "comply" with cost containment by cutting services or slowing quality improvements, we would, curiously, be "financing" NHI's health benefit improvements for some consumers through cutbacks in the benefits of other consumers. Indeed, some consumers may lose on one hand the advantages gained on the other. They may obtain improved insurance coverage (with more services reimbursed) at a lower cost, but receive a style of care when they are in a hospital that falls short of their desired treatment.

The administration also proposes relying on a process of "negotiations" to update allowable fees for doctors serving people covered by Health Care. Private plans would be encouraged to use the publicly set fee schedule for Health Care patients, and the names of physicians who adhere to it would be published by the government. Negotiations over allowable fee schedules could be expected to degenerate into a test of political strength, and it is by no means clear that the government would have the bargaining strength to achieve its targets. Moreover, by clamping a lid on allowable charges to Health Care patients, the

---

Medicare and Medicaid payments, respectively, and $6.6 billion of nonfederal savings. These figures are lower than those reported earlier by CBO because they updated their projections.

[13] CBO, *Controlling Rising Hospital Costs*, p. 30.

government may inadvertently foster a situation in which these patients have relatively less access to timely, high quality services.

In addition to savings arising from the proposed hospital cost containment bill, the administration's plan also envisions savings from "incentive effects." But, regrettably, such favorable effects are likely to be limited under the Carter proposal. The NHP's answer to a lack of consumer choice among alternative delivery systems—an important cause of health care cost escalation[14]—is further government stimulus to HMOs. This would be done through such means as requiring employers of twenty-five or more workers to offer their employees a choice between an insurance plan or participation in any HMO in the area. But, federal efforts to stimulate the growth of HMOs as alternatives to traditional fee-for-service health care delivery in this fashion have not met with much success since the passage of the 1973 HMO legislation. Requirements that HMOs maintain standards of comprehensiveness which, in some cases, exceed those typically found in private health insurance policies, along with preferences by many consumers for a fee-for-service arrangement with free choice of doctors, have limited the development of HMOs. More important, the president's NHP proposal offers little incentive for a *variety* of health delivery models— differing in one respect or another from either classical HMOs or traditional fee-for-service models—to develop and compete.[15]

Moreover, the Carter proposal would solidify the current job-centered nature of most insurance purchases, in which employers frequently provide their workers either a single insurance package or the choice between a standard package of benefits and an HMO, with no cost savings (penalty) to the worker for selecting the low (high) cost option. The administration's insistence on a standard minimum benefit package throughout the private economy tends to make the choice of insurance—one place in the health care area where the consumer clearly *could* have control over health expenditures—a rigid one (if there is any choice at all), in the name of administrative simplicity and equity. This is not to deny the advantages of group insurance emanating from reduced administrative costs. We need not thwart the effort to provide workers insurance as a group or an employee unit. What is essential is to provide such a group a meaningful choice

---

[14] See Alain C. Enthoven, "Consumer-Centered vs. Job-Centered Health Insurance," *Harvard Business Review*, vol. 57, no. 1 (January-February 1979), pp. 141–152.

[15] For an explanation of the advantages of such variety, see Walter McClure, "On Broadening the Definition of and Removing Regulatory Barriers to a Competitive Health Care System," *Journal of Health, Politics, and Law*, vol. 3, no. 3 (Fall 1978), pp. 303–307.

among *various* health packages (not just the streamlined HMO alternative), and ensure that the workers benefit from the selection of a relatively low-cost option.

The proposal does provide for equal employer contributions to alternate plans, with employees permitted to obtain the savings from selecting a low-cost plan, and this is a step in the right direction. But the favorable impact of this feature is limited by the fact that plans must provide all of the benefits stipulated in the legislation. As this "minimum package" is enriched over time, it would place a high floor on costs and thereby limit possible savings. One of the reasons that the cost of the administration's NHI proposal is likely to balloon over time is that it fails to stimulate meaningful competition, and indeed may unintentionally retard it, because of its emphasis on a standard benefit package rather than a variegated set of alternatives.

It is also worth noting that the provision for patient cost-sharing up to a maximum of $2,500 per year contemplated by this plan could act as a deterrent to the overconsumption of health services. However, this advantage may dwindle over time, as the plan envisions scaling down the cap on household cost-sharing. Another potentially positive feature in this regard is the provision enabling employers who qualify for subsidized insurance through the new Health Care fund to take the cash equivalent of the subsidy and use it to purchase private insurance.[16]

Thus, the Carter plan bows in the direction of the two market-oriented approaches to slowing down cost increases—consumer cost sharing and a more competitive environment for insurance plans and health care delivery models. But in both cases the steps taken are tentative, and their potentially favorable impact is limited by other features of the program. On balance, it seems likely that the NHP proposal would feed rather than reduce health care cost escalation.

A discussion of the run-out costs of NHP, of course, must also account for the greater program costs that will emerge in the future due to benefit enrichment and more widespread coverage. Although the current proposal does not specify the exact timing of such benefit improvements, it does suggest that minimum insurance coverage will be made more comprehensive and more widely available. First, the plan envisions covering all of the poor, whereas in Phase I only those with

---

16 There could be some negative effects from presenting employers with the option to buy into Health Care if their costs exceed 5 percent of payroll—the current HEW criterion. Employers whose health costs comprise a little less than this proportion of total costs may have an incentive to let their costs ride up so as to qualify for the Health Care subsidy. For those who do qualify, the treatment of the subsidy as a kind of voucher that can be used anywhere is a positive feature of the proposal that could promote greater variety in insurance plans. But, the NHP mandate of a standard minimum benefit package would limit this effect.

incomes below 55 percent of the poverty line will be automatically covered. In view of the HEW estimate that it will cost $5.5 billion to cover those below the 55 percent threshold and the likelihood that there are more people in the non-Medicaid poor group between this threshold and the poverty line than there are beneath the threshold, the cost of filling this gap would probably exceed $5.5 billion. Indeed, HEW estimates that Phase I coverage of that portion of the poverty group who "spend down" to the threshold would cost $3.8 billion. If this estimate assumes that about one of four households eligible for this spend-down provision use it (and that it would cost about the same per household to cover those who do not), a rough estimate of $15–16 billion—in 1980 dollars—emerges for covering the whole group between the 55 percent threshold and the poverty line.

Second, the plan envisions extending and enriching the employer guarantee. Part-time workers are ultimately to be included, and it is reasonable to assume that this will add at least $1 billion to employer costs.[17] And, according to the administration's proposals, "Cost-sharing could be reduced and deductibles eliminated, converting catastrophic coverage to comprehensive coverage."[18] This, of course, represents an immediate transfer of costs from households to employers, but could ultimately increase total outlays if consumers use more health services with a smaller cost constraint.

There are several other areas in which the Carter administration's plan contemplates broader benefits during subsequent phases of NHI. First, cost-sharing would be reduced for the aged and disabled, who would also begin to receive drug benefits. Second, the plan would ultimately extend the prenatal, delivery, and infant benefit through the child's sixth year without patient cost-sharing. Third, comprehensive coverage could be required for people outside of the labor force who are neither poor nor aged. Such people would have the option in Phase I of "buying into" the Health Care fund. This group would include people who are spouses of Medicare recipients but not eligible themselves, disabled people for whom a mandatory disability benefit waiting period has not elapsed, and single people who are not in the work force, but have sufficient income from non-working sources to be above the poverty level. Finally, administrative costs and tax effects would change as the coverage and comprehensiveness of the program changes. At the present time there are no cost estimates available for these

---

[17] Currently, part-time workers are about 20 percent of the size of the group working full-time. Since HEW estimates that it will cost employers $6.1 billion to cover full-time workers, one could begin by estimating that it would cost another $1.2 billion to cover the part-time work force (20 percent of $6.1 billion).

[18] HEW, *Fact Sheet*, p. 40.

proposed benefit changes, but they would clearly add to the out-year costs of NHP.

Other Proposals

An alternative national health plan with a more ambitious timetable for implementation has been proposed by Senator Edward M. Kennedy, and various catastrophic illness bills are being supported by other members of Congress.[19] A comparative assessment of all of these proposals is beyond the scope of this paper. It is worth noting, however, that the Kennedy plan basically represents an approach similar to the Carter plan, though there are differences in timing and substance. The Kennedy plan has somewhat broader coverage, as reflected in the figure for total U.S. spending (in 1980 dollars) for health services covered by the plan—$171.4 billion. The corresponding figure for the Carter plan is $148.0 billion. If the Kennedy plan were implemented in FY 1983, total spending for covered services would rise to an estimated $211.4 billion (in 1980 dollars), representing a projected total program cost of $40 billion for the first year,[20] as compared with the figure of $18.3 billion for the Carter plan. Much of the difference, of course, represents the phasing of the Carter proposal rather than major differences in ultimate coverage. Of the $40 billion initial cost of the Kennedy program, $28.6 billion would be accounted for by rising on-budget federal costs (which would total $79.6 billion under the Kennedy plan instead of the projected $51.0 billion for comparable services under current law).

An alternative proposal by Senator Schweiker (S.1590) would require employers with 200 or more workers to offer their employees three or more health plans from three different carriers, with at least one containing a 25 percent hospital copayment (but no more than 20 percent of family income). The tax deductions for employer contributions to insurance would be tied to offering workers at least three plans, making equal contributions to all plans, and allowing employees selecting a low-cost plan to receive tax-free rebates. The tax benefits would also be tied to a requirement that all plans contain a minimum level of catastrophic protection and coverage for preventive treatments. Schweiker's plan would also restructure Medicare to provide catastrophic coverage and encourage state risk pooling programs for employees of small firms, the self-employed, and uninsurable risks.

---

[19] Such bills have been introduced by Senator Long (S.760) and Senators Dole, Danforth, and Domenici (S.748).

[20] See *Congressional Record*, vol. 125, no. 112, 96th Congress, 1st session, September 6, 1979, pp. 60–61.

Unlike the Carter and Kennedy plans, this proposal would take steps in the direction of modifying tax incentives and stimulating broad choices among competing health plans, two changes that are vital to the achievement of lasting moderation in cost escalation.

The Problem with the Carter and Kennedy Proposals

The ultimate cost impact of either the Carter or Kennedy proposals will hinge on the capacity of their constraints on providers permanently to limit cost increases. Neither proposal would significantly alter the structural forces stimulating demand, but both would intensify the upward pressure on demand by broadening insurance coverage and making it more comprehensive. This upward pressure is to be "contained" by controls on charges and the anticipated challenge from federally qualified HMOs.

The problem with these proposals is not that they aim to extend insurance coverage to millions of Americans who currently lack coverage or that they seek to remove various limitations on the coverage that others currently maintain. Whether we want to ensure that all Americans have a comprehensive package of health insurance benefits is an important policy question, but its answer will only be a first step in evaluating the impact of NHI on private health care costs and the federal budget. The ultimate impact of guaranteeing a minimum insurance package to everyone would depend on the mechanisms established to discourage wasteful spending on health care. Starting from the premise that such waste emanates largely from providers' control over patients and their desire to increase earnings or profits by over-testing and over-hospitalizing unwary patients, these NHI proposals would attempt to "finance" NHI through a squeeze on providers. This squeeze is likely to be counter-productive, leading either to greater cost acceleration or cuts in services, while the fundamental forces leading to waste —inextricably involved with the growth and current nature of insurance—are left unaltered.

The argument over the Carter and Kennedy proposals is, in a sense, a microcosm of the controversy over government attempts to clamp economy-wide controls on suppliers while simultaneously stimulating demand in the overall economy. And the result—rapid cost and price increases, shortages, and quality problems—is likely to be the same. Past attempts to increase the rate of growth in a nation's money supply above the pace that would otherwise be considered prudent, relying on wage and price controls to ensure that this excessive growth improves real variables such as production and employment without an acceleration in inflation, have typically resulted first in various short-

24

falls in supply and "black markets," and ultimately in a spurt in inflation as controls are relaxed.

Similarly, if the demand for health services is stimulated through substantial increases in the depth and breadth of insurance coverage while supply is constrained through controls on hospital beds and charges, as well as on physician supply and fees, the result will tend to be a combination of longer waiting times for treatments, a deterioration in the quality of services, and an explosion in costs when consumers ultimately insist on a restoration of the kind of services to which they have grown accustomed.

The Carter and Kennedy proposals would convert the *carrot* of open-ended tax breaks (designed to encourage comprehensive insurance) into a *mandate*; yet they would leave the tax breaks intact, failing even to convert them into fixed-dollar credits that would limit their yield. Thus, everyone would receive automatically what the government deems minimal insurance protection, and get rewarded for doing so through tax incentives that become a kind of windfall. And, the proposals forgo an opportunity to encourage meaningful competition among a variety of alternative delivery systems by taking a "uniform package" approach, rather than stimulating the kind of heterogeneous insurance environment in which consumers can select the mix of benefits, costs, and risks that suits their own tastes.

Of course, the aim of these proposals is not simply to control health care cost increases—their primary goal is to ensure access to care for all U.S. citizens irrespective of age and income. But, both proposals allege that this assurance can be given *without* a major long-term impact on costs (through a system of strict controls on providers), and it is *this pledge* that is misleading. If we are going to insure everyone, and remove the cost consequences of major illness, we are going to have to pay for it. Through an elaborate system of provider controls it may be possible to divert temporarily some of this cost from a monetary to a nonmonetary form, but we cannot make the cost evaporate.

Efforts to freeze the share of GNP accounted for by health care expenditures by negotiating or legislating "acceptable" fees and charges fly in the face of free consumer choices. Rather, we should strive to alter those forces distorting consumer choices and feeding wasteful spending so that such growth in the health care share of GNP as occurs is simply a manifestation of consumer preferences for more health care, for which they are willing to sacrifice more of some other goods and services. Surely, we do not want to freeze permanently the shares of the economic pie accounted for by food, health, housing, etc.

Housing costs have also been rising as a share of GNP (and we provide open-ended subsidies for a significant portion of the cost of owner-occupied housing). Are we to cap this growth by controls on home builders?

There is growing evidence, both from studies of controls on hospitals[21] and from more general evaluations of cost-plus regulatory interventions, that a regulatory approach to cost containment will not provide the hoped-for results. Indeed, the increasingly complex body of federal and state regulations is beginning to be viewed as much as a *part* of the health cost problem as its *cure*. Given this mounting evidence, it becomes increasingly important that an effort to increase insurance coverage, if undertaken, be accompanied by structural modifications that hold more promise for a lasting abatement of wasteful spending.

NHP and the Federal Budget

The administration's health initiative comes at a time when the budget is being buffeted by a variety of forces, all of which are putting upward pressures on outlays. As recently as January 1979, or before NHP was proposed, the Office of Management and Budget was projecting fiscal 1984 outlays at $673.7 billion. Only six months later, deteriorating short-run economic conditions combined with the introduction of the NHP and new energy initiatives caused OMB to raise the projection by $64.3 billion, a 9.5 percent increase. Both of these budget projections are made on the basis of long-range economic assumptions that are consistent with the unrealistic goals of the Humphrey-Hawkins Act. When OMB shifts to more realistic, or what it calls "alternative economic assumptions,"[22] projected 1984 outlays are raised another $36.7 billion.

Although President Carter once had the goal of reducing federal outlays to 21 percent of the GNP by 1981 (compared with about 22 percent in 1978), the new projections based on the alternative assumptions would not attain this goal by 1982 and only bring outlays slightly below 21 percent of the GNP by 1984. This assumes, of course, that there are no new spending initiatives between 1980 and 1984 other than those that have already been announced.

---

[21] See, for example, David S. Salkever and Thomas W. Bice, *Hospital Certificate-of-Need Controls: Impact on Investment, Cost, and Use* (Washington, D.C.: American Enterprise Institute, 1979); and Frank A. Sloan and Bruce Steinwald, "Effects of Regulation on Hospital Costs and Input Use," paper presented at the Annual Meeting of the American Economic Association, Chicago, Illinois, August 29, 1978.

[22] For details, see Office of Management and Budget, *Mid-Session Review of the 1980 Budget*, July 12, 1979, pp. 72–73.

To understand the difficulty of lowering outlays relative to the GNP, it is necessary to take a brief look at the budget decisions of the past two decades. Since the Korean War, there has been an explosion in the non-defense outlays of the federal government. Between 1955 and 1978 such outlays rose from 7.5 to 16.9 percent of the GNP. Over the same period, federal tax burdens rose only slightly, because we were able to finance the increase in non-defense activities by lowering defense spending from 10.5 to 5.1 percent of the GNP and by accepting a strong upward trend in the deficit. It appears obvious that we can no longer continue along this path. A broad political consensus has developed that favors increased defense spending and many believe that it should grow faster than the GNP. An even larger proportion of the population has become hostile to budget deficits, and in the midst of a tax revolt, it is hard to imagine rapid increases in tax burdens.

The problem could be solved if the growth in non-defense programs could be halted, but this will prove extremely difficult, if not impossible. Much of the expansion in these programs in the middle 1960s and early 1970s involved the creation of new entitlement programs or vast increases in older entitlement programs, such as social security. In other words, the new and expanded programs promise a stream of benefits to precisely defined recipient groups. Those groups will fight vigorously to see that the promises are not violated. Before the 1970s, the promises were made in money terms, and it was sometimes (although not often) possible to let them erode in real terms. But in the early 1970s indexing was introduced, that is to say, the programs promised not only money but also protection against inflation. A further problem arises because a very large portion of entitlement assistance goes to the aged, and the over sixty-five population will grow more than twice as fast as the total population throughout the 1980s. Thus, the nation faces a difficult budget situation even before major new initiatives, such as NHP, are considered.

In the following discussion, the administration's own budget projections through 1984, including NHP, will be examined in some detail. It is necessary to emphasize that those projections do not reflect administration policy for all programs. They reflect decisions already made for some programs, but current services projections for all others. The administration's cost estimates for the NHP and other programs will be accepted even though they may, as we have seen, prove decidedly optimistic.

By drawing out the implications of the budget projections, we shall provide a basis for judging whether the populace wants national health insurance badly enough to accept the significant sacrifices that are implied either in the form of other program cuts, deficits, or higher

TABLE 2

ACTUAL BUDGET OUTLAYS FOR 1978 AND PROJECTIONS FOR 1984, SELECTED FUNCTIONS

(dollar amounts in billions)

	1978	1984
National defense	105.2	181.0
Energy	5.9	9.2
Health	43.7	107.0[a]
Social security	92.2	173.0
Veterans' benefits and services	19.0	23.1
Interest	44.0	68.4
Allowances for contingencies	—	29.8[a]
All other functions	140.8	183.2
Total	450.8	774.7
Total as a % of GNP	21.9	20.8[b]

[a] In Office of Management and Budget, *Mid-Session Review of the 1980 Budget*, the cost of NHP is included under "allowances for contingencies." In the above table, $27 billion has been taken out of "allowances" and put into the health function. This cost estimate assumes a lower inflation rate than in the "alternative" economic assumptions.

[b] Fiscal GNP figures were estimated from the calendar year data provided in the *Mid-Session Review of the 1980 Budget*.

SOURCE: Office of Management and Budget, *Mid-Session Review of the 1980 Budget*, July 1979.

tax burdens. We shall not attempt to make this judgment ourselves, but will, instead, leave that difficult task to the reader.

The analysis will accept the "alternative" economic assumptions of the administration. These are not unduly optimistic. For the period 1978–1984, they imply an average annual real growth rate for GNP of 2.8 percent, an average annual inflation rate of 7.5 percent, and a 1984 unemployment rate of 5.6 percent.

Table 2 provides projections of selected budget functions for fiscal 1984 and compares them to actual outlay figures for fiscal 1978.

Although these projections show outlays declining slightly relative to GNP between 1978 and 1984, it is important to note that the deficit in 1978 was equivalent to 2.4 percent of the GNP. Therefore, a balanced budget in 1984 would require about a 7 percent increase in tax burdens[23] above 1978 levels. This implies a peacetime record-high tax burden in 1984, and it is worth noting that even the 1978 tax burden was slightly above the average prevailing over the previous

---

[23] The tax burden is defined very crudely as the ratio of budget receipts to GNP.

twenty-five years. The required tax increase could be slightly more than cut in half if NHP were eliminated from the projections.

But it must be emphasized that the projections are highly optimistic.. They imply a real increase in defense spending of about 1½ percent per year in the face of the president's goal of 3 percent per annum and the requirement stipulated by numerous senators for real increases up to 5 percent per year in order to make SALT acceptable. The social security projection assumes certain cuts in the program which were advocated in the 1980 budget, but which have already been rejected in perfunctory fashion by the Congress. The projection of veterans' benefits implies a real decrease in outlays of over 20 percent despite the fact that the 1980s will see the retirement of the huge cohort of World War II veterans. The interest projection assumes a more rapid approach to a balanced budget than now seems likely, and the allowance for contingencies provides for civilian pay increases of only 5.5 percent per year over the period, whereas the President has already relented and allowed a 7 percent increase for 1979.

Despite all of these optimistic biases, it is necessary to decrease "all other functions" by 3 percent per year in real terms in order to keep total outlays as low as 20.8 percent of the GNP. Given that the "all other" category includes functions such as agriculture, transportation, education, training, unemployment, and social services, such a rapid decline seems quite implausible.

It has already been noted that if the outlay projections are accepted, the elimination of NHP could lower the necessary tax increase by more than 50 percent, or from about 7 to about 3 percent. Another way of looking at the problem is to specify the trade-off between NHP and other programs. For this purpose, it is assumed that in 1984, the public will be willing to accept a tax burden equivalent to 20.8 percent of the GNP.

First, assume that the estimated $27 billion cost of NHP in 1984 were used instead for defense. The 1½ percent annual real growth rate in defense spending under the administration assumptions could then be increased to about 4 percent. Alternatively, instead of allocating the NHP cost to defense, assume that it is used to finance "all other functions." Then, without the NHP, the decline in this category could be held to less than one percent per year instead of declining at a real rate of 3 percent per year, as it does in the administration projections.

It should again be emphasized that the budget projections described above are extremely tenuous and could be made totally irrelevant by a foreign policy crisis or a severe domestic recession. They are used here only as a base to give a crude idea of the sort of sacrifices that would be necessitated by the introduction of the first phase of NHP. These sacrifices have probably been understated because the assumed 1984 cost of $27 billion is likely to be much too low for all of the reasons discussed in the first section of this paper and because the other program projections are highly optimistic. As subsequent phases of NHP are introduced, the budget cost will soar relative to the GNP. The implied sacrifices will be mitigated somewhat, because in subsequent phases, NHP should substitute to some extent for private spending; but the net cost will still be enormous. Whether voters will perceive that the benefits of NHP are worth such sacrifices, we shall let the reader decide.

Taxation and the Cost of National Health Insurance

Edgar K. Browning and William R. Johnson

Any expenditure program undertaken by the government has a cost the public must bear, usually in the form of taxes. A balanced evaluation of the program must not only consider the effects of the expenditures but also the consequences of the required taxes. National health insurance is no exception to these general statements. Yet the differential impacts of the proposed methods of financing alternative NHI plans have been given very little attention.[1] Taxes are simply a "necessary evil" that lurk in the background of most discussions. In this paper, to foster a more balanced view, we bring financing issues to the foreground by emphasizing how taxes influence the consequences of NHI plans.

Taxes are important in an evaluation of NHI for two somewhat different reasons. One is well known: Given a specific expenditure pattern, the taxes used to finance this expenditure determine the overall, or net, effect of the entire program on the distribution of income. The second reason is less well understood: The real cost of financing a given expenditure will vary with the method of finance. More specifically, most taxes impose a cost on the public that is greater than the amount of revenue collected. The extra cost (in addition to the revenue actually collected), called an "excess burden" or "welfare cost" by economists, becomes part of the real cost of financing NHI.

This paper is divided into two main sections, to consider these two issues in turn. The first section focuses on the distributional effects of the taxes used to finance an NHI plan, beginning with an overview of the present U.S. tax system and then estimating the benefits and costs by income classes for a hypothetical NHI plan. The second section

---

[1] The significance of taxes for distributional issues, the topic discussed in section 1 of this paper, has been considered by several authors. See Martin S. Feldstein, Bernard Friedman, and Harold Luft, "Distributional Aspects of National Health Insurance Benefits and Finance," *National Tax Journal*, vol. 25 (December 1972), pp. 497–510; R. Fein, "Impact of National Health Insurance on Financing," R. Eilers and S. Moyernan, eds., *National Health Insurance Conference Proceedings* (The Leonard Davis Institute of Health Economics, 1971), pp. 75–103; and B. Mitchell and W. Schwartz, "The Financing of National Health Insurance," *Science*, vol. 192 (May 1976), pp. 621–636.

deals with the welfare cost of taxes. It explains the nature and determinants of this cost and develops estimates of the welfare cost for the hypothetical NHI plan examined.

Distribution of Benefits and Costs

Current Tax System. Since most NHI proposals envisage securing the necessary revenue from existing federal tax instruments, a brief discussion of the current tax system will prove helpful. The federal government relies largely on four types of taxes: personal income, payroll, corporation income, and excise. Since each of these distributes burdens among income classes in a different way, the exact tax or mix of taxes used to finance NHI will have a decided impact on the distribution of the cost of the program.

Table 1 gives estimates of the distribution of tax burdens for each type of tax in 1976 by income decile (each containing 10 percent of all households, and ranked from lowest income, decile 1, to highest, decile 10). The estimates are given in the form of average tax rates: the total tax burden of each decile divided by its total before-tax income. Before discussing these figures, one general point should be made.

TABLE 1

DISTRIBUTION OF TAX BURDENS
(average tax rates; percentages)

Income Decile (1)	Federal Personal Income Tax (2)	Federal Payroll Taxes (3)	Other Federal Taxes (4)	State and Local Taxes (5)	All Taxes (6)
1	0.6	3.3	3.1	4.7	11.7
2	1.6	3.9	2.7	4.4	12.5
3	2.6	5.4	3.0	5.2	16.3
4	4.0	6.9	3.1	6.0	20.2
5	5.5	8.0	3.3	6.5	23.2
6	6.9	8.5	3.2	6.9	25.5
7	8.1	8.2	3.3	7.1	26.7
8	9.1	7.9	3.4	7.7	28.1
9	10.2	7.2	4.0	8.6	30.0
10	11.6	3.8	8.5	14.4	38.3

SOURCE: E. K. Browning and W. R. Johnson, *The Distribution of the Tax Burden* (Washington, D.C.: American Enterprise Institute, 1979), tables 14 and 15.

The definition of before-tax income used here is considerably broader than that commonly used. In addition to cash income, we have included in our measure of before-tax income: cash and in-kind government transfers, imputed income of owner-occupied housing, accrued capital gains (for example, proxied by undistributed corporate profits), and business taxes paid that would have otherwise been received as income by households. The reason for using this broader measure of income is that it corresponds more closely to the economic meaning of the term income than does, for example, adjusted gross income. One result of using a broader definition of income is that the estimated tax rates are lower than generally reported. Note, for example, our finding that the national average rate under the federal income tax is only 8.5 percent. Alternatively, if measured as a percentage of adjusted gross income (what many families think of as their before-tax income), the national average rate is about 13 percent. The difference is due to our use of a broader concept of income, not to any underestimate of tax liabilities.

Returning to Table 1, it will be noted that all major federal taxes are generally progressive in their incidence. (A progressive tax is one in which the average tax rates rise with income. A regressive tax exhibits declining rates while a proportional tax imposes the same rate at all income levels.) The personal income tax is the most progressive, with rates rising from 0.6 percent for the lowest decile to 11.6 percent for the highest. Payroll taxes are less progressive, with the rate rising from 3.3 percent at the bottom to 8.5 percent for the sixth decile, then declining slightly through the ninth and more sharply for the tenth decile.

Although the payroll tax is frequently referred to as "regressive" or even "highly regressive," it is, in fact, moderately progressive throughout most of the income range. This deserves emphasis since many NHI plans propose to use the payroll tax as a revenue source. The nature of the payroll tax accounts for the pattern of rates shown in Table 1. Basically, it is a flat-rate tax on labor earnings up to a ceiling ($15,300 in 1976). Because it falls only on earnings, households receiving a large portion of their incomes in the form of nonlabor income bear a low tax rate with respect to their total incomes. Low-income households receive about 60 percent of their incomes in the form of government transfers; only the 26 percent of their income that is labor income is subject to the payroll tax. As we move up the income distribution, the fraction of income received as transfers falls, and the fraction received as labor earnings rises, which largely accounts for the rising pattern of rates for the lower deciles. The ceiling on taxable earnings, together with the increasing importance of capital income for higher-income groups, is responsible for the decline in rates beyond the sixth decile.

The figures in Table 1 give considerable insight into the importance of the taxes used to finance an NHI plan. Most proposals specify that the funds will be derived from some combination of payroll-tax revenues and general federal revenues. Assuming that "general revenues" means personal income taxes (and this is sometimes explicit), and assuming further that the revenues will be raised in proportion to existing tax burdens under these taxes, the estimates in columns 2 and 3 indicate the importance of the combination of taxes actually used. Since the personal income tax is more progressive than the payroll tax, the larger the share of the costs financed from general revenues, the more progressively will the costs be distributed.

To be more specific, if income taxes are exclusively relied on to finance an NHI plan, the wealthiest 20 percent of households will be required to pay 61 percent of the total cost of NHI, while the poorest 20 percent of households will pay only 0.7 percent. (The wealthiest 20 percent of households included all those with more than approximately $24,000 in before-tax cash incomes in 1976.) If payroll taxes are used exclusively, the top 20 percent of households will bear 37 percent of the total cost, and the bottom 20 percent will bear 2.8 percent. A combination of the two taxes used to finance NHI, with half the total revenue raised by each, will result in the top 20 percent of households paying about half the total cost, and the bottom 20 percent about 1.8 percent.[2]

These estimates presuppose that the payroll tax used to finance NHI involves a flat-rate tax on taxable earnings as defined by the social security program in 1976. In 1977, however, Congress legislated significant changes in the social security payroll tax. The most important for the purpose of this study was a sharp increase in the ceiling on taxable earnings, which makes the payroll tax more progressive, increasing the burdens on upper-income households without changing the tax burdens on lower-income households. If this change is fully implemented (it is currently being phased in), the cost of any NHI plan that relies on payroll taxes levied on taxable earnings will be more progressive than the estimates in Table 1, which are based on the 1976 program.

One other point to consider in connection with payroll taxes is that some NHI plans propose a payroll tax that does not fall on taxable earnings as defined by the social security system. The Kennedy-Corman

---

[2] Edgar K. Browning and William R. Johnson, *The Distribution of the Tax Burden* (Washington, D.C.: American Enterprise Institute, 1979), table 2, p. 36.

bill, for example, proposes a 1.0 percent tax on the employee's earnings up to 150 percent of the ceiling on taxable earnings used by the social security system, and a 3.5 percent tax on all earnings to be paid by employers (but which would, of course, be borne by the workers). Such a payroll tax would impose a substantially larger share of the total burden on upper income households than did the actual payroll tax in 1976.

Another proposed method of financing NHI is to use premiums similar to health insurance premiums. Since the premium must be paid, it can be viewed as a tax. If the premium is an actuarially fair premium so that two households with the same relevant characteristics must pay the same amount, then it would represent a regressive tax. Suppose two households are identical in all respects except that one has an income of $10,000 and the other an income of $20,000. If both are required to pay a premium of, say, $500, then the lower-income household must pay 5 percent of its income while the other pays only 2.5 percent. (Of course, the benefit of the insurance provided would also be a smaller percentage of the wealthier household's income.)

The only additional point to make about premiums is that at least one proposal specifies a premium that is not actuarially fair. Senator Kennedy's most recent proposal calls for "income-related premiums." What this means is that households with higher incomes will pay higher "premiums" for the same insurance coverage. Of course, this is not really a premium at all, at least as the term is commonly understood, but simply a new name for a tax. But if it is permissible for the social security system to call its taxes "contributions," then we suppose Senator Kennedy can call his proposed taxes "premiums." The important point is that these "premiums" are apparently nothing more than payroll taxes, and the discussion above indicates how they are likely to be distributed among income classes.

In sum, the mix of payroll and income taxes has important implications in determining who will bear the cost of an NHI program. This is, however, only part of the story. We must also consider the distribution of benefits in assessing the overall distributional effect of NHI.

Simulation of Distributional Impact of NHI. The important distributional question concerning NHI is the combined, or net, effect that both the government outlays and the taxes that finance them have on the distribution of income. As a general matter, for a *given* expenditure program, the more progressive the taxes that finance it are, the more redistributive the combined tax-expenditure package will be. It should be understood, however, that the tax need not be progressive for an NHI plan to redistribute income downward. Suppose an NHI program involves the same benefits for all households, say $500 per household. For this program to leave the distribution of income unchanged, it would have to place a tax of 10 percent on a $5,000 income, and a tax of only 1 percent on a $50,000 income. A highly regressive tax is, therefore, distributionally neutral, while a tax that is regressive, but less so than this extreme example, would still redistribute income in favor of low-income households. Since all existing federal taxes are progressive, it is clear at the outset that most NHI proposals will redistribute income downward.

In this section we will investigate the magnitude of redistribution accomplished by a specific NHI plan. We had originally intended to consider several actual proposals, but upon examination this appeared to be an impossible task. The proposals we examined were so vague and diverse that any attempt to allocate benefits and costs using the available data would have required far too many arbitrary judgments. As an expedient, we decided to consider the distributional impact of a hypothetical NHI plan that has much in common with some well-known proposals. The advantage of this approach is that we are able to develop fairly precise estimates of the distributional impact of the plan. The obvious disadvantage is that the estimates cannot be applied directly in an evaluation of any actual proposals. We hope, however, that the hypothetical plan is sufficiently similar to some existing proposals to provide valuable clues as to the likely distributional impact of other NHI plans.

Our hypothetical NHI plan will be a comprehensive health insurance plan covering all Americans and financed by a combination of payroll and income taxes. Total outlays (and taxes) are assumed to be $50 billion. This means that the program is not large enough to cover out of increased public funds all health care costs in 1976 (which would have required perhaps $75 billion), but it is still a relatively large program. Half of the cost of the program is assumed to be derived by increasing the payroll tax rate on the same base of taxable earnings that existed in 1976. The remaining $25 billion of the cost is assumed to be acquired by increasing federal income tax liabilities in proportion to existing liabilities in 1976.

The distribution of the tax costs among households under this plan can be estimated in a straightforward way. The more troublesome question is how to distribute the benefits among households. Assuming that the program provides the same degree of insurance coverage (with the same coinsurance rates, deductibles, etc.) to everyone, there will still be some variation in benefits since the value of the coverage will depend on such things as age, family size, and so on. However, there is some evidence indicating that consumption of health care does not vary significantly with income level when the same insurance coverage applies, at least for middle- and upper-income households.[3] This suggests that an assumption of equal per capita benefits may be a reasonable approach, at least for that part of the population not already covered by Medicare and Medicaid.

Households eligible for Medicare and Medicaid require special consideration since they already receive benefits from publicly provided health insurance.[4] Per capita benefits received in 1976 by these households already exceeded the benefits that would be provided them under a general NHI plan—that is, if $83 billion ($50 billion plus 1976 spending of $33 billion on Medicare and Medicaid) were divided equally among the population. It seems clear that no NHI plan would be adopted that involved reducing benefits to the Medicare-Medicaid population. Consequently, we have adopted two alternative approaches. In the first, beneficiaries of Medicare and Medicaid are assumed to receive unchanged benefits with the $50 billion allocated on an equal per capita basis among the remainder of the population. In the second, benefits to recipients of Medicare and Medicaid are assumed to be increased somewhat (we will assume by 15 percent, or about $5 billion of the NHI outlays), with the remaining $45 billion allocated to the remainder of the population. Judging from the actual NHI proposals with which we are familiar, this second alternative is probably more realistic.

One other matter deserves brief comment. We will assume that benefits and taxes are valued at their cost. In other words, if a household pays taxes of $500 and receives insurance coverage that costs the government $600 to provide, we assume the benefit and cost to the household are $600 and $500 respectively. The assumption regarding taxes is almost surely inaccurate and will be dropped in the next section. The assumption regarding benefits is also probably inaccurate, but the direction of bias is not clear. On the one hand, administrative costs of publicly provided health insurance may be less than for privately provided insurance, so households may secure benefits greater than they would by purchasing their insurance privately. On the other hand, imposing a standardized plan on a heterogeneous population is likely to mean that many households receive coverage they would not

---

[3] H. Klarman, ed., *Empirical Studies in Health Economics* (Chicago: University of Chicago Press, 1970), pp. 73–95; Karen Davis, *National Health Insurance: Benefits, Costs, and Consequences* (Washington, D.C.: The Brookings Institution, 1975).

[4] The original computer tapes contained estimates of actual Medicare and Medicaid outlays made on behalf of each beneficiary. We have reallocated these outlays among the eligible populations on an equal per capita basis since this should be a better approximation to the preferred insurance value measure of benefits.

TABLE 2

Distributional Impact of Hypothetical NHI

(no change in benefits to Medicare-Medicaid population)

Income Quintile (1)	1976 ATAT Income ($ billion) (2)	1976 Percentage Shares of Income (3)	Benefits of NHI ($ billion) (4)	Costs of NHI ($ billion) (5)	Net Change ($ billion) (6)	Net Change per Household ($) (7)	Final ATAT Income ($ billion) (8)	Final Percentage Shares (9)
First	$ 59.8	5.4	$ 2.7	$ 0.3	$ 2.4	$158	$ 62.2	5.6
Second	129.9	11.7	6.4	3.0	3.4	225	133.3	12.0
Third	187.6	16.9	11.3	8.2	3.1	201	190.7	17.1
Fourth	258.5	23.3	14.5	13.4	1.1	70	259.6	23.3
Fifth	476.2	42.8	15.1	25.2	−10.1	−658	466.1	41.9

SOURCE: Authors' calculations as described in the text using the data base developed for Browning and Johnson, *Distribution of the Tax Burden.*

choose on their own. In addition, the specific coinsurance rates, deductibles, and controls on the supply, allocation, and prices of medical resources that are contained in many NHI plans may also impair the efficiency of resource allocation in the medical sector. On balance, benefits could be worth more or less than their cost, but in the absence of evidence on this matter we will assume that benefits equal governmental outlays.

Based on these assumptions, we have developed estimates of the distributional impact of the hypothetical NHI plan. Table 2 presents the estimates for the case where the Medicaid-Medicare population receives no expansion in benefits. The results are tabulated by ranking households on the basis of their income and then aggregating them into income classes, each containing 20 percent of all households (quintiles). The second and third columns give estimates of the actual 1976 distribution of after-tax, after-transfer (ATAT), or disposable income among households. In that year, the lowest quintile of households received 5.4 percent of total disposable income, while the highest received 42.8 percent. Columns 4 and 5 give the benefits and costs of the NHI plan for each quintile. It will be noted that benefits are significantly greater for the higher-income classes. There are two reasons for this. First, Medicare-Medicaid recipients receive no new benefits under this variant, and these households are predominantly in the lower quintiles. Second, although each quintile contains the same number of households, the number of persons per household is greater in upper-income households so that a per capita distribution of benefits implies greater total benefits for the higher quintiles. The distribution of costs in column 5 follows the pattern suggested in the previous section, with about half of the total cost borne by the highest quintile.

Of greatest interest are the estimates given in columns 6–9, which indicate the net change in the distribution of disposable income brought about by the NHI plan. The lowest four quintiles gain a total of $10 billion while the top quintile loses this amount. In effect, of the $50 billion in total expenditures, $40 billion is simply returned (as health insurance) to those who pay the taxes, while the remaining $10 billion represents a net redistribution from upper-income households to lower-income households.

Table 3 presents the estimates of the distributional impact of the second variant of the NHI plan involving a 15 percent increase in the benefits to Medicare-Medicaid recipients. The results differ from Table 2 in a predictable way, with greater benefits to the lower quintiles and smaller benefits to the higher quintiles. This is understandable since the Medicare-Medicaid population is largely located in the lower quintiles. The net effect is that this variant is more highly redistributive

39

TABLE 3

DISTRIBUTIONAL IMPACT OF HYPOTHETICAL NHI

(15% increase in benefits to Medicare-Medicaid population)

Income Quintile (1)	1976 ATAT Income ($ billion) (2)	1976 Percentage Shares of Income (3)	Benefits of NHI ($ billion) (4)	Costs of NHI ($ billion) (5)	Net Change ($ billion) (6)	Net Change per Household ($) (7)	Final ATAT Income ($ billion) (8)	Final Percentage Shares (9)
First	$ 59.8	5.4	$ 4.3	$ 0.3	$4.0	$261	$ 63.8	5.7
Second	129.9	11.7	7.2	3.0	4.2	279	134.1	12.1
Third	187.6	16.9	10.9	8.2	2.7	176	190.3	17.1
Fourth	258.5	23.3	13.5	13.4	0.1	5	258.6	23.3
Fifth	476.2	42.8	14.1	25.2	−11.0	−723	465.2	41.8

SOURCE: Authors' calculations as described in the text using the data base developed for Browning and Johnson, *Distribution of the Tax Burden.*

than the previous one, with a total of $11 billion redistributed from the top quintile to the lowest four.

As mentioned earlier, we hope these estimates will provide some insights into the likely distributional impact of actual NHI proposals. In particular, we believe the second variant is likely to be similar in its distributional effects to most proposals that involve fairly comprehensive coverage for the entire population financed by payroll and income taxes. Of course, care must be taken in using these estimates when actual proposals differ significantly from the hypothetical plan assumed. Specifically, it would be a mistake to think that because this $50 billion plan redistributes $11 billion, a $25 billion proposal will necessarily redistribute exactly half as much. To take a specific example, President Carter's proposed National Health Plan is estimated to involve new governmental outlays of $18.2 billion in fiscal 1983. These outlays, however, finance benefits almost exclusively for low-income households, rather than spreading benefits over the entire population as does our hypothetical plan. Moreover, these outlays are to be financed totally out of "general revenues." As a consequence, Carter's proposal will involve much more net redistribution per dollar of government outlay than does our hypothetical example.

One common characteristic of most NHI proposals is that they would effect a substantial redistribution of income. This makes an evaluation of these proposals susceptible to confusion about two markedly different policy questions. One issue concerns whether a mandatory tax-financed health insurance plan will solve any of the problems that exist in the allocation of medical-care resources. A second issue is whether it is desirable to expand the role of government in achieving a more equal distribution of income.

It is possible to deal with these two issues with separate policies: An NHI plan can be financed in a way that does not significantly redistribute income (by using actuarially fair premiums), and income can be redistributed by other means without expanding the government's involvement in the health care sector. This is an important point to understand because, to approve unreservedly of almost any of the existing NHI proposals, one must be prepared to defend both greater income redistribution by government and an increased role of government in the health care field.

Most people familiar with the ongoing debate over NHI are aware that most proposals will produce a substantial redistribution of income. Whatever the merits of combining redistribution and tax-financed health insurance, it is our impression that the general public has not been made aware of the redistributive content of these proposals. If this is so, then perhaps the emphasis on the distributional effects of NHI in this section has not been misplaced.

The Welfare Cost of Financing NHI through Taxes

It is frequently argued in discussions of NHI that government provision of health insurance coverage to the population involves no real cost. The reasoning behind this position notes that the public is already bearing the costs of consuming medical care, either in premiums paid to insurance companies or in out-of-pocket expenses. When the government finances the medical care, the public's taxes go up but its premiums and out-of-pocket expenses go down, so there is no net cost. This reasoning has an element of truth in it, but it ignores an important difference between using taxes to finance some service, and financing the service by paying for it directly. Using taxes to finance any good or service will distort the economic behavior of households in a way that leads to a misallocation of resources. Direct payment for goods and services avoids this cost. Taxes are, in general, a more expensive way to provide a given service than paying for it directly.

Understanding how taxes distort resource allocation to produce a welfare cost is important because this welfare cost is part of the real cost of government spending. A clear distinction must be drawn between the direct cost of a tax, represented by the revenue it raises, and the welfare cost of the tax which results from the inefficient use of economic resources caused by the tax.

To help illustrate the difference between these two costs produced by taxation, we shall begin with an extreme example. Suppose the government places a tax of 100 percent on all earnings in excess of $5,000 (that is, an exemption of $5,000). No matter how much a taxpayer earns, no more than $5,000 can be kept. Clearly, we can expect the taxpayer to reduce his actual earnings to $5,000 since he does not gain anything by working to earn more.

In this example, the government collects no tax revenue because the taxpayer only earns $5,000, so the 100 percent rate applies to a zero tax base. There is no direct cost of the tax because no funds are transferred from the taxpayer to the government. The taxpayer, however, is clearly worse off, and this cost is the welfare cost of the tax. The full reduction in his earnings from, say, $15,000 to $5,000 is *not* a measure of how much worse off he is, however, because he has gained additional leisure time that is worth something to him. The welfare cost must be measured as the difference between the $10,000 in sacrificed earnings and the value of additional leisure time. We know there is a net loss to the taxpayer because he chose to earn the extra

$10,000 in the absence of the tax, implying that the additional $10,000 was worth more to him than the leisure time he had to give up to earn it.

Our extreme example was designed to illustrate that a tax imposes a real cost on taxpayers quite apart from the revenue it raises. The same general principle applies to more realistic taxes that do not lead people to behave in extreme ways to avoid payment of the tax entirely. All real world taxes raise revenue, and to that extent result in a direct cost to the public, but they also distort economic behavior in ways that produce a welfare cost. For example, a 60 percent tax on earnings means that a taxpayer whose market wage rate is ten dollars an hour can keep only four dollars an hour. His productive behavior will then be guided by the four-dollar net wage he receives, so he will work only as long as four dollars adequately compensates him for the cost of supplying his time to the job. But since the value of his labor services to society is ten dollars per hour, he will be working less than the efficient amount. As a result, this tax has both a direct cost—the revenue it actually raises, and a welfare cost due to the inefficiently low labor supply. The real cost of the tax is the sum of these two costs and it always exceeds the direct cost of the revenue the government collects.

These examples have focused on the way a tax on earnings produces a welfare cost. Payroll and income taxes are likely to affect labor supply and produce a welfare cost of the same type as in our examples. In addition, personal income taxes can affect the total supply of capital resources, distort the use of the taxpayers' incomes through the use of special provisions (tax "loopholes"), and adversely affect resource allocation in other ways. Other taxes can distort economic behavior in different ways. Without minimizing these other effects, we think it is most helpful to conceptualize the way these taxes produce a welfare cost as one affecting the total supply of productive services (labor and capital).

Of paramount concern, of course, is how large the welfare cost of a tax will be. Two factors interact to determine the size of the welfare cost. The first is how responsive taxpayers are to a given change in the net rate of pay. The more labor supply falls in response to a given tax, the greater the distortion in resource allocation and the larger the welfare cost. We will have a good deal more to say about this later. The second factor is the level of the marginal tax rate applicable to a change in earnings: The higher the marginal tax rate, the larger the total welfare cost. It is important to understand that the marginal tax rate of a tax produces the welfare cost. When a person is considering working more or less, his marginal tax bracket determines how much his net earnings will vary if he changes his gross earnings. Under a proportional tax, the average rate of tax equals the marginal rate of tax, but for all other types of taxes the marginal rate differs from the average rate, and it is the marginal rate that is crucial.

One final point is also important. The present tax system distorts resource allocation in a variety of ways, and so has a welfare cost. But when we consider the financing of NHI, the welfare cost of the present system is not relevant. Instead, we must be concerned with the additional, or marginal, welfare cost produced by the increased taxes required to finance NHI. It is this additional welfare cost, along with the additional direct cost, that represents the real cost of financing NHI. As it turns out, the marginal welfare cost of increasing taxes is generally much larger than the average welfare cost of pre-existing taxes.

Having made these preliminary observations about the nature and determinants of the welfare cost of taxation, let us turn to the empirical estimation of the additional welfare cost of the taxes used to finance NHI. The first step is to determine the current level of marginal tax rates on earnings imposed by the present system. Table 4 presents our estimates of the effective marginal tax rates on households that result from the combined impact of the tax and transfer system. These estimates are developed by simply ranking households on the basis of their before-tax-and-transfer incomes and using the variation in disposable income from decile to decile to calculate the marginal tax rates. While there are several problems associated with this method of esti-

TABLE 4

1976 MARGINAL TAX RATES
(percentages)

Income Decile (1)	MTR of Transfer System (2)	MTR of Tax System (3)	Effective MTR (4)
1 & 2	37.1	14.9	52.0
3	36.3	26.2	56.5
4	27.1	27.2	54.3
5	15.4	30.3	45.7
6	10.4	31.3	41.7
7	4.5	33.0	37.5
8	0.7	35.5	36.2
9	0.6	40.8	41.4
10	0.0	45.8	45.8

SOURCE: Authors' calculations as described in the text using the data base developed for Browning and Johnson, *Distribution of the Tax Burden.*

mating marginal rates, we feel the resulting figures give a reasonably good picture of the pattern of rates among income classes.[5] The rates are generally quite high, and the taxes that finance NHI will push them still higher.

The highest marginal rates fall on low-income households, with the bottom 40 percent of households facing rates in excess of 50 percent. Both tax and transfer programs interact in determining a household's marginal tax rate, and for low-income households the impact of transfer programs is especially important. When a transfer program operates (as several do) to reduce a household's transfer income when its own earnings increase, this is equivalent to placing a marginal tax rate on the additional earnings since disposable income will rise by less than the extra earnings. Low-income households also pay taxes on extra earnings, and together the tax and transfer systems produce extremely high effective marginal tax rates. Marginal tax rates are lower for middle-income households and then are higher again for the upper-income classes. As a point of interest, it might be mentioned that taxes were about 32 percent of net national product in 1976, so as Table 4 makes clear, all households confront marginal tax rates well in excess of the overall average rate for the nation.

The taxes that finance an NHI program will lead to increases in these already high effective marginal tax rates, and these increases will further distort the economic behavior of households. To estimate the welfare cost of the required taxes, two further principal ingredients (in addition to the initial level of marginal tax rates) are necessary. First, we must know how much the effective marginal tax rate will vary for each income class, and second, we must know how much earnings change in response to the higher marginal rates. The second factor will be considered first.

Although economists have studied the effects of taxes and transfers on labor supply and saving behavior for years, we do not yet possess sufficiently accurate estimates to allow us to determine with any precision the way households would respond to a tax-financed NHI. To develop estimates of welfare costs, however, we must specify the magnitude of the response. In the absence of firm empirical evidence, we have decided to consider a range of alternative responses which we think spans the outcomes that existing evidence suggests are plausible. Specifically, we will assume that the supply of productive services of households is inversely related to the effective marginal tax rate: The

---

[5] Our data did not permit separate estimation of marginal tax rates on labor income and on capital income, so the figures presented here should be considered as a weighted average of the two. In general, taxes on capital income are substantially heavier than taxes on labor income.

TABLE 5

RESPONSES OF EARNINGS TO MARGINAL TAX RATES
(percent of no tax earnings)

MTR (1)	Case A (2)	Case B (3)	Case C (4)	Case D (5)
0	100	100	100	100
10	99.7	99.9	100	100
20	98.2	99.2	99.6	99.8
30	95.1	97.3	98.5	99.2
40	89.9	93.6	96.0	97.4
50	82.3	87.5	91.2	93.8
60	72.1	78.4	83.3	87.0
70	59.0	65.7	71.3	76.0
80	42.8	48.7	54.1	59.0
90	23.2	27.1	30.8	34.4
100	0	0	0	0

SOURCE: See note 6.

higher the marginal tax rate, the lower will be the gross earnings of the households. Four alternative functional relationships[6] will be used to specify the magnitude of the assumed responses to a change in marginal tax rates.

Table 5 gives the four cases we will consider. The figures are given as a percentage of what earnings would be with a zero marginal tax rate. For example, case A implies that a household with a 40 percent marginal tax rate will earn 89.9 percent as much as it would if the tax rate were zero. An increase in the rate to 50 percent will reduce earnings to 82.3 percent, or by 8.5 percent of their level when the rate is 40 percent [(89.9 − 82.3)/89.9 equals 8.5 percent]. Case A obviously represents the largest responses to marginal tax rates we are assuming, while case D represents the smallest responses.

While these four relationships present only our best-informed guesses as to the range of plausible alternatives, they were chosen to conform to three bits of information we have about the responsiveness of resource supply to taxation. First, it is generally agreed that the present tax system has not resulted in any significantly large reduction in resource supply. Since the bulk of taxpayers now face 35 to 45 per-

---

[6] The four cases are calculated from the expression $E = 100(1 - MTR^x)$, where E is earnings as a percentage of earnings when the marginal tax rate is zero, and MTR is the marginal tax rate. The exponent x is 2.5 for case A, 3.0 for case B, 3.5 for case C, and 4.0 for case D.

cent marginal tax rates, we chose relationships with relatively small reductions over that range. Indeed, the reductions are small enough, especially in cases C and D, that it would be understandable if empirical investigation were unable to estimate any reduction at all. Second, experimental investigations of negative income tax transfer programs suggest that low-income households will reduce labor supply significantly when confronted with a 50 percent marginal tax rate, but generally the reductions are estimated to be in the 5 to 15 percent range. Our relationships encompass this range, but it must be admitted that results for low-income households may not be reliably applied to middle- and upper-income households. Finally, the relationships in Table 5 all embody the theoretical presumption that resource supply will fall more sharply as the marginal tax rate approaches 100 percent, and fall to zero when the rate reaches 100 percent. In other words, each additional increment in the marginal tax rate can be expected to lead to a greater reduction in supply, although of course we will not be dealing with rates that are anywhere near 100 percent.[7]

We invite the reader to examine the four cases in Table 5 to determine which, if any, appears to embody a reasonable set of responses to marginal tax rates. For what it is worth, we think that case C is probably the most plausible case, although admittedly it would be difficult to defend it against the other alternatives shown in the table.

We return now to the other basic ingredient needed for an estimate of the welfare cost of the taxes required to finance NHI, namely, how much the taxes in question will increase the effective marginal tax rates for each income class. For purposes of developing these figures we will consider the hypothetical $50 billion NHI plan described in the last section (the variant with Medicare and Medicaid benefits increased by 15 percent). The calculation of the increases in marginal tax rates resulting

---

[7] As a theoretical matter, economists do not expect there to be a unique relationship between the marginal tax rate and earnings. It is recognized that any change in the tax and transfer structure will affect earnings in two distinct ways: A higher marginal tax rate encourages people to work less since the cost of not working (consuming leisure) is reduced, but a higher average tax rate, by reducing disposable income, can induce people to work more. These two theoretically distinguishable effects, called the substitution and income effects, together determine the net effect on labor supply. We have glossed over this distinction by emphasizing the substitution effect; in effect, we are assuming that the income effect would be small enough to ignore. Note that when a net transfer is made to a household, the income effect also encourages less work, so the net effect is unambiguously to lower work effort. This is true for the tax-transfer combination we are examining for the lowest four quintiles. Only for the top quintile is there an income effect that would encourage more work. (See Table 3.) It is, therefore, possible that households in the top quintile might not reduce labor supply. Even in this case, however, there would still be a welfare cost since the distorting effect of a tax reflects only the substitution effect and this does depress work effort.

from a combination of payroll and income tax changes to produce $50 billion in additional revenue is straightforward, though tedious. The difficulty is that the increase in rates that will produce $50 billion in new revenue when there is no change in gross earnings (as we implicitly assumed in the last section) will not yield that much when gross earnings fall in response to the higher tax rates. Consequently, several iterations had to be calculated for each of the four cases to identify the change in tax rates that would produce the necessary $50 billion. Generally speaking, the final result for most income classes was an increase of three or four percentage points in the effective marginal tax rate.

Before presenting the actual estimates of welfare costs, we will explain briefly how the information and assumptions described above are used to calculate the welfare cost borne by each household. From the computer simulation, we can estimate the increment in the marginal tax rate for each household. The relationships in Table 5 then allow us to calculate how much gross earnings fall in response to the higher marginal tax rate. As mentioned above, this reduction in earnings is not the welfare cost since households place a value on the additional leisure time they consume when labor supply is reduced. By assuming that people work up to the point where the net marginal rate of pay just compensates for the last hour of leisure sacrificed, we can estimate the value of additional leisure consumed.[8] For example, if a household's marginal tax rate is 40 percent and a slight increase induces it to earn $100 less, then the additional leisure gained is valued at $60—equal to the after-tax earnings given up. Thus, the additional welfare cost is $40, $100 in sacrificed earnings less the $60 gain in leisure. While the actual calculations proceeded in a slightly different way, this illustrates the general way in which the assumptions and data are used to calculate the additional welfare cost of higher marginal tax rates.

Table 6 presents the estimated welfare costs (along with the other information) for each of the four cases representing different degrees of supply response. Column 2 gives the actual 1976 disposable income for each quintile, while the third column gives the disposable income after the distributional effects of the hypothetical NHI when there is no reduction in earnings. (These figures are from Table 3.) The remaining columns incorporate the relevant supply responses in calculating the costs borne by households.

Consider case C first. The total welfare cost of the higher taxes summed over the population is estimated to be $10.2 billion. The sig-

---

[8] Although our discussion in the text proceeds as if all income were labor income, actually about 25 percent of total factor earnings is capital income. Of course, a higher marginal tax rate distorts the allocation of resources devoted to saving and also produces a welfare cost.

TABLE 6

Welfare Cost of Hypothetical NHI Plan
($ in billions)

Income Quintile (1)	1976 ATAT[a] Income (2)	Final ATAT[b] Income (3)	Case A		Case B		Case C		Case D	
			Welfare cost (4)	Net change (5)	Welfare cost (6)	Net change (7)	Welfare cost (8)	Net change (9)	Welfare cost (10)	Net change (11)
First	$ 59.8	$ 63.8	$ 0.0	$ 4.0	$ 0.0	$ 4.0	$ 0.0	$ 4.0	$ 0.0	$ 4.0
Second	129.9	134.1	2.3	1.9	1.4	2.8	0.9	3.3	0.7	3.5
Third	187.6	190.3	3.4	−0.7	2.0	0.7	1.3	1.4	0.9	1.8
Fourth	258.5	258.6	4.9	−4.8	3.0	−2.9	1.9	−1.8	1.2	−1.1
Fifth	476.2	465.2	12.6	−23.6	8.5	−19.5	6.1	−17.1	4.4	−15.4

[a] From table 3, column 2.
[b] From table 3, column 8.
SOURCE: Authors' calculations as described in the text using the data base developed for Browning and Johnson, *Distribution of the Tax Burden.*

nificance of this figure is straightforward. It means that the taxes which finance the NHI plan would place a burden of $60.2 billion on the public—$50 billion in revenue collected and an additional welfare cost of $10.2 billion. The relevance of this in evaluating NHI is also straightforward: Ignoring the redistributional content of the plan, each dollar the government spends costs the public $1.20, so if the plan is to represent a productive investment, each dollar of spending must confer benefits of at least $1.20. In other words, it is not enough for the government to simply provide a service people could purchase for the same outlays themselves, for they would then receive benefits of $50 billion from the government outlays, but bear a cost of $60.2 billion.

In short, the size of the welfare cost indicates how much more productive government spending must be than the private spending it replaces for the tax-expenditure package to produce a net improvement. The existence of this welfare cost does not necessarily mean that this type of NHI plan is undesirable; it only identifies the real cost of the program. The benefits have not been considered here. As we mentioned earlier, it is conceivable that the public expenditures will be more valuable than private outlays of the same magnitude.

As expected, the welfare costs of the other three cases vary widely since they reflect the wide variations in supply responses among the cases. In all cases, however, the magnitudes are significant. In case D, the welfare cost is 14 percent of the $50 billion in tax revenues, while it is 46 percent in case A. As already stressed, we do not feel that the available empirical evidence is sufficient to identify one of these cases as the most plausible, but the variation in the estimates suggests the importance of considering this question carefully. An NHI program that would represent a net improvement if case D is the appropriate assumption could produce a large net loss if case A is appropriate.

Recognizing the welfare cost of the taxes that finance NHI also modifies the distributional consequences considered in the first section. When the program was imposed, with no change in earnings assumed, the gain to lower-income households exactly equalled the loss to upper-income households. But the welfare cost is a net loss which does not represent a gain to anyone, so when it is included the loss to upper-income households is greater than the gain to low-income households. Consider case C again. Column 9 gives the net change in real income when the welfare cost is included. (This equals the gain or loss when earnings remain unchanged minus the welfare cost when they do change.) The upper two quintiles now lose a total of $18.9 billion while the lower three quintiles gain only $8.7 billion. Each dollar of net benefit to lower-income households results in a net cost of more than two dollars for upper-income households. Note that the fourth quintile, which appeared to be a small net gainer when we ignored the welfare cost, is a net loser under all four variants when it is included. Indeed, in case A the top three quintiles (which, while containing 60 percent of all households, contain 70 percent of all persons) lose on balance, and these combined losses are five times as large as the net benefits to the lowest two quintiles.

These estimates are all based on an assumed $50 billion increase in taxes, half of which comes from payroll taxes and half from income taxes. For NHI plans that utilize this mix of taxes, these estimates should be a fairly good indication of the likely range of welfare costs that will be involved. A different mix of taxes would, however, lead to a different welfare cost. For example, if the revenues are derived entirely from income taxes, the welfare cost would be higher because income taxes are more progressive than payroll taxes and marginal tax rates would increase more sharply. By contrast, if actuarially fair premiums are used, there would be no welfare cost because premiums are in effect lump sum taxes that remain unchanged as earnings increase (that is, they place a zero marginal tax rate on any change in earnings). In general, the more progressive the financing instrument, the larger the welfare cost will be. A larger welfare cost, however, does not rule out the use of progressive taxes since these taxes also result in greater redistribution, and if that is desired it has to be weighed against the greater welfare cost.

To summarize briefly, the welfare cost of the tax that finances NHI is part of the real cost the public bears in financing the program. While we do not know the exact size of the cost, the estimates developed here suggest that it will probably add significantly to the cost of NHI. In evaluating any NHI proposal (or other expenditure proposal, for that matter), it is important to recognize that unless this extra cost is fully offset by benefits that cannot be obtained through private sector alternatives, the proposal must result in a net loss to the public.

National Health Insurance
by Regulation:
Mandated Employee Benefits

Charles E. Phelps

Social issues have often been solved, at least in part, by requiring that certain activities be undertaken by businesses on behalf of their employees. The entire social security system, workmen's compensation plans, and affirmative action for hiring of minorities are cases in point. The concept of using mandating as a portion of a national health insurance (NHI) plan arose during the Nixon administration and has been periodically (though not necessarily currently) embraced by such diverse entities as the administrations of Presidents Nixon and Carter, the U.S. Chamber of Commerce, and prominent members of Congress of a variety of political persuasions from both major political parties.

The broad political appeal for using mandated insurance appears to rise from several roots. First, it is "off budget." That is, a national health insurance plan can be structured without giving the appearance of affecting federal spending. Second, it gains the political support of a potentially powerful interest group: Because it retains an active role for the private insurance industry, it retains a market-oriented structure generally appealing to those desiring to minimize the appearance of government intervention. Finally, because the mandating provides a "floor" on coverage for the employed and their families, it is easy for persons who desire more insurance than the floor to fulfill their desires —the private employer package is substantially more flexible than a single government plan. Indeed, many employers now offer a variety of insurance packages to employees, reflecting the ease with which variety in insurance coverage can be sustained.

While desirable aspects of mandating insurance do indeed exist, one cannot conclude that the technique is without problems. The central theme of this paper is that many of the apparently desirable features of mandated insurance possess intrinsic liabilities as well. We have not yet

NOTE: The research on which this paper was based was supported by the Health Insurance Study of The Rand Corporation under a grant from the Department of Health, Education, and Welfare. The opinions and conclusions reached are solely those of the author and do not necessarily reflect the opinions or policies of any sponsors of Rand Corporation research.

52

found the proverbial free lunch. Some of these problems are correctible. if dealt with, but some appear to be inescapable. On net, it still appears plausible to me that, if national health insurance is to be enacted, mandated insurance for employees and their families may be the most desirable way to finance and operate such a plan.

The central issues of mandated insurance are relatively simple. First, the belief that mandating health coverage does not affect the federal budget is false. Because employer payments towards health insurance are tax deductible as a business expense by employers, but are not counted as taxable income by the IRS against employees, there is invariably an effect on tax revenues, and hence the federal budget, when mandating is used. Under the hypothesis that premium payments are (at least in the long run) offset by reductions in wage payments (which would be taxable), federal tax receipts would fall by billions of dollars annually under most mandated plans. In some plausible cases, the loss in tax receipts can be one-quarter to one-half of the size of direct outlays for complementary parts of NHI packages.[1]

Second, use of private insurance carriers for a significant part of the NHI plan makes more difficult any insurance-based efforts to control costs of care through provider incentives or payment mechanisms, because of the diverse source of payment and the lack of coordination of information about such things as fee schedules, double billing, et cetera. However, the technique of mandating still leaves open prospects for innovative private financing schemes and alternative delivery of care systems, such as health maintenance organizations, independent practice organizations, or novel approaches providing both consumer and provider incentives for cost control.[2] However, those favoring a centrally administered NHI plan to provide the most favorable opportunity for centralized cost control find mandating a dissatisfying approach. Because I do not number myself among such groups, I do not generally view with alarm the prospect of having a large and diverse set of carriers for a NHI plan.

Third, one must consider the effects of the mandated plan on the firms involved. The economic effects of mandating national health insurance through employers are driven in a large part by the size

---

[1] Bridger M. Mitchell and Charles E. Phelps, *Employer-Paid Group Health Insurance and the Costs of Mandated National Coverage*, R-1509-HEW (Santa Monica, California: The Rand Corporation, September 1975); also in abbreviated form: "National Health Insurance: Some Costs and Effects of Mandated Employee Coverage," *Journal of Political Economy*, vol. 84, no. 3 (June 1976), pp. 553–71.

[2] Many of these approaches are discussed in Alain C. Enthoven, "Consumer-Choice Health Plan," *New England Journal of Medicine*, vol. 298, nos. 12 and 13 (March 23 and 30, 1978), pp. 650–58.

distribution of firms in the United States. As a general statement, most large firms will be only trivially affected by a mandated NHI plan, unless it is considerably towards the extreme of NHI proposals of today. Nearly every large firm has some sort of employee health insurance plan, and many already have existing employer contributions at or near the generally considered mandated levels. On the other hand, relatively few of the small firms in the country have such plans, so mandating not only requires new direct (marginal) labor costs, but also requires a possibly large fixed cost associated with acquiring and managing a health insurance plan for only a few employees. Table 1 portrays the size distribution of firms and employees in the United States. It is striking that the smallest firms (under 20 employees) account for less than one-quarter of the nation's employees, yet constitute seven-eighths of the firms in the country. At the other extreme, firms with 100 or more employees account for over half of all U.S. employees, yet are just over 2 percent of the number of firms.

There are sound economic reasons for the existing pattern of insurance across firm size. First, the smaller groups are (because of the law of large numbers) riskier to the insurer, so there is a higher price charged for a given package of insurance than for larger firms. Small

TABLE 1

Size Distribution of U.S. Firms

Firm Size (number of employees)	Percent of All Employees[a]	Percent of All Firms
1–3	5.4	50.1
4–7	6.5	20.5
8–19	12.4	16.8
Subtotal	24.3	
20–49	14.4	7.7
50–99	10.8	2.6
Subtotal	25.2	
100–249	13.6	1.5
250–499	10.0	0.5
500 or more	26.9	0.3
Subtotal	50.5	

[a] 57,265,292 employees, 1970.

Source: U.S. Department of Commerce, *Country Business Patterns*, Washington, D.C., 1971.

firms also present the possibility of true "adverse selection" due to asymmetric information between the insurer and the insured group. For example, a small employee group may opt for complete coverage if it is believed that a member of the group has contracted cancer. The benefits versus costs of such an action are considerably different in a small group than in a large group.

There are also substantial fixed costs of transaction and management of the plan for each firm, making it a less attractive form of compensation for small firms. Finally, I suspect that there is considerably higher turnover in small than large firms (although I do not have data to support this belief). If true, this further adds to the costs of administration of any health plan.

Mandating of NHI solves only a few of these problems for the small firm. Because every employee (indeed, every person) in the country will have some form of insurance, insurers will be able to substantially ignore problems of differential information between insureds and insurer.[3] Any problem of turnover and high fixed costs will only partly be mitigated through a mandated plan. Each new employee requires re-registration for eligibility of the employee with the insurer, requiring both employer time and insurer time to modify eligibility records. Completion of the cycle also requires decertification of the employee at the former place of employment. All of these could contribute to the higher cost, and hence lower distribution of health insurance as a form of compensation in small firms, and all will remain with mandated plans. The ultimate effect of mandating employer plans as a part of NHI may not be so much on employment itself, but rather on the size distribution of firms. Without special compensation, it seems possible that the optimum size of the firm may increase with mandated NHI. The mandating method has an effect comparable to requiring a fixed-cost license for doing business for every firm in the country, independent of size. (This is not to say that most of the costs of a health plan are fixed, but rather that there are nontrivial fixed costs associated with any plan.)

Finally, one must consider how the increased costs of labor implied by mandated national health insurance will be dealt with by the firms, at least in the short run. In concept, mandating health insurance plans is akin to requiring a minimum level of employee compensation in addition to wage payments. Theory of the firm suggests that the

---

[3] Some adverse selection problems will still exist. One insurance company has reported to me that a small group of psychotherapists acquired an insurance plan which included coverage for psychotherapy. A considerable fraction of the firm's business was then spent with the therapists treating one another, while billing their newly found health insurance plan for the services.

equilibrium wage payment (in total) will be set to the marginal revenue product of the employee, regardless of the composition of the wage payment. Thus, in general, increased mandated insurance coverage should lead to reduction in wages where the mandating has increased the amount of insurance provided. In a long-run general equilibrium context, it is possible that some of the incidence of the higher cost falls on capital, rather than labor, but empirical estimates show this amount to be very small,[4] as might be expected if the elasticity of supply of capital is large.[5]

In the short run, however, the incidence may be somewhat different. With capital immobile in the short run, part of the incidence may fall on capital, and part may fall on customers of the affected firms, *if wages are sticky downward* but prices are immediately flexible. Simple considerations suggest that the period of adjustment for wages is likely to be short—probably less than half a year.[6] With such a short period of adjustment, massive revision of pricing practices by firms seems unlikely, and there seems to be even less likelihood that relative demand between industries would change markedly in response to any product price changes that occur.

Several features of the problem lead to this conclusion. First, the change in wages required by a mandated plan is not likely to be large (proportional to wages) in many firms. An increase in premiums of, say, $500 per worker is at maximum for most firms an increase of under 5 percent in wage payments. One of the few side-benefits of a 12–15 percent inflation rate may be that it minimizes any adjustment problem associated with such things as mandated NHI. Freezing nominal wages for an added four to six months beyond customary practice should return real wages to equilibrium, even after the shock of mandated NHI.[7]

Second, the firms with the largest increases in premiums from man-

---

[4] Martin S. Feldstein, "The Incidence of the Social Security Payroll Tax: Comment," *American Economic Review*, vol. 62, no. 3 (September 1972), pp. 735–38.

[5] There is an important exception. Kip Viscusi has pointed out in his discussion of this paper that there may be a permanent effect on demand for some labor. For those workers near or at the legal minimum wage, there will be no possibility of shifting back the costs of the health insurance premium to the worker. Thus, in effect, mandated NHI has the effect of placing a lump-sum tax on the annual employment of such workers, relative to more highly skilled workers. For such workers, there could be a permanent decline in demand for labor, and hence a permanent decline in the levels of employment. So long as health care costs increase at least as rapidly as the legal minimum wage, this phenomenon would not be reversed through any inflationary pressures.

[6] Mitchell and Phelps, *Employer-Paid Group Health Insurance*.

[7] Labor contracts with built-in inflation adjustment will not provide this self-correcting feature.

dated NHI are likely to be (a) small, and (b) nonunionized. If turnover is largest in such firms (which, I have argued, is one of the reasons for lower levels of insurance coverage currently), then that turnover itself will facilitate rapid adjustment of the real wage to equilibrium levels. Firms with collective bargaining agreements will find it more difficult to make nominal downward adjustments, but they are also much more likely already to have significant health plans, and thus would be little affected by the mandated plan.

Taken together, these considerations make me believe that the adjustment proposed in Mitchell and Phelps's *Employer-Paid Group Health Insurance and the Costs of Mandated National Coverage*[8] is the one that would predominate—firms would in the short run substitute overtime work for added workers, allowing natural turnover rates to adjust the magnitude of the labor force as desired. That, coupled with significant rates of inflation in the economy, lead to the belief that equilibrium can be obtained within six months to a year with considerable certainty.

The pertinent published research on mandated national health insurance is small. While a variety of federal studies have been published which include estimates of the employer costs of mandated NHI, virtually none has made its methodology open for critique, nor are those studies amenable to simple adjustment from one time period to another, or yet adjustable to account for new data superseding preliminary data and assumptions employed by the researchers. One 1975 study, of which I was coauthor, contains a methodology with which I am sufficiently familiar to make adjustment as required to forecast 1980 effects of mandated NHI. That study made several key assumptions about events which had (nearly) transpired at the time it was published, but for which no data were available. Some of those assumptions have retrospectively turned out to be significantly in error. In this paper, I will modify the work presented in the earlier paper, and present tentative conclusions regarding the current effects of NHI mandated through employee benefit plans.

Any attempt to forecast with fine precision the current effects of mandated NHI are dangerous. To identify the effects of mandated NHI in great detail requires a set of data not commonly available. Mitchell and Phelps employed a survey conducted in 1970 by the Center for Health Administration Studies (CHAS) of the University of Chicago, which contained the minimum data required to conduct such an analysis carefully. While new data are being collected currently by the National Center for Health Services Research of the Department of Health,

---

[8] Mitchell and Phelps, *Employer-Paid Group Health Insurance.*

Education, and Welfare, they are not currently available, so forecasting the effects of mandated NHI in 1980 requires extrapolation of a data set a decade old. Finally, the reader should be aware that the updating used in this paper is as yet tentative. I have not actually performed a resimulation of the effects of mandated NHI, but rather I use aggregate data to rescale results from the previous simulation using 1970 survey data. Such a resimulation would not be likely to produce answers differing in serious magnitude from the more crude adjustments of Mitchell and Phelps's results which I make in this paper. The most prominent problems of any such study is the enforced reliance on a data base ten years out of date, in a period when employer insurance premiums have tripled in nominal value.

Capsule Summary of Mitchell and Phelps's Methodology and Results

The 1970 survey employed by Mitchell and Phelps provided a stratified random sample of households in the United States in that year. Among other things, the survey gathered data from families on each health insurance plan held by them and then obtained directly from the insurer or employer data on the total cost of the plan, the employer's share, the employee's share, and the extent of coverage of the plan (both in terms of services covered and in terms of the family members covered). These data, when scaled to 1975 levels through use of aggregate data ratios, provided the basis for our past simulation. (Premium contributions were scaled upward by the ratio of estimated 1975 aggregate premiums to known 1970 premiums. Labor force increases were projected from contemporaneous rates of labor force increases.) For the key simulation, Mitchell and Phelps compared the (estimated) 1975 premium contribution of the employer of each worker in the 1970 sample against a variety of mandated standards under consideration. The added premium costs (above estimated 1975 contributions) were added across the sample, and rescaled to match the national population projected for 1975. From these data, estimates can be made for virtually any proposed mandated NHI plan in terms of cost, potential unemployment effects generated (by industry), and increased losses of federal tax receipts (when combined with knowledge of family income and externally estimated marginal tax rates for each family).

In brief summary, Mitchell and Phelps estimated new employer premium costs in 1975 ranging from $5 billion per year for a "low level" proposed mandated NHI plan through $9 billion for a plan approximating that of the Nixon administration to over $21 billion for the most generous plan under consideration at that time involving mandated NHI. The increased premiums per worker were found to vary by a factor of two across industries, the lowest being in manufacturing and retail trade, and the highest being in agriculture, mining, service, finance, real estate, and the construction industries, that is, industries typically dominated by smaller firms. Relying on estimates by Ehrenberg[9] we forecast transitory increases in unemployment ranging from 0.3 percent for the "low level" plan to 1.4 percent for the most generous plan. Again, effects varied across industry, by a factor of three or more, with the largest effects being predicted for the service industry (up to 2.1 percent unemployment for the most generous plan) and lowest in the manufacturing sector, as might be expected. It was shown that these unemployment effects could be substantially mitigated through temporary subsidies to employers to offset payroll increases, but that subsidies sufficient to be effective at minimizing employment loss would range, in some cases, into multiple billions of dollars. Finally, when premium data were combined with family income and estimated marginal tax rate data, an estimate was obtained of the loss in federal tax receipts associated with the mandating. This calculation was based upon the assumption that the long-run incidence of the mandated premium cost is on the worker and that employer-paid premiums would continue not to be counted as taxable income for employees. The "low level" plan had tax expenditures of over $1 billion; the intermediate plan had tax expenditures of $2.5 billion, and the "high level" plan had tax expenditures of $6 billion annually.

Actual 1975 Premiums, 1978 Premiums, and Forecasts of 1980 Premiums

There has been a veritable explosion in employer-plan health insurance benefits and premiums in the past decade. In 1970, such plans had $13.65 billion in premiums, $9.1 billion of which was paid by employers (67 percent). Mitchell and Phelps extrapolated these data to 1975 and predicted total premiums of $22 billion, $14.6 billion of which would be paid by employers (a 60 percent increase above 1970). Actual data now available show the increase in total premiums to have been substantially larger. Data from Gibson[10] show total health insurance benefits in 1975 of $30.9 billion, corresponding to about $34 billion in premiums. If 1970 ratios hold in 1975, some 80 percent of those premiums, or $27 billion, would be employer-group related. A similar methodology provides an estimate of $36 billion for 1978, and

---

[9] Ronald G. Ehrenberg, *Fringe Benefits and Overtime Behavior*, (Lexington, Massachusetts: Lexington Books, 1971).

[10] Robert M. Gibson, "National Health Expenditures, 1978," *Health Care Financing Review*, vol. 1 (Summer 1979), pp. 1–36.

extrapolation of contemporaneous growth rates provides a crude forecast of $47 billion for total employer-group premiums in 1980.

Changes in Employer Contributions and
Employer Share of Premiums

No direct data are available to ascertain the magnitude of employer contributions, although the *Survey of Current Business* (SCB) provides data that indicate employer contributions for health *plus* disability premiums.[11] The 1970 survey used in Mitchell and Phelps's *Employer-Paid Group Health Insurance and the Costs of Mandated National Coverage* revealed an average employer share of 67 percent, with 41 percent of the observed policies receiving 100 percent payment by the employer. One can *infer* the growth patterns in employers' share so long as the fraction of all full-time employees covered by some insurance is known. The most recent data available allow such a calculation directly for 1975. By comparing the growth rate in per-employee contributions by employers against the growth rate in per-capita health care benefits, one can infer the proportion paid by employers. Extrapolations must be employed for later years. The steps required to make this inference are: (1) compute the growth rate in premiums per employee in the economy; (2) adjust for the growth rate (if any) in the proportion of employees in the economy with some health coverage through employer work groups; (3) adjust for any changes in per-capita insurance benefit payments (preferably per-enrollee benefits payments in employer-group plans, but such data are not available). This is equivalent to adjusting for premiums if loading fees are constant during the period; use of benefit data allows more use of actual data, rather than extrapolation, for periods past 1976. The logic is that any differential growth rates in employer contributions beyond growth rates in overall premiums (benefits) must be accounted for by changes in the proportion paid by employers.[12]

In 1975, the data suggest that employers' share of existing pre-

---

[11] Direct inquiry at the SCB could not clarify the exact content of the data, but simple calculations demonstrate that the reported levels are inconsistent with the belief that only health premiums are directly reported in the category described as "group health insurance." Adjustment for apparent premiums on disability insurance makes these data consistent with direct measures of employer contributions towards pure health insurance.

[12] The 1975 data required for this are found in Martha Remy Yohalem, "Employee-Benefit Plans, 1975," *Social Security Bulletin*, vol. 40, no. 11 (November 1977), pp. 19–28 (for proportion of workers covered); U.S. Department of Commerce, *Survey of Current Business*, July issues of 1973 through 1979, tables 6.13 (for employer contribution levels); and Gibson, "National Health Expenditures," pp. 1–36 (for aggregate health insurance benefit payments).

miums had increased to 72 percent, rather than the 67 percent observed directly in 1970.[13]

Projections of employer payment proportions to 1978 and beyond require assumptions regarding any changes in the fraction of workers covered by health insurance. As noted, the data show a remarkable stability in this fraction from 1970 to 1974, hovering near 70 percent. In 1975, that proportion jumped to 72.2 percent, a 3 percent growth rate in one year. Is this a new equilibrium level (responding, say, to the tax reform act of 1975), the beginning of a new growth pattern not yet in equilibrium, or a mere aberration from a long-term equilibrium near 70 percent? Inferences about proportions of premiums paid by employers are sensitive to assumptions made about this number, as will be demonstrated momentarily. Several things suggest that it is probably a permanent, if not complete move. First, the *number* of worker covered by health insurance through employment groups actually increased by 1 percent in 1975, despite a decline in aggregate employment of wage and salary workers by 2 percent. Those laid off were almost certainly overrepresented among those workers with no insurance, so a part of the increase in the rate of coverage was due to decline in the base work force, and a part was due to increases in numbers covered. Second, the data contain a correction factor for multiple coverage obtained from a 1972 survey. That survey, drawn during a period of relative economic growth, will show a relatively high fraction of multiple-worker households, and hence will provide a relatively large downward correction from total number of insureds to obtain coverage levels. (The correction is to avoid double counting of persons covered not only by their own work group policy but by a spouse's.) Multiple coverage almost certainly declines during a recession, so that the 1972 figure will overstate the desirable downward correction in coverage. Thus I am prone to accept the 72 percent coverage level as a useful datum, until direct measures are published. Extrapolation to 1978, 1980, or beyond is obviously risky. Reentry of marginal workers back into the ranks of the employed during a recovery will slightly lower the overall ratio, but general income growth should have an opposing effect. My best guess, and it is nothing more, is to use a coverage rate of 72 percent for the years through 1980.

---

[13] During this period, the fraction of all workers covered by some form of employment-group related insurance was stable at 70 percent until 1975, when it increased to 72.2 percent. See Yohalem, "Employee-Benefit Plans," pp. 19–28; employer contributions increased by 119 percent (U.S. Department of Commerce, *Survey of Current Business*); the labor force increased by 5 percent (U.S. Department of Labor, Bureau of Labor Statistics, *Employment and Earnings*, published monthly); and per-capita benefits increased by 96 percent (Gibson, "National Health Expenditures," pp. 1–36).

We are now in a position to estimate the fraction of all premiums paid by employers during 1978 and to make a forecast for 1980. From 1975 to 1978, per-employee contributions towards health insurance premiums by employers rose by 60 percent.[14] Per-capita health insurance benefits rose by 43 percent.[15] If the assumption about a 72 percent worker coverage rate is correct, this implies an astonishing increase in employer share of 12 percent during this three-year period (1.60 ÷ 1.43 = 1.12). The estimated average employer's share for 1978 is therefore estimated to be 0.72 × 1.12 = 80.6 percent.

Is such a dramatic increase in a three-year period believable? I offer tentative evidence to support my belief that it is. First, general inflation, pushing (particularly) higher-wage workers into higher marginal tax brackets, offers incentives to increase employer payments in lieu of wage increases. Increases in the social security maximum taxable income provide the same incentive for workers with incomes near the current maximum. Second, direct measures of the proportions of workers receiving 100 percent payment by employers shows that measure to have increased from 41 percent in 1970[16] to 57 percent in 1977.[17] We can infer that the distribution of employer share has shifted markedly towards full-payment by employers from the 1970 distribution (see table 4 below). These, coupled with the lack of persuasive evidence that the proportion of workers covered by some sort of insurance has increased markedly during this period, lead me to acceptance, at least tentatively, of the 80.6 percent employer's share.

The cumulative effects of growths in various factors are summarized in table 2. The premium increases per se are totally explained by changes in labor force levels and by changes in medical expenses per person, *if* changes in medical prices have little effect on proportions of medical bills covered by insurance. Econometric analysis of demand for insurance as a function of medical prices shows no persistent effects,[18] suggesting this to be a relatively benign inference.

The growth in employer contributions is accounted for by labor force growth of 12 percent, increases in the fraction of workers covered of 3 percent (author's very rough estimate), and an apparent 20 percent

[14] U.S. Department of Commerce, *Survey of Current Business*, various issues.

[15] Gibson, "National Health Expenditures," pp. 1–36.

[16] Mitchell and Phelps, *Employer-Paid Group Health Insurance.*

[17] Health Insurance Institute, *Source Book of Health Insurance Data 1977–78* (New York, 1978).

[18] Charles E. Phelps, "Demand for Reimbursement Insurance," in Richard N. Rosett, ed., *The Role of Health Insurance in the Health Services Sector,* Universities-National Bureau Conference Series No. 27 (New York: National Bureau of Economic Research, 1976).

TABLE 2

Growth of Factors In Employer-Group Premium Increases, 1970–1978

Factor	Total Employer-Group Premiums (1978 ÷ 1970 levels)	Employer Contributions (1978 ÷ 1970 levels)
Premiums	2.71[b]	3.77[a]
Labor force (full-time)	1.12	1.12
Proportion of workers covered	1.03[b]	1.03[b]
Per-capita medical expense	2.40	2.40
Benefits per person	2.80	2.80
Employer's share of premiums	—	1.20[b]

[a] Excludes growth of $2 billion in employer contributions in dental insurance, estimated from benefit data.

[b] These ratios based on the author's very rough estimates.

Sources: Robert M. Gibson, "National Health Expenditures, 1978," *Health Care Financing Review*, Summer 1979, for medical expense data; Martha Remy Yohalem, "Employee-Benefit Plans, 1975," *Social Security Bulletin*, November 1977, for worker coverage data; U.S. Department of Commerce, *Survey of Current Business*, various issues, for employer contributions. Calculations by author.

increase in the employer's share of premiums, from a rate of 0.67 to a rate of 0.81. (Notice also that these data are slightly inconsistent in the following way. I calculated the increase in *total* premiums for employer work groups by assuming that a constant fraction [80 percent] of all private health insurance derived from work groups. But this is inconsistent with the datum that rates of coverage were growing in the employment sector faster than the population was growing, which in fact was true. Thus I have not attempted to calculate the implicit employer's share of premiums directly from my estimate of total premiums for employer work groups, which derives entirely from aggregate benefit data.)

Finally, table 3 summarizes what my best estimates of employer contributions and employer share might be in 1975, 1978, and roughly extrapolated, 1980. For 1975, 1978, and 1980, the entries associated with the highest proportions of premiums paid by employers are those in which I hold the highest confidence, but the reader should again be reminded of the substantial level of assumption required to reach these estimates.

Revision of 1975 Estimates by Mitchell and Phelps

We have now reached a position where we can provide some level of correction to the estimates by Mitchell and Phelps regarding required premiums for 1975 mandated insurance.[19] The important question to be answered here is, "What portion of the added premium (beyond those considered by Mitchell and Phelps) will actually reduce employers' liability for new premiums if an NHI of certain cost characteristics is mandated?" In our forecasts of 1975 employer premiums, it now appears that we ignored some $4.8 billion in employer premium payments. Some of these contributions merely extended upward the fraction paid by the employer (for example, from 85 percent of the premium to 100 percent of the premium). No such premiums will offset liability of mandated NHI which requires only a 75 percent sharing by employers. Alternatively, some of the $4.8 billion increase must be attributed to payments for newly enrolled workers, much or all of which does reduce employer's liability under an NHI plan. Intermediate cases can readily be conceived as well. For lack of any other alternative, I have arbitrarily used the 1970 distribution of employer share to settle the issue: I will "allow" these added contributions to reduce employer liability by the same fraction as was the 1970 proportion of employers with contributions *below* a given mandated rate of sharing. Pertinent data are presented in table 4; a clarifying example follows. I will also divide the added $4.8 billion in 1975 employer contributions between individual and family unit policies proportional to their 1970 ratios of individuals and families (20 percent for individual policies, 80 percent for family policies).

This fixed amount of added premiums will be assumed to reduce the liability stated in tables in Mitchell and Phelps's report.[20] For example, those results show a liability of $1.11 billion in 1975 for individual insurance policies, if the employer is required to pay at least

---

[19] Since 1975 has departed us, this exercise may best be viewed as an attempt to improve, if not set straight, the record. More interestingly, the methodology employed is identical to that which I shall use to forecast effects and costs of mandated NHI for 1980; hence, it can be viewed as a learning exercise by the reader, if nothing else.

Bridger Mitchell has not reviewed this effort. Thus he should be held completely blameless for errors, while still receiving credit for his share of whatever merit the original work possesses.

[20] Mitchell and Phelps, *Employer-Paid Group Health Insurance.*

TABLE 3

EMPLOYER GROUP INSURANCE PREMIUMS FOR HOSPITAL,
PHYSICIAN INSURANCE

Year	Total Premiums (billions)	Employer's Share	Employer-Paid Premiums (billions)
1970	$13.65	0.67	$ 9.1
1975 (estimate by Mitchell/Phelps)	21.80	0.67	14.6
1975 (recent data)	≈27.00	0.67[a] 0.72[b]	18.1[a] 19.4[b]
1978	≈36.00	0.67[a] 0.72[b] 0.81[c]	24.0[a] 26.0[b] 29.0[c]
1980 (projected)	≈47.00	0.67[a] 0.72[b] 0.81[c,d]	31.0[a] 34.0[b] 38.0[c]

[a] Assumes that 1970 employer's share of 67 percent remains constant.

[b] Assumes employer's share increased at same rate aggregate as per-worker employer contributions to health and disability insurance from 1972 to 1975, scaled by per-capita benefit increase rates.

[c] Same as note (b), except growth to 1978 included. For 1980, assumes same rate as 1978.

[d] Based on the author's very rough estimate.

SOURCES: Yohalem, "Employee-Benefit Plans, 1975," and *Survey of Current Business*, various issues.

50 percent of the premium. The method of allocating the $4.8 billion in added payments (above those in Mitchell and Phelps) is to presume that 20 percent of the $4.8 billion (= $0.96 billion) is potentially available to reduce the liability on individual policies. Since 72 percent of "individual" workers already receive at least a 50 percent contribution on individual policies, I allow only the remaining 28 percent as a reduction of employer liability estimates. Thus the entry in the revised table would be $1.11 − ($4.8 × 0.20 × 0.28) = $1.11 − 0.27 = $0.84 billion. For a plan with this specific requirement, the estimated employer liability is reduced by 24 percent (0.84 ÷ 1.11 = 0.76). This same fixed reduction in liability of $0.27 billion occurs for all entries in the 50 percent employer share column, for calculation of the liability for individual policies. An entirely analogous calculation is made for

TABLE 4

DISTRIBUTION OF EMPLOYER PREMIUM SHARE IN 1970

Employer Share of Premium (%)	Individual Policies (% of total)	Family Policies (% of total)
0	9	12
1–25	4	8
26–50	15	21
51–75	12	13
76–99	8	10
100	52	37

NOTE: Totals may not add to 100 percent because of rounding.

SOURCE: Bridger M. Mitchell and Charles E. Phelps, *Employer-Paid Group Health Insurance and the Costs of Mandated National Coverage*, R-1509-HEW (Santa Monica, California: The Rand Corporation, September 1975), table 3, p. 6.

family policies, and for required sharing rates of 75 percent as well as 50 percent by the employer. Tables 5 and 6 provide the revised estimates for individual and family policies.

In Mitchell and Phelps,[21] three prototype plans, dubbed "low," "intermediate," and "high" mandated plans (taken from the range of proposals put forth in the Congress then), had estimated premium increases of $4.88 billion, $10.7 billion, and $18.19 billion respectively.[22] Using the revised tables, these same bills would cost $3.07 billion (63 percent of the original estimate) for the low plan; $8.3 billion (78 percent of the original estimate) for the intermediate plan; and $18.83 billion (87 percent of the original estimate) for the high plan.

While these estimates are diminished somewhat, the required premiums now estimated for the 1975 mandated NHI plans are still of considerable importance, and would still have the adverse effects on the economy noted in the original estimates.

Because the estimated unemployment effects from mandated NHI are linearly related to the implied new premiums, the revised estimates of temporary unemployment are simply the scaled down estimates of the original ones. The low plan was estimated to have a 0.3 percentage point increase in the unemployment area. I would now revise that estimate to 63 percent of that, or a 0.2 percentage point increase in unem-

---

[21] Mitchell and Phelps, *Employer-Paid Group Health Insurance.*

[22] The $10.7 billion figure is for the long-run 75 percent employer's share, rather than the initial 65 percent share planned for the first three years of the program.

TABLE 5

REVISED ESTIMATED INCREASES IN 1975 EMPLOYER
PREMIUM PAYMENTS FOR MANDATED NHI PROPOSALS—
INDIVIDUAL POLICIES

Total Premium Per Individual Policy	50% of Total Premium from Employer		75% of Total Premium from Employer	
	Level (billions)	% of original estimate	Level (billions)	% of original estimate
$200	$0.84	76	$1.37	78
220	0.96	78	1.57	81
240	1.09	80	1.78	82
260	1.21	82	2.00	84
280	1.34	83	2.22	85
300	1.48	84	2.45	87
320	1.61	85	2.68	88
340	1.75	86	2.91	88
360	1.89	87	3.15	89
380	2.04	88	3.40	90
400	2.18	89	3.64	91

SOURCE: Revision of estimates by Mitchell and Phelps. See text for a description of the method of calculating entries in the table.

ployment. For the intermediate plan, the estimated unemployment rate increase was 0.6 percentage points; an estimate of 0.5 percent is now implied. For the high plan, the original unemployment effect estimate was 1.4 percentage points; the revised estimate remains high at 1.2 percentage points. These estimates are all made on the assumption of no offsetting payments to employers. In our original estimates, we calculated the offsetting effects of various subsidies, but the methodology I am employing here is not well suited to undertake such estimates.

Finally, I turn to the question of revising the estimated reductions in income tax associated with mandated NHI. For the three prototype plans, the estimated tax revenue losses were $1.3, $2.4, and $5.9 billion respectively. Since tax revenue reductions are essentially linearly related to the additions to employer premiums, the same scaling factors can be applied for revised estimates. In 1975, the revised tax revenue reduction estimates would now be $0.84 billion for the low plan, $1.89 billion for the intermediate plan, and $5.12 billion for the high plan.

In a capsule summary, inclusion of the added $4.8 billion in

TABLE 6

REVISED ESTIMATED INCREASES IN 1975 EMPLOYER PREMIUM PAYMENTS FOR MANDATED NHI PROPOSALS— FAMILY POLICIES

Total Premium Per Family Policy	50% of Total Premium from Employer		75% of Total Premium from Employer	
	Level (billions)	% of original estimate	Level (billions)	% of original estimate
$ 400	$1.24	45	$ 2.80	58
450	1.72	53	3.65	64
500	2.23	60	4.56	69
550	2.76	64	5.52	73
600	3.30	68	6.52	76
650	3.84	71	7.58	79
700	4.45	74	8.68	81
750	5.06	77	9.84	83
800	5.70	79	11.03	84
850	6.35	80	12.27	86
900	7.02	82	13.54	87
950	7.73	83	14.83	88
1000	8.44	85	16.15	89

SOURCE: Revision of estimates by Mitchell and Phelps. See text for a description of the method of calculating entries in the table.

employer premiums known to have arisen by 1975 (in addition to those considered in Mitchell and Phelps's study) diminishes somewhat the adverse effects predicted previously, but they remain large and significant. In general, between two-thirds and seven-eighths of the previously predicted increase in employer premiums and their attendant effects would now be predicted to arise under mandated NHI in 1975.

Forecasts of Mandated NHI Effects in 1980

I now turn to a more difficult, but more interesting, task, namely extrapolating these results to a forecast of 1980 mandated NHI effects. I construct revised tables similar to those established for 1975. However, reading them must be done slightly differently. A plan that was forecast to cost $240 for an individual and $600 for a family in 1975 will be significantly more expensive in 1980. Actual per-capita personal health expenses increased by a factor of 1.4 between 1975 and 1978.

TABLE 7

ESTIMATED INCREASES IN 1980 EMPLOYER PAYMENTS
FOR MANDATED NHI—INDIVIDUAL POLICIES

Total Premium Per Individual Policy	Employer Share Required	
	50% (billions)	75% (billions)
$200	$0.7 ($0.4)	$1.1 ($0.9)
240	0.9 ($0.7)	1.3 ($1.3)
280	1.1	1.7
320	1.2	2.2
360	1.5	2.6
400	1.8	3.1
440	*2.1*	*3.6*
480	*2.4*	*4.1*
520	*2.7*	*4.6*
560	*3.0*	*5.2*
600	*3.3*	*5.8*

NOTE: Italicized entries reflect simple numerical extrapolation of other results in the table in order to extend its range. Two alternative methods for estimating some values are employed, with minimum estimates shown in parentheses. See text for details.

SOURCE: Revision and extension of estimates by Mitchell and Phelps. See text for a description of the method of calculating entries in the table.

Having been caught once by underprediction, I am loathe to do so again; therefore, I am assuming a 15 percent annual rate of increase in such expenses in 1979 and 1980. Even this may be foolhardy—the annual rate of inflation in general during 1979 has approached 12 percent, and medical expenses have exceeded most other expenses in cost increases annually since the passage of Medicare. Nevertheless, this suggests that the "intermediate" plan of our 1975 article, one requiring $240 for individual plans and $600 for family plans, would now require $440 and $1010 respectively, or some 80 percent more than in 1975.

According to my (tentative) estimates, 1980 employer contributions could be as high as $38 billion, or some $23 billion above the levels used in Mitchell and Phelps's tables. (See table 3 and associated discussion.)

Using that increase, I construct tables 7 and 8, showing estimates of the newly required premiums for individual and family policies in 1980, taking into account the increased 1980 employer contributions. The lower end of the tables' range is deleted; an upper end increased *through simple extrapolation* to make the tables more useful for 1980 cost levels. I allocate the $23 billion in additional 1980 premiums (above those used in Mitchell and Phelps's report), 20 percent to individual plans, and 80 percent to family plans, as before.

A decision is also required as to how much of the added premiums are to be allowed to reduce employer liability estimates for 1980. For example, those employers now paying 100 percent of the premium for an employee will have his payments escalate sharply (by a factor of 1.8 approximately) between 1975 and 1980 simply for increases in medical costs. Using a recent (if scanty) Health Insurance Association of America report that at least 57 percent of the work-group contracts are now paid for 100 percent by employers, the arbitrary decision employed here is to reduce the "allowable increase" fractions for a 50 percent required sharing plan to 15 percent for individual plans, and 20 percent for family plans. (Compare these numbers with 28 percent and 41 percent, respectively, chosen for 1975.) For a plan requiring 75 percent employer payment, the arbitrary choice is to allow 20 percent of the increases on individual plans, and 35 percent for family policies. (Compare with 40 percent and 53 percent for 1975.) The primary

---

TABLE 8

ESTIMATED INCREASES IN 1980 EMPLOYER PAYMENTS FOR MANDATED NHI—FAMILY POLICIES

Total Premium Per Family Policy	Employer Share Required	
	50% (billions)	75% (billions)
$ 500	$ 2.1 ($0.1)	$ 3.2 ($2.9)
600	2.6 (1.1)	4.9
700	3.0 (2.3)	7.0
800	3.5 (3.5)	9.3
900	4.9	11.9
1000	6.3	14.5
1100	7.7	17.2
1200	9.1	20.0
1400	10.5	23.0

NOTE: Italicized entries reflect simple numerical extrapolation of other results in the table in order to extend its range. Two alternative methods for estimating some values are employed, with minimum estimates shown in parentheses. See text for details.

SOURCE: Revision and extension of estimates by Mitchell and Phelps. See text for a description of the method of calculating entries in the table.

source of new employer cost under mandating in 1980 will be provision of insurance to those currently without coverage, rather than upgrading coverage of existing employees. This is particularly true given the significantly higher fraction of premiums now covered by employers, and the large proportion of plans for which the employer pays 100 percent of the premium. The numbers chosen are defensible only in that they are not implausible, and that they allow continuation of the exercise to estimate 1980 mandated NHI effects.

Independently, a lower bound can be established on new added costs. In 1980, there will be over 80 million full-time wage and salary workers, or over 72 million when the self-employed are excluded. The 1970 CHAS survey showed 47 percent of individual (unmarried) workers, and 81 percent of workers in other types of families to be covered by existing insurance. These can be rounded up to 50 percent and 85 percent for conservatism. Recall that about 20 percent of all wage earners are individuals, and 80 percent of all workers are in other types of families. These data provide reasonable estimates for the minimum new premiums required. For example, with a 50 percent sharing and a $240 individual worker premium, the minimum new amount required is $120 per worker for some 7.2 million workers (72 million total $\times$ 20 percent individual units $\times$ 50 percent currently uninsured). The lower bound for such a policy is therefore approximately $0.9 billion in 1980.[23] Tables 7 and 8 show the effective minimum required whenever that minimum exceeds the value that is calculated using the standard methodology employed in construction of these tables (which value is shown in parentheses beside the minimum number entered in the tables). The necessity of this adjustment demonstrates the potential for error associated with the crude extrapolations being undertaken here.

Two examples will be used to demonstrate the use of the 1980 tables. For the first example, I will use the "intermediate" plan discussed earlier, which in 1975 required an employer share of 75 percent, an individual premium of $240, and a family premium of $600. In 1980, such plans would cost $430 and $1100, respectively. (This plan approximated the Nixon administration's Comprehensive Health Insurance Plan.) For the second example, I will use the Carter administration's proposed NHI plan, which is reported to require *initially* a 75 percent employer share and have premium costs in the neighborhood of $630 per worker in 1980.[24] Since family premiums are approximately 2.5

---

[23] $240 $\times$ (0.5) $\times$ 7.2 million = $0.9 billion.

[24] U.S. Department of Health, Education, and Welfare, *Lead Agency Memorandum on National Health Program*, Washington, D.C., April 3, 1978.

times individual premiums, this is akin to a plan requiring $280 individual premium, and $700 family premium. The Carter concept is to phase in NHI to higher levels in later years.

The intermediate plan, using tables 7 and 8, would cost about $3.6 billion for the individual component, and $17 billion for the family component, or $20.6 billion. It resembles the final phases of the Carter plans.

The estimated required new premiums for the initial Carter proposal are taken directly from tables 7 and 8 as $1.7 billion for individuals, and $7.0 billion for families, or a total of $8.7 billion, considerably above the "official" estimates of about $6 billion for the Carter plan in 1980. These estimates accept uncritically the estimated per-worker premium for the Carter plan. If actual costs exceed those envisioned by HEW analysts, then employer premium costs also rise. It is precisely for this reason that I provide tables 7 and 8. They allow the reader to estimate required new premiums for nearly *any* conceivable mandated plan, with per-worker costs chosen at the discretion of the analyst.

The direct unemployment calculations made for 1975 data cannot be readily derived using the methodology presented here. The most reliable approach would be to translate loosely any proposed 1980 plan into 1975 cost levels and use estimates in the original Mitchell and Phelps report to predict unemployment levels. Since premium contributions were underestimated in the Mitchell and Phelps assumptions, and have increased since then in intervening years to 1980, those predicted unemployment effects must be adjusted towards zero. The proportional adjustments shown in tables 5 and 6 of this paper provide a useful method of adjustment for the 1975 premium corrections. Roughly doubling the indicated downward percentage adjustment for 1980 is probably appropriate. For example, if table 5 or table 6 shows a 15 percent decline in new employer costs relative to Mitchell and Phelps, then 1980 estimates are probably not too far from a 30 percent downward adjustment to the estimated unemployment costs. This must be true because the approximate decline in *real* liability to employers is about the same between 1975 and 1980 as were the adjustments made herein to modify the original Mitchell and Phelps estimates.

Tax revenue reduction estimates are slightly more complicated. Premium contributions by employers have grown dramatically, as shown, and these have had their associated tax receipt-reducing effects already! Although mandating will not have as large an effect per se, the hidden costs to the government in maintaining the tax deductibility of employer premium payments has already partly increased, even without mandated insurance. Also, general inflation has markedly increased the marginal tax rates of many individuals, thereby increasing the estimated tax revenue reductions from either mandated insurance or continued maintenance of the health insurance exemption from taxation. Simple extrapolation of the tax revenue losses from current (1980) employer contributions (using the data from table 3) suggest that the 1980 tax expenditure will be at least $12.3 billion, even if there has been no change in marginal tax rates of individuals due to inflation. Inflation-derived increases in marginal tax rates could readily increase this estimate to above $13 billion. Mandated NHI would increase these amounts from $3 to $7 billion for the prototype plans discussed above.

Concluding Remarks

The estimates and tables provided herein should be treated only as crude approximations of potential reality. A ten-year-old data base is being used for analysis of phenomena that have undergone substantial change during the decade. Nevertheless, these tables should serve as a useful indicator of the level of new employer costs associated with various health insurance plans. The concomitant effects on employment (in the short run) and on tax receipts can be inferred from these estimates. The pertinent message to ponder is that, even with the substantial increases in premium contributions by employers on behalf of their employees, there remain significant new costs associated with mandating of NHI, and the associated effects of employment and tax receipts will be substantial for many proposed plans. These effects should be taken into account when legislation considering the imposition of mandated national health insurance is debated.

Commentaries

Glenn R. Markus

Many of the excellent points made in the papers in this section underscore the importance of the political environment in which some of the economic aspects of alternative approaches to national health insurance are being considered. The Meyer/Penner paper in particular makes several significant observations in this regard.

The first of these is that most national health insurance proposals would affect health care spending primarily by shifting the composition, source, and direction of much of the spending now occurring in the economy. Despite the rhetoric about additional spending for the benefit of the "have nots" in our society—those not protected by insurance or by other programs—political reality focuses the policy-making process on some of the more sensitive issues, such as who will pay for whom and how much? Federal budgetary concerns and impact, which is the focus of the Meyer/Penner paper, are certainly parts of this process. But, insofar as national health insurance is concerned, the budgetary impact of alternative decisions seems, at this juncture, to be far more important to the executive branch of the federal government and to economists than it does to the Congress. Though concerned with the flow of health dollars to and from the national budget, the current debate has not focused on budgetary considerations per se. Congress seems to recognize quite clearly that decisions relating to a national health plan will have broad economic impact—far beyond consequences for government budgets alone.

The Meyer/Penner paper also notes, with some concern, that there is little assessment of the long-range economic implications of passage of a major national program. This, however, is a common indictment of the public policy-making process, and I do not fully understand what the authors suggest needs to be undertaken in order to ease their concerns. Long-range forecasting and assessment, it seems to me, rarely appear to have much of an impact on the ordinary political decision-making processes of the Congress. I would be especially surprised if

74

such an analysis—were it to be done—would have much significance for current NHI discussions.

Nevertheless, Meyer and Penner raise some tough and troublesome questions. What, for instance, will be the impact of a national health insurance plan on the supply and distribution of health resources? How will any additional stimulus of demand affect the increasingly serious inflation pressures in the health care field? Some of these critical questions may be dealt with politically as discrete policy issues, rather than as parts of any coherent review of national health alternatives. Cost containment, for example, is being considered in the Congress separate from various financing and coverage issues. There are also a number of so-called incremental health benefit proposals before Congress, which have more modest coverage or financing goals than do the comprehensive proposals that are regularly labeled as national health plans. Some of these bills look only to the aged, others to the poor or to mothers and children. Passage of such piecemeal legislation makes rationalization of our national health resources even more difficult to bring about.

NHI-watchers on Capitol Hill have also learned to pay careful attention to the reactions of the institutional constituencies who have an important stake in alternative health insurance actions. The views of the business community and of organized labor about employee fringe benefits, and their costs, are especially critical in this regard. So, too, are the views of states and local governments, whose changing fiscal fortunes will most assuredly shape answers to the questions Meyer and Penner have asked about the impact of NHI proposals on the budget.

Robert P. Inman

This paper gives us two often neglected facts regarding the financing of any national health insurance (NHI) plan. First, NHI is likely to involve important redistributions of income from the rich to the poor. Second, if financed from general taxation, NHI may generate significant tax costs in excess of the dollars of revenues raised and this "excess burden" of taxation may be as high as twenty cents per tax dollar. What are we to make of these findings when designing an NHI proposal?

It is important to realize, first of all, that any health insurance program involves a redistribution—from the healthy to the sick—and the simple facts of disease incidence imply a high negative correlation of this redistribution with family income. The poor get sick, and the sick are poorer.[1] This fact, however, does not negate the potential social

---

[1] Disentangling the income-health relationship is problematic to be sure, but for recent evidence that seeks to establish the linkages from income to health and from health to income, see S. Rosen and P. Taubman, "Changes in the Impact

value of the insurance program. A simple example makes the point. Imagine one group in society is initially rich (average income equal to $20,000) and another relatively poor (average income of $10,000) with families in the rich group facing probability of chronic illness of 0.02 and families in the poor group facing higher probability of 0.04. Assume the population is divided equally between the two groups. If the chronic illness imposes a (present value) cost of $100,000 on those who happen to get sick, then the expected costs to the rich families will be $2,000 (= 0.02 × $100,000) and the expected costs to the poor families will be $4,000 (= 0.04 × $100,000). It seems likely that both groups would like to purchase insurance to cover these large potential losses. If the two groups could be easily identified—that is, if the causal relationship between "observed" income and the generally "unobserved" illness probability were known—private insurers could write insurance contracts which in the long-run could cover these expected losses and make both groups better off. In fact, the true illness probabilities for chronic illnesses or an identifying characteristic related to these probabilities are not likely to be known. In this instance, it can be shown that (1) no stable, competitive insurance equilibrium need exist (with no insurance as one possible outcome), and (2), if so, a pooled government-enforced insurance contract may be preferred by both groups.[2] This government-run "catastrophic" health insurance program would charge each citizen a common $3,000 premium equal to the expected pooled expenses of insurance, the average of each group's expected losses of $2,000 and $4,000.[3] Note, however, the resulting distribution of dollar benefits. When all is done, the rich have paid a $3,000 premium per family and received, on average, $2,000 per family in benefits for a *net dollar loss* to the group of $1,000 per family. The poor families on the other hand have paid their $3,000 per family premium and received, on average, $4,000 per family in benefits for a *net dollar gain* to the group of $1,000 per family. Clearly, dollars have moved from the rich to the poor, but this redistributional fact is *only an incidental outcome of a unanimously preferred catastrophic*

---

of Education and Income of Mortality in the U.S.," unpublished paper, Department of Economics, University of Pennsylvania, 1979; A. Bartel and P. Taubman, "Health and Labor Market Success: The Role of Various Diseases," *Review of Economics and Statistics*, vol. 61 (February 1979), pp. 1–9, and H. Luft, "The Impact of Poor Health on Earnings," *Review of Economics and Statistics*, vol. 57 (February 1975), pp. 43–57.

[2] See M. Rothchild and J. Stiglitz, "Equilibrium in Competitive Insurance Markets: An Essay on the Economics of Imperfect Information," *Quarterly Journal of Economics*, vol. 90 (November 1976), pp. 629–51.

[3] These large premiums need not be paid all at once, for this is a lifetime insurance contract. Premiums can be spread over each family's working years with an interest charge for deferred payments.

insurance program in response to a market failure. In this example, the observed redistribution of dollars has no bearing whatsoever on the desirability of the proposed health insurance plan. Put simply, the dollar transfers are all part of a mutually acceptable agreement which offers both groups better risk coverage.

While a simple counting of dollar flows between income groups can therefore be extremely misleading—"NHI should not be a redistribution program, therefore any observed redistributions negate the value of the policy"—there is no doubt that NHI contains within it the potential for significant redistributions beyond that justified by an efficiency-motivated extension of insurance coverage. Professors Browning and Johnson are right to call our attention to this matter. But the important task is to separate the aggregate dollar flows reported by Browning and Johnson into those transfers which are pure redistributions unrelated to improved coverage.[4] To do so, one must have a clear prior notion of what is the allocatively preferred NHI package. That decision involves a subtle balancing of risk coverage, health care costs, and population health improvements;[5] no mean task to be sure, but a necessary one if we are to interpret the Browning-Johnson redistribution numbers properly.

More to the point is Browning and Johnson's fact number two: NHI imposes a cost of $1.20 for each new dollar of tax revenues required.[6] This $0.20 added ("excess burden") cost per dollar revenue raised is an efficiency loss quite in addition to any allocative efficiency

---

[4] We might suspect that a major source of non-insurance-related redistribution within any NHI proposal comes from the progressive tax financing of insurance coverage. In general, that is probably correct, but we still need a careful analysis of the issues before concluding that proportional or progressive tax financing is totally unwarranted. It is perfectly reasonable that under certain circumstances the preferred catastrophic insurance scheme should pay "pain and suffering" in addition to medical expenses. See, for example, S. Shavell, "Theoretical Issues in Medical Malpractice," in S. Rottenberg, ed., *The Economics of Medical Malpractice* (Washington, D.C.: American Enterprise Institute, 1978). If for administrative reasons only medical expenses are explicitly covered by insurance, then "pain and suffering" compensation can be offered through tax relief for certain illnesses, making the overall tax package potentially progressive when illness and income are inversely related.

[5] See, for example, J. Harris, "The Aggregate Coinsurance Rate and the Supply of Innovations in the Hospital Sector," unpublished paper, Massachusetts Institute of Technology, Department of Economics, July 1979.

[6] As Professors Browning and Johnson emphasize, their estimate of a $0.20 marginal excess burden for new taxation is at best a first guess. Their table 5 is only briefly described and references to the relevant supporting literature are not provided. It is therefore difficult to judge the accuracy of their numbers. Yet calculations of this sort are an extremely subtle business; see, for example, J. R. Green and E. Sheshinski, "Approximating the Efficiency Gain of Tax Reforms," *Journal of Public Economics*, vol. 11 (April 1979), pp. 179–95.

losses in the health care sector itself prompted by NHI. How shall we use this important fact in the debate over NHI? The answer turns largely on how that debate is placed within the general budgetary deliberations of Congress.

The advice of Browning and Johnson is to require that each dollar spent on NHI generate at least a net social benefit (loosely, the gains from risk coverage and improved health minus added health care costs) which exceeds the $1.20 marginal social costs of raising that dollar through the existing tax structure. The advice is sound, but only within a particular, though perfectly reasonable, budgetary setting. First, Browning and Johnson take the existing tax structure as given and assume NHI will be financed from such taxes. Second, they assume all existing public programs will continue to be funded; thus, NHI is truly the marginal public program. Third, they assume NHI itself is being debated incrementally so that the marginal NHI dollar can indeed be balanced against its marginal tax cost. Dropping any one of these three assumptions about the form of the NHI debate will require a change in the Browning-Johnson rule.

First, instead of relying on the payroll tax and the current income tax, potentially more efficient taxes are available whose excess burden losses may be below the $0.14 to $0.46 margins estimated by Browning and Johnson. There is no irrevocable reason why NHI need be financed by existing taxes; fixed premiums are always an option, as are any slightly less regressive variants. There is good reason to believe that such lump-sum charges will have lower efficiency losses than the existing tax system.[7] Importantly, an NHI proposal which fails the $1.20 marginal social benefit requirement might well pass the test of a lower cut-off made possible through a more efficient financing structure. In any case, it is important to look for new financing strategies before ruling against NHI as a necessarily inefficient policy.

Second, if NHI is considered within a more general budget context than simply being counted as the last, or marginal, public policy, then the relevant marginal tax cost for NHI may not be Browning and Johnson's $1.20. Specifically, a wide range of existing public programs may, after time, have been revealed to offer marginal social benefits significantly less than NHI's.[8] Such existing programs ought then to be

---

[7] Another option now debated in the tax policy literature is to move the entire tax structure away from our current income tax and towards a broad-based consumption tax. It has been estimated that such a move would significantly reduce the excess burden of our tax structure, but these estimates are now best seen as preliminary. See, for example, Green and Sheshinski, "Approximating the Efficiency Gain."

[8] Public programs can outlive their usefulness, or policies which were thought before funding to have a high pay-off may prove to be ineffective once in place.

considered as inferior to NHI. Placing NHI ahead of these inferior programs in the line for public funding, we may find that the relevant marginal tax costs for funding NHI is not now $1.20 but say $1.15 or $1.10. (I am assuming that the marginal tax costs rise as we increase the size of the public budget, and the best programs ranked by marginal social benefits now get the first public dollars.) An NHI proposal which might have failed the $1.20 limit might pass when properly ordered within the ranking of public programs. Note, however, that the many existing public programs inferior to NHI would then be phased out as they fail to generate marginal benefits in excess of their marginal tax costs. This is as it should be.

Third, the design of NHI is an exceedingly complex problem and fine-tuning its level of funding may be impossible. Thus, as a political matter, NHI decision making may reduce to a series of decisions to accept or reject three or four very different proposals, rather than considering the appropriate incremental expansion of a favored plan. If so, then the choice should not be based on a comparison of the social benefits of a plan's marginal NHI dollar with the costs of its marginal tax dollar. Rather, the criterion should be to select that proposal with the largest positive difference between aggregate social benefits and aggregate tax costs. Against this criterion, we might well prefer an NHI package whose marginal social benefits are less than its marginal tax cost. This preferred program might be too large (marginal benefits less than marginal costs), but it is still better than all the alternatives, including no NHI at all.

How NHI is to be considered within the budgetary process therefore plays a crucial role in determining how we ought to judge alternative proposals. Browning and Johnson have assumed one budgetary model which places each NHI dollar at the margin of the public budget, and they rightly ask that that dollar generate benefits to compensate for its high marginal tax costs. Alternative scenarios of how NHI will be decided are possible to imagine, however, and these different budgetary settings may demand less of the marginal NHI expenditure. Again, a simple fact may be misleading unless understood within the broader context of its proposed use.

Professors Browning and Johnson have placed two new hurdles before those who search for the holy grail of NHI. They have asked us to justify the observed dollar redistributions within any NHI proposal on the grounds of improved risk coverage or better health, or else to stand up and make the case explicitly for any additional income redistribution which an NHI proposal might entail. They also want us to be sure that NHI's benefits exceed the explicit and hidden costs of public financing. Neither challenge can be ignored.

COMMENTARIES

W. Kip Viscusi

Phelps's assessment of the impact of mandated employee health insurance benefits is a careful analysis. He uses a large set of data on past employer health insurance costs to estimate the likely increase in costs due to national health insurance. The cost projections entail a variety of assumptions that appear reasonable and are also delineated clearly so that the underpinnings of the analysis can be scrutinized. The sensitivity of the findings to the most crucial assumption—the extensiveness of the national health insurance plan—is also addressed through consideration of low, high, and intermediate plans. Since the analysis throughout the paper is of consistently high quality, the emphasis of the discussion below will be on the relationship of these findings to several broader issues raised by mandated compensation.

The first issue pertains to the nature of the financing of national health insurance. In particular, why is the program to be funded by the equivalent of a payroll tax rather than an income tax? The structure of the financing closely resembles that of the social security payroll tax with deductions from worker earnings and a division of the tax between the employer and employee. The principal difference of mandated compensation is that the tax would probably be a fixed amount per worker rather than an increasing function of one's earnings.

The parallels with the social security payroll tax not only reflect the political advantage of having an off-budget expenditure, but also may be an attempt to replicate the success of social security. That program is the most successful remnant of the New Deal, in part because there is widespread perception that beneficiaries have an earned right to benefits. Although the link between contributions and benefits under social security is not as strong as it should be to preserve work incentives fully, there is a substantial relationship between the two. Unless national health insurance taxes and benefits are also linked, it is doubtful that the program image will be enhanced. The widespread awareness by female spouses of the lack of a link between their social security taxes and benefits suggests that taxpayers have a sufficient understanding of program incentive structures to distinguish policies that reward one on the basis of one's financial contributions from those that do not.

A second concern pertains to the effect of mandated compensation on employment. One side effect of the tax is that wages will rise. Consider the following simplified example. Suppose initially that only workers at Firm X receive health insurance, but after national health insurance all individuals in society will receive these benefits. Coverage of all individuals diminishes the relative attractiveness of jobs at Firm X since they are no longer receiving additional health coverage not received by others. As a consequence, the wage must rise to attract these workers in the future.

Viewed somewhat more generally, there will be a long-run negative effect of mandated benefits on labor force participation rates (that is, the employed and the searching unemployed). An increase in the costs of hiring workers will not only have short-run unemployment effects but will also diminish the size of the labor force.

The employment effects of the tax do not hinge on the division of the employer and employee shares. If one ignores the differential tax status of the payments, there will be no difference in the impact of the tax whether it is labeled an employer contribution or a tax to be borne by workers. In competitive contexts, the effects will be identical. This argument does not involve any complicated analysis of short-run or long-run tax incidence, but rather stems from the irrelevance of labels in assessing the economic consequences of a financing system. The wage plus nonwage costs imposed by workers will be identical regardless of the formal division of the burden, if markets function in the conventional fashion.

In assessing the incentive effects of the policy, one must know not only the tax rate but also the link between the taxes and the benefits. To the extent that the mandated-compensation approach permits a linkage between taxes and benefits, there will be greater preservation of work incentives than if there were no such relationship. Tax payments are expected to be in terms of a levy per worker rather than in terms of a percentage of one's earned income throughout a broad range, as in a standard payroll tax. The primary effect of preserving a link between taxes and benefits will not relate to the worker's hours-of-work decision (although employer attitudes toward overtime will be altered), but will pertain instead to the discrete choices of whether or not to work, which enterprise to select, and which occupation to pursue.

The mandated-compensation concept also offers an additional advantage in terms of increasing the diversity in health insurance coverage. Plans with different degrees of coverage can better match individual needs, such as different levels of health insurance demand for different income groups. Unless the array of plans offered becomes too broad, it is doubtful that any major economies of scale will be forgone. Moreover, a diverse approach offers potentially large gains in terms of creating an environment that will encourage innovative responses to health care needs, such as new institutional responses and various kinds of health maintenance organizations. The motivation for permitting additional coverage of individuals above some minimal insurance level can be traced to several economic advantages of this approach and need not be attributed to the tax breaks that can be potentially reaped by arranging the compensation package in this fashion.

It should be emphasized that even Phelps's dramatic estimates of the impacts of national health insurance are likely to be quite conservative. A critical input to ascertaining the increase in employer costs is the likely cost to be imposed by national health insurance—a figure that was not calculated by Phelps. If there is any lesson from the Medicare experience, it is that the imposition of increased demands on the health care system will boost prices and diminish quality.

What we can reasonably expect is that national health insurance will be costly and will have a profound effect on the medical care system. The principal missing input is some assessment of the likely benefits of this effect. More specifically, what effect will national health insurance have on medical care received and, more importantly, on the health status of the beneficiaries? How would health insurance coverage of different groups in the economy differ, and what would be the change in the level of coverage and morbidity and mortality distributions? In view of the substantial costs of this policy, it seems ill-advised to make a major commitment of resources to this area without ascertaining the answers to such fundamental questions.

Part Two

Solving the Problem of
Underinsurance

Rationales for Government Initiative in Catastrophic Health Insurance

Bernard Friedman

Introduction

When a family has catastrophic health insurance (CHI), it is assured that financial consequences of health care will be no more than a modest loss in relation to net worth. This feature of an insurance contract is sometimes called a "stop-loss," which limits a family's direct payment for covered services to a maximum of, for example, $2,000 per year. Universal stop-loss protection is a shared objective of most proposals for new federal government intervention in health care and insurance markets.

The purpose of this paper is to assess a variety of arguments for a federal CHI program. A government CHI program might be advocated because insurance markets fail to create contracts that people are willing to purchase or because existing public regulatory and subsidy programs promote inefficient insurance holdings and other undesirable effects. This study finds the latter rationale the more persuasive.

This introductory section will review the availability and the growth of CHI in the private sector, the evidence on the marginal cost of adding a stop-loss in conventional coverage, and the reasons for thinking of CHI as protecting family wealth rather than health.

The recent growth in stop-loss protection might be the insurance industry's response to the threat of government intervention or simply a response to the growth in demand. For a better understanding of the prevalence of CHI, alternative theories must be formulated and tested. Theoretical analyses of potential inefficiency in insurance markets have not previously been subjected to much empirical testing. Theoretical models of the demand for insurance, with very few exceptions, presume that the demand for CHI at fair premiums would be universal. How-

NOTE: I am grateful to the Center for Health Services and Policy Research at Northwestern University for financial assistance, to Cynthia Alessis for highly productive research assistance, and to the National Bureau of Economic Research for supporting an analysis of insurance data used in the paper. Editorial comments by Mark Pauly were helpful in clarifying the rationale for reform of existing public-financed health insurance.

ever, it will be argued, beginning in the section "Does CHI Protect Wealth or Health," that demand analysis has previously omitted important considerations.

The section entitled "Indicators of Market Failure" will consider whether the problem of adverse selection and associated transaction costs may account for the absence of CHI until recently. It is found that this type of conceivable market failure is not consistent with either important detailed characteristics of the uninsured population or the slow growth of conventional HMOs since 1973. The section "Consumer Demand for Stop-Loss Insurance" will consider whether an appropriate model of the consumer and social institutions in health care can account for the uninsured population, the late historical growth of CHI, and the slow growth of HMOs.

Availability and Growth of CHI. Before 1967, virtually no one except subscribers of HMOs and those already impoverished had stop-loss protection for health care. This is no longer true. The pace of innovation, however, has been so rapid that data are rather fragmentary.

In 1967, Aetna Life & Casualty (the second-largest private underwriter) initiated a stop-loss provision for federal employees, reimbursing 100 percent of covered family expenses over $10,000. Today, their high-option policy has an annual stop-loss of $1,000 per person and $2,000 per family. These are the most common stop-loss parameters found in unpublished surveys by the Health Insurance Association of America. According to that organization, some 95 million persons in 1977 held "major medical" contracts with private insurance companies, and half of these contained stop-loss provisions.[1] In 1972, by comparison, only about 10 percent had a stop-loss.

Currently, thirty-five of sixty-nine Blue Cross Associations offer various stop-loss provisions in their major medical contracts. This fraction perhaps underestimates catastrophic protection by Blue Cross Associations, since "basic benefits" sometimes cover full hospital costs for 120 or even 365 days.[2] Considering the coverage of Blue Cross Associations, private companies, and HMOs, it seems conservative to say that at least half of insured persons have CHI.

Stop-loss provisions first appeared in employer group contracts,

---

[1] Major medical coverage is tabulated in Health Insurance Institute, *Source Book of Health Insurance Data 1977–78* (Washington, D.C., 1978). The definition of "catastrophic insurance" in this publication is a high maximum benefit. David Robbins of Health Insurance Association of America supplied unpublished survey information on stop-loss provisions.

[2] This information was obtained from actuary Carl Madrecki at the National Blue Cross headquarters.

but they are now available in individual contracts. Prudential Insurance Company of America is the largest private insurer and second only to Mutual of Omaha in individual contracts. Prudential has offered a stop-loss in group contracts since 1969 and in individual contracts since 1973. The stop-loss is $1,000 per family in their principal plan, and there is no maximum benefit.

Even a casual attempt to become informed about the non-group-insurance market is enough to dispel extreme views about the unavailability of options and the consequences of the problem of adverse selection. The Prudential plan for individuals, for example, is available nationwide and does not require a medical exam. Premiums are based on the insured's age and sex, and every state has allowed four levels of surcharge based on medical history. Company executives say that about 16 percent of all contracts are written with a surcharge. The standard premium for a family headed by a thirty-five-year-old man is only about 20 percent above the cost of comparable coverage in large employer groups.[3]

Mutual of Omaha does not offer a stop-loss in their contracts, but this company and others refute the notion that an individual cannot buy a stand-alone major risk contract. A policy with a $2,000 deductible and 20 percent coinsurance up to a benefit of $250,000 would cost a thirty-year-old man about $80 per year.[4] The Equitable Life Assurance Society offers a $2,000 deductible with a stop-loss at $3,000. The annual cost for a thirty-five-year-old man is about $187. Companies newly entering the market, such as State Farm, offer a stop-loss, so Mutual of Omaha's failure to do so is perhaps only complacence as a result of its large market share. The three companies cited do not find much demand for high deductibles, which is perhaps not surprising in view of tax incentives for the purchase of health insurance.

One persistent problem in the individual contract market is the differentially higher cost of accommodating applicants with temporary demands for insurance. Prudential, Aetna, and others are screening out the unemployed and students into separate plans with special restrictions. To save on commissions and other initiation costs, these plans are being written with exclusions of preexisting medical conditions and

---

[3] Information on Prudential's Comprehensive Health Insurance Plan was provided by Richard Drake, vice-president and associate actuary. The premium quotation for the text illustration was $110 per month in the Chicago area, compared with the Aetna High Option plan for federal employees at $87 per month. Blue Cross groups paid as much as $140 per month in the same area for more complete insurance, and Northwestern University employees have a Prudential option with a bit higher copayment costing $85 per month.

[4] The premiums quoted in this paragraph also apply to the Chicago area, where costs are above the national average.

lower maximum benefits. Brokerage fees and the costs of medical evaluation are reduced.

Differential costs of stop-loss protection are averaged in group insurance plans, so that older people or those in poorer health, who would pay high individual rates, receive a relative subsidy in large employer groups. An interesting research question is whether these differential costs are fully arbitraged in the labor markets, especially if lifetime rather than annual earnings and benefits are considered. For example, age discrimination would be expected to be more prevalent in the hiring practices of large employers and the length of their employees' careers shorter.

Extra Premium Cost of a Stop-Loss. The cost of adding stop-loss protection to a more conventional plan can be estimated from a variety of sources. This section will review some experience for federal employees under age sixty-five and for residents of the states of Rhode Island and Maine.

In 1977, the Aetna High Option plan for federal government employees included about 274,000 contracts for families headed by an enrollee under age sixty-five. A total of about 730,000 persons were covered under these contracts.[5] Our analysis shows that average health care expenses for this sample are only slightly lower than for more nationally representative insured groups; the proportional importance of large bills is perhaps slightly higher than for other large insured groups.

Claimants faced the following approximate parameters on effective coverage: a deductible of $60 and coinsurance of 15 to 20 percent depending on the composition of services. The stop-loss would be invoked when family covered expenses reached $10,000. A family with two children would therefore have a maximum out-of-pocket risk of about $2,000. The expenditure distribution for such a family was synthesized from the distribution of claims for adults and children and from exogenous estimates of unclaimed expense. Families of four who incurred more than $10,000 in medical expenses accounted for about 22 percent of the expenses incurred by all families of four. The extra benefits received from the stop-loss were only about $25 per family, or some 2.6 percent of the family premium of $960.

It is likely that this benefit of $25 per family is an underestimate of the marginal cost of adding the stop-loss. The existence of this provision has probably induced some increased spending. For example, if

---

[5] The extent of selection bias and other characteristics of this sample that may lead to unrepresentative expenditures have been analyzed in a technical note available from the author.

half of all expenses over $10,000 could be attributed to the availability of the stop-loss, the marginal premium cost would have been $77, still a modest fraction of the total premium.

The marginal cost of government CHI would be less than the amount suggested by insurance claims statistics because it would partly replace other redistributive transfers. This result is illustrated in the experience of state-financed CHI in Rhode Island since 1975. The Rhode Island plan has a stop-loss of $5,000 or 50 percent of allowable income for families with no insurance, and $500 or 10 percent of income for families with a conventional package of basic and major medical coverage. Benefits are paid as a "last-resort" program, subordinated to Medicaid and free care of various sorts.

In 1977, total benefit payments and administration cost were less than two dollars per state resident.[6] The subpopulation with qualified private insurance received benefits of about $2.80 per family. This differs from the Aetna claims experience by an order of magnitude, presumably partly because there are other avenues for care and payment than the last-resort CHI. This possibility will be further examined in the section "Does CHI Protect Wealth or Health?"

The state of Maine has also had a tax-supported CHI program for five years. The stop-loss is $1,000 per person, regardless of insurance coverage. Provided that many persons do not drop their private contracts (and this apparently has not occurred), it would not be surprising if there were fewer beneficiaries in Maine per capita because family expenses are not aggregated. The more generous coverage of the uninsured, however, seems to outweigh the individual eligibility, and there are more recipients per capita than in Rhode Island. The cost per resident is again less than two dollars for a program with benefit payments about 1 percent as much as Medicaid assistance.[7]

A federal CHI program would not be as cheap as those of Rhode Island and Maine because states would not treat it as a last resort. The Aetna experience cited above would also underestimate the cost of a federal program, once private contracts are rewritten. The marginal premium cost of $25 per family of four was the difference between 80 percent and 100 percent reimbursement of losses over $10,000. With a *federal* stop-loss of $2,000 and 80 percent reimbursement, the family would not want to pay any premium for private insurance coverage of gross expenses over $10,000. The average federal cost of paying

---

[6] Detailed experience of the Rhode Island plan is available in James Cooney et al., *Analysis of Rhode Island Catastrophic Health Insurance Program*, Final Report on grant 1-R01-HS-02786-01 (Hyattsville, Md.: National Center for Health Services Research, 1978).

[7] These unpublished data were obtained from the Maine Bureau of Social Welfare.

100 percent of the larger losses would have been about $130, or 13.5 percent of total premiums.

The marginal cost of CHI in existing private contracts is evidently rather low. This presents some puzzles for microeconomic analysis. This low marginal cost does not by itself justify mandating CHI as the desirable first step in a comprehensive federal insurance plan. Reasons should be offered for compelling people to make such purchases. The state experience suggests that people have other avenues of support for large bills. If a federal CHI is to replace these other supports, an analysis of the prospective benefits should be undertaken.

Does CHI Protect Wealth or Health? Customarily, theoretical models of the demand for health insurance ignore other social institutions in medical care. Such models often assume that bankruptcy would prevent a family from receiving desired care, but this assumption ignores price discounts by hospitals and doctors, free care in state institutions, and means-tested assistance such as Medicaid. These alternatives may seriously affect the demand for CHI.

Price discrimination in medical care has a long history, going back at least to the Code of Hammurabi. Today we still observe this discrimination in hospital financing, despite the growth of reimbursement insurance and the formalization of public assistance. Nonfederal short-term hospitals in 1976 did not collect 15 percent of their "gross revenue"—billable services at standard rates. Obviously, standard rates tend to be high enough to offset the shortfall in collections, allowing for philanthropic gifts. The shortfall is greater in the larger hospitals, reaching 19 percent for hospitals with over 500 beds.[8]

The shortfall in collections can be broken down into three categories. The first category is composed of patients who have not payed their bills but may eventually make some payment and are judged able to pay. This accounts for only about one-third of the total shortfall. A second category called "charity care" involves mostly patients who use outpatient clinic services where all prospective charges are waived at the initial encounter. The final and largest category is contractual discounts for individual patients, adapted to their particular situations.[9]

In 1976 there were about 24.4 million individual recipients of

---

[8] These crude data are published by the American Hospital Association in their *Hospital Statistics*, 1977 edition, p. 184.

[9] One study of 130 hospitals in seven states in 1971 was reported in *Hospital Financial Management*, December 1972. Total deductions from gross revenue were found to be about 11 percent throughout a ten-year period. Bad debts were declining to just over 4 percent. A second study, appearing in the same journal in May 1973, covered nine states and found that between 25 percent and 60 percent of bills to "self-paying" patients went uncollected.

Medicaid payments for health care. Some of this group are eligible for assistance solely because of health problems and costs, and not because of conventional poverty definitions. About 2.8 million were disabled persons under age sixty-five, who were often previously employed. Another 2 million were eligible solely because the family had large medical bills relative to income and size. Availability of this assistance in many states tends both to reduce financial barriers to medical care and to formalize redistributive financing of major expenses by all taxpayers.

In view of public and private redistributive arrangements in medical care, it may be rational for people to believe that exhausting their wealth will not lead to total deprivation of care. They may nevertheless wish to provide for the option to demand more than the standard. Such a decision, if based on expectations of utility, would display very complex information requirements.

The literature on medical ethics and critical care decisions suggests that most physicians are biased toward aggressive treatment of all "salvageable" patients, even those with permanent damage. In a major empirical study of current practices in hospital settings, Crane found that, while physicians do use a variety of plausible criteria for withholding or withdrawing therapy in some critical cases, the financial burden of care upon society is by far the least important consideration. The wishes of patients and families were not even as powerful as one might expect (or hope), partly because of the diffusion of authority in the hospital setting. In this study and other reports, physicians express particular discomfort in accommodating the requests of families or their own conceptions of duty to terminate care that is expensive and largely fruitless.[10]

The above observations are offered to justify a model of the demand for insurance in which family disposable wealth is the ultimate stop-loss. It is not implied that demand for care is independent of wealth, prices, or tastes. Instead, what is important is that unpredictability about charges for health care is only one aspect of uncertainty related to health. The unpredictability about the outcomes of illness and accident, the quality of care, or the timely availability of resources motivate a variety of existing market arrangements and interventions. For example, we observe programs that intensively screen new providers,

---

[10] Diana Crane, *The Sanctity of Social Life: Physicians' Treatment of Critically Ill Patients* (New York: Russell Sage Foundation, 1975). Additional references are more anecdotal than the work by Crane. There have been some articles in popular magazines and notes in medical journals on a patient's right to die. The various interviews and surveys on physician opinion on this particular subject suggest that the social cost of "heroic" care is largely irrelevant, and the family cost may have some weight for the fraction of doctors who follow the wishes of the family and patient under critical circumstances.

triage selections in emergency and outpatient care, and frequent lawsuits for nonconformity with standards of care.

Health insurance contracts have a value that depends on the context of these other arrangements. Families with relatively low disposable wealth may attach a low value to CHI because of other redistributive and quality assurance practices. This may help to explain the pattern of demand for CHI in the marketplace. A more formal model will be presented in the section "Consumer Demand for Stop-Loss Insurance."

Indicators of Market Failure

Market failure may be defined as the nonoccurrence of mutually advantageous transactions. This is sharp enough for useful empirical investigation, although Arrow argues that a more insightful general concept is the inefficiency in the size of transactions as a result of transaction cost. One should not presume that transaction cost is largely avoidable by government programs; this point has been argued by Pauly in the case of health insurance.[11] It would seem that market failure, narrowly defined, presents more of a *prima facie* case for intervention.

The first question to be addressed in this section is whether the existence of a meaningful number of persons holding no health insurance contracts is evidence of market failure. Survey analyses of insured and uninsured populations have been presented by Aday and Andersen and the Congressional Budget Office (CBO).[12] Predictions about the characteristics of uninsured persons in the case of market failure can be derived from theoretical studies by Pauly[13] and by Rothschild and Stiglitz.[14]

The theoretical papers partition a population into groups with a low or high risk of monetary loss to be insured. Each competitive firm offers some dollar benefit in the event a loss occurs and charges a premium that in equilibrium is equal to expected benefit per contract.

---

[11] Mark V. Pauly, *The Role of the Private Sector in National Health Insurance* (New York: Health Insurance Association of America, 1979), pp. 20–28.

[12] Lu Ann Aday and Ronald Andersen, "Insurance Coverage and Access: Implications for Health Policy," *Health Services Research*, vol. 13 (1978), 369; U.S. Congressional Budget Office, *Profile of Health Care Coverage: The Haves and Have-Nots*, Washington, D.C., 1979.

[13] Mark V. Pauly, "Overinsurance and Public Provision of Insurance," *Quarterly Journal of Economics*, vol. 88 (February 1974), pp. 44–62.

[14] Michael Rothschild and Joseph Stiglitz, "Equilibrium in Competitive Insurance Markets: An Essay on the Economics of Imperfect Information," *Quarterly Journal of Economics*, vol. 90 (November 1976), pp. 629–49.

Although the individual knows his risk class, the firm cannot distinguish the risk class of a particular individual.

In Pauly's model, there is a single market-clearing contract and premium, with a premium greater than actuarially fair for low-risk buyers. Thus, consumers choosing not to buy insurance should belong to the low-risk group. Rothschild and Stiglitz show that a firm might find it profitable to offer a contract with low benefit and low premium to attract only the low-risk buyer. An equilibrium with multiple types of contract, however, can be unstable. As more people are attracted into a low-benefit contract, premiums for the higher-benefit contracts increase, possibly leading high-risk individuals to switch to the low-benefit contract, driving up the costs of the premium there. At a given time, if there are multiple contracts, one should find relatively more low-risk persons in the low-benefit contract.

If a firm can invest in information and discriminate among risk classes, it may offer the same benefit at different premiums, different benefits at the same premium, or some combination of these extremes. Nevertheless, all premiums are raised above actuarially fair levels because of the transaction cost. If these costs are equally distributed across contracts, low-risk individuals should again be relatively more prominent among the low-benefit or uninsured populations.

According to the survey by Aday and Andersen, 12 percent of the population under age sixty-five in 1976 had no insurance and were ineligible for public assistance. Compared with the 10 percent of the population holding individual contracts, the uninsured cannot be considered as a relatively low-risk class. Because insurance takes the form of reimbursement for expenses that are partly optional, the observed difference in use of services according to insurance status should be considerable. Yet there was virtually no difference in the probability of hospitalization or in the mean number of physician visits between persons with no insurance and those in individual plans. The uninsured were less likely to have a regular source of medical care or to purchase preventative examinations, but this was not because they had fewer serious symptoms or a more favorable perception of their health status.

Uninsured persons, compared with those holding individual policies, were slightly more likely to be young adults, to live in the South, and to be nonwhite. But primarily the uninsured were less wealthy in terms of family income and occupational status of the household head. If these characteristics are to be reconciled with market failure, it might be argued that an insurance firm rationally uses these rather arbitrary criteria for nonprice rationing, or that less wealthy persons are also less risk averse and therefore unwilling to pay the transaction costs of risk classification.[15] Unfortunately, the surveys do not reveal whether the uninsured person was rejected upon application for insurance or has risk-averse preferences. If the absence of coverage is because higher selling costs of "temporary" policies exceed consumer willingness to pay, this is not market failure.

Young adults and persons in families in which the head is temporarily unemployed may be subject to nonprice rationing in the market. Many policies do have age limits for dependent children, and there is informal evidence about rejection of the unemployed by some firms. These two characteristics account for at most 26 percent of the uninsured (there is some overlap in the two categories) in an analysis prepared by the Congressional Budget Office. Nonetheless, it would be surprising if no firms were willing to offer policies to these groups, with premiums reflecting the differential cost of high turnover; in fact such policies are available. Perhaps the problem is that people are willing, but unable, to purchase longer-term contracts to guarantee the continuance of coverage and smooth out the premiums over time and employment contingencies. Social policies encouraging employer-based coverage may inhibit longer-term contracting.

The CBO found that 45 percent of uninsured persons were members of families in which the family head had private or public coverage. If the family head were eligible for Medicare, veterans' benefits, or workmen's compensation, he or she would not have the option to purchase coverage for dependents. In other cases, the option to purchase coverage for dependents, except for children over age nineteen who were not students, must have been nearly universal.

A theoretical aspect of family demand for insurance can plausibly account for family heads' being more frequently covered than dependents. Occasions when the family head incurs medical expense may also be occasions when family income is reduced. Therefore insurance on the head is more valuable to the entire family than it would be on dependents suffering illness or injury. This hypothesis implicitly, and perhaps innocuously, assumes imperfection in capital markets. It does not explain why dependents are uninsured.

Beyond the question of why some people have no private insurance, we should consider why a substantial number of insured persons do not have stop-loss protection. We have seen that the marginal actuarial cost of a stop-loss is low. However, moral hazard (extra demand for care, caused by insurance) may be especially important for large expenses. The proportional increase in premium due to moral hazard

---

[15] An alternative hypothesis that wealth is a strong independent factor in demand for expensive care is not easy to justify empirically.

may be for care that is proportionally much less valued. Another possible consideration is that the insurance firm is somewhat risk-averse. If these two considerations were important, they would encourage the growth of HMOs. The full-service HMO is a form of catastrophic health insurance with a management incentive structure that counteracts the moral hazard in reimbursement insurance.

Before proceeding to examine the trend in HMO enrollment, there is a special feature of the insurance market that may deserve further investigation. Blue Cross Associations are tax-exempt, not-for-profit firms with a large market share, whose management may not be rewarded for providing an efficient insurance plan. It might be detrimental to their management to offer stop-loss protection if consumers would drop first-dollar coverage and thereby lower the volume of total administrative cost.

A national survey of seventy-seven HMOs in 1973 asked HMO executives about their perceptions of the obstacles to growth.[16] The most frequent obstacle cited was marketing. About three-quarters of the replies cited severe or moderate problems in "obtaining access to new employed or other groups." Beginning with a congressional act in 1973, the government has attempted to mandate that consumers have the option to purchase HMO coverage with the same employer subsidy given to conventional insurance. If market failure did account, in part, for the low enrollment in HMOs, enrollment should have grown markedly since 1973.

There are some problems in interpreting HMO enrollment data. Some enrollees are Medicaid recipients who already have a sort of stop-loss protection. Enrollees of an individual-practice association or even some group practice plans may not have catastrophic insurance for hospital care. Finally, a build-up of excess demand may be required to recruit capital and physicians and to permit growth after a time lag.

Restricting attention to prepaid group practice, with 6.4 million enrollees and 86 percent of total HMO enrollment in 1978, we find a compound growth rate of 2.4 percent for the period 1973–1978. By contrast, the compound rate for 1967–1973 was 4 percent annually.[17] This trend does not support market failure as an explanation of the historical HMO marketing problem. Recently, there has been a rapid growth in individual-practice associations. In 1978, there were 1.1

---

[16] Robert E. Schlenker et al., *HMOs in 1973: A National Survey* (Minneapolis: Interstudy, Inc., 1974).

[17] Marjorie Smith Caroll, "Private Health Insurance Plans in 1976: An Evaluation," *Social Security Bulletin*, vol. 41, no. 9 (September 1978), pp. 3–16. Also see U.S. Public Health Service, "National HMO Census of Prepaid Plans, 1978," mimeographed.

million enrollees. This seems to be the only tidbit of information supporting the view that moral hazard and risk aversion on the part of insurance firms may have prevented the offering of catastrophic protection.

Consumer Demand for Stop-Loss Insurance

This section will consider how family wealth affects the demand for insurance even if wealth does not affect expenditure on health care, and why the past decade has seen a dramatic growth in demand for CHI. These issues are not easily treated in models of demand for health insurance such as those of Arrow[18] and Phelps.[19]

Suppose that a family has disposable wealth w, and is assured that it will obtain at least a minimum standard of care in the event of any illness or injury regardless of whether the cost is greater than w. The family is offered a contract which limits out-of-pocket losses to a level D that, for convenience of analysis, is also a deductible.

By purchasing this contract, the family can reduce uncertainty in its financial position and maintain an option to demand more than the standard of care in the event of serious health problems. The information requirements for an exact evaluation of the demand option are extreme. To ignore this value, however, is to make an unacceptable assumption that demand and consumption of care are inelastic with respect to insurance coverage. In a previous model, Feldstein and Friedman[20] evaluated gains from a reimbursement contract by assuming that the demand for care is a function of the direct price with the same functional form and elasticity in every state of nature. That model did not consider that the minimum standard of care for some health problems may be more expensive than people would wish to purchase indirectly through insurance premiums.[21]

---

[18] Kenneth J. Arrow, "Uncertainty and the Welfare Economics of Medical Care," *American Economic Review*, vol. 53 (December 1963), pp. 941–73.

[19] Charles E. Phelps, "Demand for Reimbursement Insurance," in Richard Rosett, ed., *The Role of Health Insurance in the Health Services Sector* (New York: National Bureau of Economic Research, 1976).

[20] Martin Feldstein and Bernard Friedman, "Tax Subsidies, the Rational Demand for Insurance and the Health Care Crisis," *Journal of Public Economics*, vol. 7 (1977), p. 155.

[21] The author, in a 1971 dissertation, and Zeckhauser show that if health positively affects the marginal utility of consumption, and if large expenses occur for conditions that are often not remediable, then even though the care would be demanded at the time of illnesses, insurance against these costs would not be attractive at a fair premium. This possibility is ignored in the text. See Bernard Friedman, "Uncertainty and Health Insurance" (Ph.D. dissertation, Massachusetts Institute of Technology, 1971), chap. 2; and Richard Zeckhauser, "Coverage for Catastrophic Illness," *Public Policy*, vol. 21 (Spring 1973), pp. 149–72.

Consider the financial position of the family with no insurance. Let x be the uncertain expense, with $f(x)$ the probability density and $P(w)$ the probability that x exceeds w. Then expected utility is where $u(w - x)$

$$V_0 = \int_0^w u(w - x)f(x)dx + P(w)u(0) \tag{1}$$

has positive but diminishing marginal utility. Should wealth be exhausted, standard care, x_m, is obtained with expected resource cost $P(w)\bar{x}_m$. If the family were to purchase a stop-loss with $D = w$ and still plan to consume x_m, the premium would be at least $\pi = P(w)\bar{x}_m$, and the family is clearly worse off. The family would be better off only if the *marginal* increase in consumption to $x_i > x_m$ is expected to be so beneficial as to outweigh the *total* premium $\pi = P(w)\bar{x}_i$. A relatively high standard x_m makes the contract with $D = w$ unattractive.

Even with a high standard x_m, people may desire insurance with $D < w$. The expected utility of the financial position with insurance is

$$V_i = \int_0^D u(w - \pi - x)f(x)dx + P(D)u(w - \pi - D). \tag{2}$$

The higher the standard x_m, the more appropriate it is to predict insurance choice solely by a comparison of (1) and (2). Define $\hat{\pi}$ as the premium equating $V_i = V_0$. This is the most that would be offered for insurance. It is easy to show that $\hat{\pi} = 0$ at $D = w$, that $\dfrac{d\hat{\pi}}{dD} < 0$, and at $D = w$, $\dfrac{d\hat{\pi}}{dw} > 0$. The interpretation of the last result is straightforward. The marginal value of a new dollar of wealth is greater when, with insurance, one can spread it over all the states with higher losses. One could not do this in equation (1).

The foregoing propositions are illustrated in Figure 1. Curve $\hat{\pi}_f$ represents what the consumer with wealth w would offer for the stop-loss contract D, considering only the expected utility of his financial position. The curve is drawn concave under a presumption of declining absolute risk aversion. But the total amount that would be offered depends also on the expected difference between the benefits of standard care and the enriched care one could demand if insured. The offer when standard free care is spartan, $\hat{\pi}_1$, is greater than when free care is similar to what one would buy if insured, $\hat{\pi}_2$. As w increases, there are fewer contingencies when the free care is relevant, so $\hat{\pi}_f$ becomes a better approximation to $\hat{\pi}_2$. The fair premium for the contract at D may be some amount such as π_s. In the case of relatively generous free care, the only purchasers would have wealth greater than w^*.

This analysis does not imply that there is a D low enough that

FIGURE 1
Hypothetical Offers for Stop-Loss Insurance Depending on Wealth and Free Care

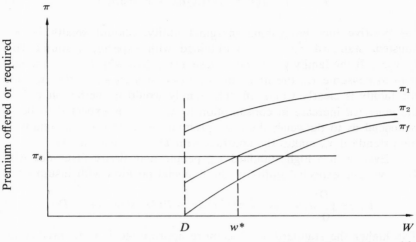

everyone would purchase stop-loss insurance. At lower D, π_s is higher and always by more than the reduction in preexisting average expense, because people are induced to demand more care. Some further questions that might be addressed are how the optimal D varies with w, and whether partial first-dollar coverage might be chosen by those who would not purchase catastrophic protection. The present analysis suggests only why people with low wealth might not purchase catastrophic insurance. If people with low wealth cannot find policies offered *only* to cover small losses (and here the overhead margin would be higher), then they may not hold any insurance.

It is possible to interpret the connection between low wealth and absence of insurance coverage as market failure. Some people do not purchase even a small contract that they might find advantageous if the regulation of medical care, hospital finances, and public assistance were designed differently than they are at present.[22] If the community

---

[22] This interpretation was suggested to the author by Mark Pauly. The statement implicitly assumes that the design of public assistance and enforcement of "medical ethics" have incentive effects that may not have been fully perceived in political exchange. The use of the term "market failure" for the insurance behavior depicted in Figure 1 should not be interpreted to mean that there is an *inherent* property of insurance contracting that inefficiently inhibits transactions.

establishes a high standard of care for those who exhaust their disposable wealth, then the foregoing analysis shows that people with low wealth may not be willing to pay the actuarially fair premium for any insurance. There is no way for such consumers to reveal that they are willing to pay *part* of the cost for the assurance of standard care and the option of higher quality care.

This observation suggests that a redesigning of all-or-nothing assistance programs such as Medicaid would be socially beneficial. Some people will purchase more partial protection that they value to supplement the protection implicit in public assistance eligibility. Taxpayers who wish to subsidize the availability of standard care will be able to do so with more net value obtained per tax dollar. (The case for redesigning existing assistance will be expanded in the next section.)

In view of these observations, one may speculate on why the demand for stop-loss protection may have developed rapidly since the late 1960s. The expansion of formalized aid to the elderly and poor in the mid-1960s would seem to be the kind of development inhibiting private catastrophic contracts. A suggestion may be developed along the following lines. The development of transplantation, dialysis, and expensive heart surgery techniques began receiving wide attention in the late 1960s,[23] but it seemed fairly obvious then they would not be available as standard care in the near future. The insurance option to demand such services may have therefore grown in value to the typical consumer. By the same reasoning, later enactment of Medicare coverage for renal dialysis and the decline of heart transplants may have eased the demand for CHI. It may also be observed that this source of rising demand for CHI does not imply a rising demand for HMOs, where consumers do not have similar demand options. It is well known, for example, that persons enrolled in HMOs have less expensive surgery than those in similar insured populations.

A National CHI as a Policy Reform

The purpose of this section is to consider more fully why a federal CHI program might be desirable even if traditional concerns over market failure are rejected.

One consequence of a family's decision not to purchase CHI is that hospital charges to other patients are higher than they would have been, given a constant total budget. These redistributive policies are

---

[23] For example, the first major publicized heart transplant was in 1967, and more were performed in 1968 than in any year since then. For other similar trends in these areas, see Jay Katz and Alexander Capron, *Catastrophic Diseases: Who Decides What?* (New York: Russell Sage Foundation, 1975).

part of a hospital's claim to tax-exempt status. Private philanthropy accounts for only about 20 percent of the difference between gross and net patient revenue. The burden of the implicit transfer program falls on self-paying patients and holders of private insurance other than Blue Cross. Purchasers of care through Medicare, Medicaid, and Blue Cross benefit from negotiating leverage and obtain stricter cost-based rates. Two aspects of this situation are noteworthy. First, redistribution among those unfortunate enough to need hospital care is less desirable than general redistribution through all premiums and taxes. Secondly, the preference given to Blue Cross and government buyers promotes the competitive viability of their "first-dollar" approach to insurance.

A federal CHI program would reduce the above type of discrimination. If coverage were compulsory, fewer discounts would be necessary. Holders of private insurance would also achieve at least partial parity in bargaining.

Medicaid is an explicit transfer program that formalized a variety of preexisting government and private aid programs to alleviate family poverty and medical needs. The program can be credited with expanding health care in targeted populations, but structural flaws are widely noted. A major observation is that because of the all-or-nothing eligibility definitions, families face high implicit tax rates on earnings to lift themselves out of poverty. Because of policy makers' concerns about work incentives, the Medicaid program has been an obvious obstacle to general reform of public assistance.[24]

Davis and Schoen express several additional criticisms of Medicaid.[25] They argue that there is regional inequity in coverage. They find little encouragement of innovations such as comprehensive health centers, since the program is designed for full payment of covered services under conventional medical practices. Finally, they observe that the regulatory efforts to control fraud, eligibility, and prices may perpetuate a second-class status for recipients.

A federal CHI program with mandated employer plans (or tax support), a sponsored risk pool for holders of individual insurance plans, and an income-related premium subsidy would offer some likely advantages over Medicaid. Compulsory coverage with income-related subsidy would increase the protection "purchased" by some low-wealth consumers who presently are disinclined to such purchases by Medicaid

---

[24] For an analysis of implicit tax rates, see Henry Aaron, "Why Is Welfare So Hard to Reform," *Studies in Social Economics* (Washington, D.C.: The Brookings Institution, 1973), pp. 33–8. Eligibility for Medicaid and other in-kind transfers were widely cited in debates of the Senate Finance Committee in the early 1970s as a reason to oppose welfare reform.

[25] Karen Davis and Cathy Schoen, *Health and the War on Poverty: A Ten-Year Appraisal* (Washington, D.C.: The Brookings Institution, 1978).

eligibility rules and ethical standards of medical practice. Earnings incentives would be improved, and status distinctions in the eyes of providers reduced. Regional equity in the basic plan would prevail in terms of coverage, if not in federal dollars spent. A flat federal per capita grant, such as the most recent Canadian innovation, could be offered to local governments to add services or reduce copayment.

There is a general reluctance to advocate that poor families be exposed to *any* health care costs. But to put this proposal in a different light, consider that poor families would benefit from shopping around for appropriate cost/quality offerings of service, once they are able to use a fractional copayment for moderate expenses. Involving the poorer consumer more directly in health insurance reimbursement would also reduce the potential for fraud and the weight of regulations promoting a second-class status.

A secondary advantage of federal CHI as a major policy reform, rather than an "add-on" program, is that it might be acceptably packaged with a removal of the tax subsidy of employer contributions for health insurance. The tax subsidy can be effectively challenged on grounds of both efficiency and distribution; other authors at this conference will take up these matters. We can expect that revisions in the tax laws might meet substantial resistance. A federally financed CHI program would increase protection for some workers and save money for others. This might sway labor leaders to a package deal involving the reduction of subsidy to other health insurance.

A major aspect of the rationale for federal CHI as a policy reform is that other programs would be replaced and consumer copayment for smaller expenses would be preserved and even increased. Whether this copayment would be significant in preserving or improving competitive cost restraint and quality incentives is an important research question. Zeckhauser[26] and Schroeder et al.[27] have expressed reservations about CHI. They anticipate a greater expansion of medical resources expended than patient benefits obtained in cases of severe illness.

Zeckhauser suggests that physicians would have less incentive to develop more cost-effective therapies under CHI, and there would be an ethical environment unfavorable to recruiting patients for such therapies. He also suggests that explicit rationing procedures for expensive care would be inevitable and would be a source of social tensions. It should be interesting to compare Zeckhauser's concerns with the experience in Canada and in the United Kingdom. Despite comprehensive

---

[26] Zeckhauser, "Coverage for Catastrophic Illness."

[27] Steven Schroeder, Jonathan Showstack, and H. Edith Roberts, "Frequency and Clinical Description of High-Cost Patients in Seventeen Acute-Care Hospitals," *New England Journal of Medicine*, vol. 300 (June 1979), pp. 1306–1309.

reimbursement coverage, Canadians are apparently still spending about 7 percent of GNP on personal health care, a share that has fallen relative to the United States in the last few years. This preliminary aggregate observation argues for caution in presuming that medical cost borne by the family is still a significant constraint in catastrophic illness in the United States.

Schroeder et al. report that between 4 percent and 24 percent of the patients in San Francisco hospitals in 1976 incurred costs exceeding $4,000 each. These costs represented about 60 percent of the total billings in large referral hospitals. Of 933 sampled high-cost patients, 13 percent died during the year studied. The adults had an average age in the late fifties, about half were admitted for chronic conditions, and fewer than one-quarter were admitted for the reason "restore to normal health." The authors assert, on the basis of this data, that "a large portion of national catastrophic health insurance resources will be devoted to persons who will die soon after receiving high-cost medical treatment."

The usefulness of the above empirical conclusion is imperceptible. Apparently, a large amount of resources are *already* devoted to high-cost terminal care. Somebody pays. Schroeder et al. offer no evidence in terms of differential coverage that financial considerations served to ration this care. Nor do they offer evidence of a reservoir of potential demand for this care that is denied or deterred on account of lack of insurance coverage.

No one would argue that expanded CHI would not have inflationary potential, largely perhaps through induced technological change. But it is also conceivable that inefficient technological enrichment could be tolerably constrained by government in a society that gives growing attention to scarcities in other areas.

One reservation about expanded CHI is a general issue in all third-party arrangements and in the acceptability of HMOs. If the patient is no longer paying even a fraction of the physician's charge, because the stop-loss has been exceeded, why should the physician continue to have an attitude of responsibility to the subjective tastes of the patient? Paradoxically, resource intensity may increase while caring attitudes are eroded. Or, in other words, instead of second-class charity status being upgraded to mainstream care, a leveling-down of care may occur. This is more appropriately a reservation about the desirability of federal CHI as an incremental program that would increase third-party coverage overall. If CHI is designed in part to replace coverage of smaller expenses, then there need be less concern about deterioration in consumers' ability to reward better service.

This study of reasons for advocating federal CHI weighs against the enactment of an incremental program. The hypothesis that insurance markets fail to provide CHI contracts that people are willing to buy at fair premiums is empirically weak. Contrary evidence has been developed. However, a hypothesis that current social regulatory and subsidy programs have limited the demand for CHI and induced inefficient contract holdings is empirically plausible. A variety of additional criticisms of Medicaid and tax subsidy of employer benefits contribute to the case for advocating federal CHI as a major reform and replacement for these programs.

Reforming National Health
Programs for the Poor

Thomas W. Grannemann

Introduction

Any plan for national health insurance, whether it calls for a completely new system of universal coverage or merely a restructuring of current programs, must deal with the problem of financing medical care for the poor. In formulating future policy in this area we are able to draw on more than ten years of experience with the federal-state Medicaid program. Dissatisfaction with current programs has been an important stimulus for consideration of more comprehensive national health insurance proposals and, as the nation's largest medical care program for the poor, Medicaid has been the source of much of this dissatisfaction. The purpose of this paper is to identify factors that have contributed to the problems of Medicaid and suggest how such problems might be avoided in future national health insurance programs.

We first describe some of the more significant problems with Medicaid, including some commonly recognized ones and others that are less familiar. Next, we describe a voter-choice model of public expenditures for medical care, and use it to explain the wide variation in Medicaid benefits across states. We also use this model to show that many of Medicaid's difficulties can be attributed to deficiencies in the incentive system embodied in federal laws and regulations. We next discuss some specific means of reforming Medicaid. We consider alternative means of controlling Medicaid costs, and show how the Medicaid matching rate formula could be modified to achieve specified national policy goals. Finally, we suggest some general guidelines for future national health programs for the poor, and use these guidelines as a yardstick to compare current legislative proposals in the health area.

NOTE: Part of the research supporting this paper was conducted at the Northwestern University Center for Health Services and Policy Research under grant number 1 R03 HS 03146 from the National Center for Health Services Research.

104

THOMAS W. GRANNEMANN

Problems with Medicaid

Historically in the United States, provision of medical care to the poor has been handled by charitable organizations and government at the local or state level. The adoption and rapid growth of the Medicaid program has brought about an expanded federal role in financing this care. But, in keeping with historically assigned responsibilities, Medicaid was designed as a program to assist state and local governments in their efforts; it was not structured to insure the attainment of any well-defined national policy goals. It is therefore not surprising that, when looked at from a national point of view, the current program falls short of what one might reasonably expect of a national medical care program for the poor. Among the more significant problems with Medicaid are the following:

High Cost. The Medicaid program costs more than $18 billion annually. Although state and local governments pay less than half of the cost of the program, it has been perceived as a burden by many state policy makers. As a provider of public health insurance under Medicaid, the government must deal with the same problem of adverse market incentives that is faced by private sector insurers. That is the problem of moral hazard which results when third-party payment eliminates incentives for efficient use of resources. Two aspects of the cost problem will be considered in this paper. The first is why some states may perceive the burden of the program to be greater than other states; the second is how the costs of this governmental program can be reduced without denying the poor access to essential medical services.

Horizontal Inequity. The term "horizontal inequity" has been used to refer to unequal treatment of potential Medicaid recipients across states. That is, two otherwise identical individuals could be treated very differently under the program if they happened to live in different states. As a federal-state program in which federal policy makers have only indirect control over the services ultimately provided, Medicaid gives states considerable latitude in determining eligibility, range of services covered, and provider reimbursement rates.

Acting within a framework of federal laws, regulations, and matching grants, states have used their freedom to establish programs that vary widely in eligibility requirements and the amount and type of services provided. For example, in fiscal year 1976, recipients as a percentage of state population ranged from over 22 percent in Pennsylvania to less than 5 percent in eight other states. Total (state and federal) Medicaid payments per capita ranged from over $185 in

TABLE 1

FEDERAL MEDICAID PAYMENTS PER CAPITA,
BY REGION, FISCAL 1977

Northeast	$62.07
North Central	37.01
South	32.97
West	37.13
25 high-income states	45.04
25 low-income states	33.67

NOTE: Figures do not include District of Columbia, Puerto Rico, or Virgin Islands.
SOURCE: U.S. Department of Health, Education, and Welfare, Health Care Financing Administration, *Medicaid Statistics, Fiscal Year 1977*, Washington, D.C., April 1978.

New York to less than $18 in Wyoming. Average payments for recipients over age sixty-five ranged from a high of $3,477 in Connecticut to a low of $451 in South Carolina.

Redistribution Effects. Associated with the variation in Medicaid benefits across states are disparities in the distribution of federal funds. Table 1 shows the regional variation in federal Medicaid payments per capita. The Northeast receives more federal Medicaid payments per capita than other regions. When states are grouped by personal income per capita, it can be seen that high-income states receive more federal Medicaid dollars per capita than low-income states.

Because high-income states pay more in federal taxes, these taxes must be considered to obtain net redistribution effects. Table 2 shows the interregional redistribution effects of Medicaid under the assumption that the costs of the program are borne in proportion to federal personal income taxes. There is virtually no net redistribution from high-income to low-income states, but Medicaid produces a sizable net redistribution of resources from the West, South, and North Central regions to the Northeast. The observed interregional redistribution is arbitrary and is probably not necessary for the attainment of health policy goals. There is no evidence that Medicaid has been effective in providing greater federal assistance to low-income states where the needs of the poor are greater and state taxpayers are less able to support the program alone.

Underprovision of Care for Children. About 18 percent of Medicaid funds are devoted to services for children. This has been viewed as too little by federal policy makers, who have encouraged states to implement

TABLE 2

INTERREGIONAL REDISTRIBUTION EFFECTS OF MEDICAID,
FISCAL 1977
(dollar amounts in millions)

	Benefit (Federal Payments)	Cost (Federal Tax)	Difference	Benefit-Cost Ratio
Northeast	$3,066	$2,171	$ +895	1.41
North Central	2,136	2,530	−394	0.84
South	2,251	2,510	−259	0.89
West	1,432	1,693	−261	0.85
District of Columbia	59	40	+ 19	1.48
25 high-income states	6,658	6,659	− 1	1.00
25 low-income states	2,228	2,227	+ 1	1.00

NOTE: Figures do not include Puerto Rico or Virgin Islands.
SOURCE: Computed from Health Care Financing Administration, *Medicaid Statistics, Fiscal Year 1977*. Tax data are from *Statistical Abstract of the United States.*

early periodic screening, diagnosis, and treatment (EPSDT) programs to identify and treat eligible children in need of medical care. Disagreements on this issue between federal officials and cost-sensitive state policy makers have led some federal policy makers to accuse the states of a "basic unwillingness . . . to provide poor children with adequate services."[1] The cause of this apparent divergence of federal and state priorities is worthy of investigation and will be examined below.

Arbitrary Limits on Services. In trying to control Medicaid costs, many states have limited the services covered by Medicaid. Limiting hospital stays to fourteen days and physician visits to one per month is not uncommon.[2] Such limits apply without regard to the medical needs of the individual and can result in denial of care to those who need it most.

Gaps in Coverage. To be eligible for Medicaid benefits, a low-income person must typically qualify as aged, blind, or disabled or as a member of a family with dependent children. Low-income persons in two-parent

[1] Karen Davis and Kathy Schoen, *Health and the War on Poverty* (Washington, D.C.: The Brookings Institution, 1978), p. 86.

[2] U.S. Department of Health, Education, and Welfare, Institute for Medicaid Management, Health Care Financing Administration, Medicaid Bureau, *Data on the Medicaid Program: Eligibility, Services, Expenditures Fiscal Years 1966–1978*, Washington, D.C., 1978.

families and single persons under age sixty-five usually cannot qualify for Medicaid benefits. As a result, many poor persons are not covered by Medicaid. This has led to a disparity between the use of medical services by Medicaid recipients and by ineligible poor and near-poor persons.[3]

Having identified some of the problems with Medicaid, we will turn to a discussion of some factors that affect voter preference for the Medicaid program and thus indirectly influence state Medicaid expenditures. We can then analyze Medicaid policy in the context of a model of the behavior of state policy makers.

Voter Preferences for Publicly Financed Medical Care

To be politically successful, any national health plan must satisfy, at least approximately, the desires of the voters. In research supporting this paper, I have analyzed state Medicaid expenditures to identify factors that motivate voters to support medical-care programs for the poor, and thereby explain the wide variation in Medicaid benefits across states.[4]

The model I use views state policy makers as responding to the desires of a representative voter (or state taxpayer).[5] I assume that voters value the use of medical services by others and so are willing to pay for governmental programs that promote the use of medical services. Just how much a typical voter is willing to pay for such programs will depend on the needs of the poor in the state, the taxpayer's income, and the cost to the taxpayer of providing services under Medicaid. The voter's demand for publicly financed medical care will thus depend on income and prices in a manner similar to the demand for other goods and services. If the actions of state and local policy makers respond to the desires of voters, as we hope they do, state Medicaid expenditures can be expected to reflect the influence of taxpayer income and prices.

A number of implications of this model have been tested using data on state Medicaid programs for fiscal years 1973–1977. Ordinary least squares and three-stage regressions were used to estimate voter

---

[3] Karen Davis and Roger Reynolds, "The Impact of Medicare and Medicaid on Access to Medical Care," in Richard Rosett, ed., *The Role of Health Insurance in the Health Services Sector* (New York: National Bureau of Economic Research, 1976), pp. 391–435.

[4] Thomas Grannemann, "The Demand for Publicly Financed Medical Care: The Role of Interdependent Preferences" (Ph.D. dissertation, Northwestern University, 1979).

[5] For a similar model see Larry Orr, "Income Transfers as a Public Good: An Application to AFDC," *American Economic Review*, vol. 66, no. 3 (June 1976), pp. 359–371.

TABLE 3

Summary of Price and Income Elasticities

Category	Donor Price Elasticity	Income Elasticity	Recipient Price Elasticity
Total Medicaid	−.779 (.180)	1.233 (.435)	.921 (.449)
Medicaid for the elderly[a]	−.884 (.232)	−.507 (.569)	−.969 (.582)
Medicaid for children[a]	−.667 (.203)	2.436 (.498)	.991 (.510)
Medicaid for AFDC adults[a]	−.568 (.190)	2.810 (.465)	.675 (.476)
Medicaid inpatient hospital services	−.412 (.180)	1.185 (.425)	1.086 (.371)
Medicaid physician services	−.305 (.212)	2.342 (.523)	−.647 (.489)

NOTE: Standard errors in parentheses.
[a] See appendix for regressions.

demand functions for Medicaid. The results, some of which are presented in the appendix, reveal a number of important determinants of state Medicaid expenditures.

Price to the Taxpayer. The price to the taxpayer of providing Medicaid depends not only on the local price of medical services, but also on the taxpayer's state tax share and the relevant federal matching (subsidy) rate that reduces the effective price to the state taxpayer. This effective price of providing Medicaid benefits was found to be inversely related to Medicaid expenditures. The first column of Table 3 shows the estimated taxpayer (donor) price elasticity of demand for Medicaid benefits. This sensitivity to price indicates that states do respond to federal incentives in the form of subsidies and that control of the federal matching rate formula could be an effective means of influencing state Medicaid expenditures.

Taxpayer Income. The income of state taxpayers was also found to be an important determinant of state Medicaid benefits. Column 2 of Table 3 shows the estimated taxpayer income elasticity of demand for

109

Medicaid. States with high taxpayer income tend to provide greater Medicaid benefits. The income elasticity is higher for physician services than for hospital services. This suggests that voters in low-income states place a higher priority on the provision of hospital services. Physician services are more freely provided in high-income states. An alternative explanation of this difference in elasticity is suggested by results below, which indicate that federal minimum benefit standards require low-income states to provide more benefits per recipient than they would choose to provide on their own. If this is the case, then the difference in elasticity may simply reflect the greater ability of these states to limit use and cost of physician services through controls on physician reimbursement rates. These states may have less control over use of hospital services.

Price to the Recipient. In locations where the price of medical care is high, poor persons have greater difficulty obtaining care on their own. It is reasonable to suppose that people would be more willing to provide medical care to the poor in areas where high cost limits access. In fact, the positive coefficients in column 3 of Table 3 indicate that voters have responded to the special needs of the poor in high-cost areas. The appendix provides additional evidence that, controlling for other factors, states with high medical-care prices tend to provide Medicaid benefits to relatively more recipients.

The Dual Relationship between Benefits and Recipients. A simple but important concept involving the benefits per recipient and the number of recipients is useful in explaining public demand for medical care programs for the disadvantaged. It is: Each incremental increase in the benefit level increases the cost to the taxpayer of expanding the number of recipients, and each incremental increase in the number of recipients will make it more costly to raise the benefit level. This dual relationship between benefits and recipients implies that an increase in one will raise the effective price (to the taxpayer) of the other. From this we would expect to observe an inverse relationship between Medicaid benefits and number of recipients across states. This relationship has been verified empirically. Controlling for other factors, states with relatively large numbers of poor tend to have relatively more recipients but lower benefit levels (see appendix). These states, in effect, spread medical-care transfers thinner than states with relatively few poor persons.

Another implication of the recipient-benefit relationship becomes important if a state is constrained to provide a higher benefit level than it would otherwise desire. This occurs where the federally required minimum set of services is greater than the benefit level desired by the

110

state. A high benefit level could also occur because, as noted above, recipients and providers have no incentive to limit use of services. In either case, the high Medicaid benefit level raises the cost to the state of each recipient and the state will choose to serve fewer recipients than if a lower benefit level were established. Under these circumstances, if an effective means can be found to reduce the cost per recipient, taxpayers would be willing to extend Medicaid benefits to a larger number of recipients.

Availability of Medical-Care Resources. One might suppose that voters would be more willing to support public provision of medical care to the poor where they perceive that use by the recipients will not crowd out or interfere with the voters' own use of medical services. Medical resource availability as measured by number of hospital beds and physicians per capita was found to be directly related to the number of Medicaid recipients. The relationship is not simply due to regional differences in average length of hospital stays and number of physician visits, because hospital beds and physicians are related to the number of recipients but not to benefits per recipient.

An Illustrative Comparison. A picture of what has led to the wide interstate variation in Medicaid benefits emerges from this analysis. As specific examples, consider the states of Mississippi, Minnesota, and New York. Mississippi has a high incidence of poverty, but the low level of taxpayer income means that the state cannot afford a generous Medicaid program. As a result, this state spreads its resources thinly by providing a relatively low level of benefits to a comparatively large fraction of the population. In contrast, Minnesota has both a higher level of taxpayer income and relatively few persons below the federal poverty level. As the dual relationship would suggest, Minnesota can concentrate its Medicaid benefits on a few recipients and offer a high-benefit program. In New York, a variety of factors combine to produce incentives for voters to support a program with both a high benefit level and a large number of recipients. Because New York has both high-income taxpayers and a sizable low-income population, it has not only the need for services but also the fiscal capacity to pay for them. The high income elasticity of demand for care for Aid to Families with Dependent Children (AFDC) amplifies the effect of high taxpayer income. In addition, medical care prices in New York are nearly twice those in Mississippi. This means that low-income persons in New York would have greater difficulty obtaining care on their own. This fact provides an incentive for the state of make Medicaid available to many persons, even those with income above the federal poverty level.

This section has provided evidence that, when comparisons are made across states, aggregate Medicaid benefits are found to be directly related to taxpayer income and inversely related to the price to the taxpayer of providing care. States can therefore be expected to respond to federal subsidies that reduce this price.

Medicaid benefits are also directly related to the needs of the low-income population, as measured by the number of poor and the price the poor would have to pay for medical care if purchased without governmental assistance. Voters thus appear to be more willing to provide medical care at public expense where economic factors prevent or discourage individuals from obtaining care on their own.

Economic factors such as income and prices can explain much of the interstate variation in Medicaid benefits. Interregional differences in attitudes toward the poor may play a much smaller role in determining Medicaid benefits than is commonly believed.

Medicaid's Defective Incentive System

Using the model of voter preferences and policy makers' behavior developed above, we can trace many of the problems with Medicaid to deficiencies in the federally established incentives facing state policy makers. Each of the problems with Medicaid identified above is linked to an incentive system which inadvertently has diverted the program from its goals.

High Cost. Under the Medicaid program, the federal government provides matching funds at a rate that can vary from 50 to 83 percent of total expenditures, depending on state per-capita income. The subsidy effectively reduces the cost to the state of providing medical care to the poor. It is, however, a subsidy on care delivered in the same costly system that has led voters to complain about the cost of their own care. The government reimburses providers for services delivered at the request of the recipient. As would be the case with full private insurance coverage, neither the provider nor the user bears any of the cost and there is an incentive to use services that have only small value without concern for the expense. Recipients have little incentive to obtain care through cost-saving health maintenance organizations (HMOs) when services are available in the fee-for-service market at no out-of-pocket cost.

States that have tried to limit use of low-value care through small copayments on basic services have been prohibited by court order from doing so. Federal laws and regulations have limited the states' ability to control the amount of care delivered to Medicaid recipients, and many states have been required to spend more per recipient than would be the case without federal restrictions. Taxpayers and policy makers observe the cost per recipient of providing care, some of which is of low value to the recipient. As a result, the Medicaid program is perceived as having a high cost relative to the value of services delivered.

Horizontal Inequity. The federal subsidy on high-cost forms of medical care has also contributed to the wide variation in Medicaid benefits across states. Consider the following hypothetical situation. Suppose the government offered to pay half the purchase price on all Rolls Royce automobiles, but prohibited buyers from reselling them. Many Cadillac drivers probably would move up to the more prestigious car while many Volkswagen drivers would continue with their present make. Similarly, many low-income states have found it too expensive to make Medicaid benefits widely available despite favorable federal matching rates. The result is that poor persons located in these states must meet more stringent Medicaid eligibility requirements and receive fewer benefits than persons located in more wealthy states.

The federal matching rate formula has not been sufficiently weighted in favor of low-income states to overcome this effect. In the low-income states, the difference between the desired benefit level and federal minimum standards is greatest. So, because of the dual relationship, these states have the greatest incentive to keep the number of Medicaid recipients below the level that would be desired if cost per recipient were lower. The current incentive structure, which does not discourage use of costly low-value care, has thus contributed to the problem of horizontal inequity.

Redistribution Effects and Taxpayer Equity. State responses to Medicaid's incentives have unequal impacts on taxpayers as well as on the poor. Low-income states tend to spend less on Medicaid because they have lower income taxpayers and because such states typically have lower medical-care prices, which reduces the need for Medicaid. But by choosing low levels of Medicaid expenditures, low-income states forgo federal matching funds. As noted above, this means that high-income states receive more federal Medicaid dollars per capita than do low-income states. The benefit to low-income states of higher matching rates is offset by federal taxes that support more extensive Medicaid programs in high-income states. Taxpayers in low-income states have been faced with the burden of supporting large numbers of poor without much net federal assistance. But the taxpayers in such states have avoided assuming this burden to some extent by limiting Medicaid eligibility, leaving many poor persons unserved.

Contributing to this situation is the federal incentive system embodied in the Medicaid matching rate formula. The current formula is inconsistent with equal benefits for the poor and equal tax shares for taxpayers. Consider the effect of requiring every state to provide $200 in Medicaid benefits to every poor person in the state. Using data for 1975 and computing the state share from the matching rates then in effect, such a plan would require only 0.126 percent of state taxpayer income in Connecticut and 0.155 percent in Indiana, but would require 0.295 percent in New Mexico and 0.392 percent of taxpayer income in Mississippi. Thus, if benefits were equalized and current matching rates were maintained, taxpayers in low-income states would end up devoting a much higher share of income to Medicaid than those in high-income states.

Anyone who advocates equal Medicaid benefits across states with the existing matching rate formula in effect advocates financing one of the nation's major welfare programs with a highly regressive tax! It is only because low-income states have established more modest Medicaid programs that this situation has been avoided. If the federal-state nature of Medicaid is maintained, even in the short run, revision of the matching rate formula should be a top priority for reform.

Medical Care for Children. Federal policy makers have also been disturbed that states have been reluctant to implement EPSDT programs for AFDC children and have tended to neglect the needs of children relative to those of aged Medicaid recipients. This is not a surprising outcome when we observe the incentives facing state policy makers and note the greater effective federal subsidy for providing for the aged. States are able to use Medicaid funds to "buy into" the Medicare program when providing for the elderly. State funds are thus matched twice—once through Medicaid and once through Medicare. States have responded to this double subsidy by devoting a greater share of resources to the elderly than might otherwise be the case.

Low-income states are particularly prone to provide low benefits for children. Table 3 indicated a relatively high income elasticity of taxpayer demand for Medicaid for AFDC recipients when compared with benefits for the elderly. States tend to provide for the elderly as a necessity, then expand benefits for AFDC children only as state taxpayer income rises.

An additional factor may be that states have a greater degree of control over benefits provided to children. Care for children is more likely to involve clinic services, dental care, and eyeglasses. These fall into the category of optional services, which a state may choose not to offer. Although the EPSDT program for children is mandatory, implementation requires a large state administrative effort and states have been able to limit EPSDT services when they desire to do so. The elderly are more likely to need required medical services such as hospital care, where existing institutional standards rather than taxpayer preferences determine the amount of care provided. Thus low-income states, which as we have seen are likely to desire lower benefit levels, have been able to enforce their preferences with children more easily than with care provided to the elderly. Federal incentives and constraints have thus tended to favor care for the elderly over care for children.

Arbitrary Benefit Limitations. In attempts to limit the cost per recipient, states have often resorted to benefit limitations on hospital days, physician visits, other services, and provider reimbursement rates. Such limits can reduce the availability of medical care without regard for the individual recipient's needs. Medicaid's structure as an open-ended provider reimbursement program has led states to find indirect ways to control costs.

Our analysis has indicated that the Medicaid benefit level in many states is probably higher than desired by taxpayers and that voters would prefer to serve more recipients at a lower level of benefits. Arbitrary benefit limitations are simply a crude attempt by states to control costs in an environment where federal rules and incentives discourage control of Medicaid expenditures by more rational means.

Gaps in Medicaid Coverage. The Medicaid program provides federal subsidies only for care delivered to persons who meet specific requirements such as an aged, blind or disabled person, or member of a one-parent family with dependent children. The federal subsidy of high-quality care for these persons, with no subsidy for others, has resulted in prominent differences in the use of medical services by Medicaid recipients and by the noneligible poor and near poor. Even if voters perceive some poor as more deserving than others and are less inclined to pay for care to persons outside specific eligibility categories, the disparity in use of medical services does not simply reflect preferences of state voters. The federal incentive structure has contributed to this sharp division in medical services provided at public expense.

This section has shown that many of the shortcomings of the Medicaid program are a direct result of federal incentives confronting state policy makers. The behavior of these policy makers, in most cases, has been a logical response to established incentives. Decisions regarding how much of a state's resources to devote to Medicaid have reflected underlying voter preferences for publicly financed medical care, in response to economic factors such as income, prices, and federal incentives.

Controlling the Cost of Medical Care for the Poor

The analysis above suggests that the limited ability of states to control Medicaid benefits has led to a situation where the benefit level is too high and the number of recipients is too low, relative to those desired by voters. An important implication of this analysis is that voters are likely to be willing to extend medical services to more recipients if ways can be found to reduce the cost of each recipient.

Currently, federal subsidies apply only to high-cost forms of care, making it expensive for states to deliver care to many recipients. This is particularly true of the low-income states, which must provide care of some kind to a large percentage of the population. It may be necessary to abandon high-cost forms of health care financing and delivery for the poor in order to obtain voter support for extending benefits to those who fall between the gaps and outside the bounds of Medicaid. Eliminating medical care of low marginal value may be necessary to obtain public support for extending eligibility.

The cost per recipient could be reduced in a number of ways. Among the possibilities are:

- eliminating fraud and abuse
- limiting the type, amount, or duration of the services
- limiting provider reimbursement rates
- controlling hospital beds or revenues
- employing utilization controls
- requiring copayments or cost sharing by recipients
- delivering care through HMOs

The first of these possibilities falls outside the scope of this study, but control of fraud and abuse should be recognized as possibly having a disproportionate impact on public support for the program. The second option—limits on length of hospital stays or number of physician visits—may reduce costs but will also limit care available without regard for the needs of the individual recipient. Such limits are not always targeted to reduce care that is of low marginal value to the recipient.

The third item—limits on provider reimbursement rates—has been employed in a number of states and is a feature of the Canadian medical-care system. In the absence of universal rate controls, such limits on rates for Medicaid providers can be expected to reduce the quality of care provided. This may be desirable if it is believed that the quality lost is of low value and not worth the price. But where such limits apply, recipients should be permitted to purchase higher quality care if they are willing to pay the amount in excess of the standard Medicaid fee. This provision would widen the range of choices for Medicaid recipients and could promote competition among potential Medicaid providers.

The model of the behavior of state policy makers also has some important implications for hospital cost-containment strategies, such as limiting hospital beds or revenues. The empirical results reveal a direct relationship between hospital beds per capita and inpatient hospital services provided under Medicaid. But, as is shown in the appendix, the number of hospital beds per capita is directly related to numbers of Medicaid recipients but not to the benefit level. It is by no means clear that controlling hospital beds would reduce care with low marginal value, such as unnecessarily long hospital stays, provided to Medicaid recipients. Reducing hospital beds may, however, induce states to tighten Medicaid eligibility requirements in order to ensure access to care for the more wealthy voters. Limits on hospital revenue could have a similar effect. Thus it is possible that states may respond to hospital cost containment by reducing the number of Medicaid recipients. The incentives facing state policy makers should be considered in developing a hospital cost-containment strategy.

The fifth alternative—utilization controls—has been discussed by Holahan and Stuart.[6] Review before or after treatment by professional standard review organizations or other groups may be effective in reducing costs and eliminating the care of lowest marginal value as evaluated by the reviewers. The decision criteria of such bodies, however, are not likely to be uniform across locations or over time and this would produce a different kind of horizontal inequity. Also, such decisions may not reflect the preferences of the individual recipient for types of care.

The remaining means of controlling costs per recipient—cost sharing, copayments, and HMOs—offer perhaps the best hope of eliminating care with low marginal value while preserving freedom of choice for recipients. Copayments and HMOs would provide incentives for the recipient or the provider, respectively, to avoid using services of low marginal value. The desirable incentives of HMOs will only exist in a competitive market with informed consumers (recipients). If Medicaid recipients have, or believe they have, no alternative source of care, providers will have an incentive to drastically limit care for Medicaid recipients. Where HMOs are employed, government should

---

[6] John Holahan and Bruce Stuart, *Controlling Medical Utilization Patterns* (Washington, D.C.: The Urban Institute, 1977).

ensure that recipients are informed of the alternative sources of care available.

An attractive means of limiting governmental cost of care for the poor is proposed by Alain Enthoven as part of his Consumer Choice Health Plan (CCHP).[7] Through CCHP, the government would provide low-income families with a voucher whose value would be determined by the actuarial cost of basic medical benefits for the family. The value of the voucher would be inversely related to family income as well. Under this plan, recipients would be able to choose from among several HMO-type plans that would deliver care for an annual fee. Recipients would have an incentive to seek out the plan that delivered the most value for the voucher. The recipient would be permitted to augment the voucher to purchase more costly care if desired, or could use the savings for other purposes if a low-cost plan were chosen. The government would thereby ensure that all persons had access to a plan with minimum benefits, but providers and recipients would have incentives to control costs. The open-ended commitment of funds that exists with Medicaid would be ended.

Matching Rate Formulas

Previous sections have indicated that states respond to the effective price to the taxpayer of providing medical care to the poor. The federal matching rate for state Medicaid expenditures is an important determinant of this price. Thus manipulation of the matching rate structure could be an effective means of influencing state Medicaid spending to achieve national goals.

Although the matching rate system is a potentially powerful policy tool that could be used to equalize Medicaid benefits across states or redistribute the costs of the program, the matching rate formula has remained unchanged since the program began. The federal share of Medicaid payments varies with state income and is computed according to the formula:

$$\text{Federal Share} = 1 - \frac{(\text{state per-capital income})^2}{(\text{national per-capita income})^2} \times 0.45$$

with an upper limit of 83 percent and a minimum of 50 percent. There seems to be little economic rationale for this particular formula. It indicates a desire that the federal government pay at least 50 percent of Medicaid costs and that the federal share should be larger for

[7] Alain Enthoven, "Consumer Choice Health Plan," *The New England Journal of Medicine*, vol. 298, no. 12 (March 23, 1978), pp. 650–658 and no. 13 (March 30, 1978), pp. 709–720.

low-income states, but the current formula is not designed to achieve any particular policy goal.

Although there are definite limits to what can be accomplished through manipulation of matching rates, it is possible to design a matching rate formula with a specific policy objective in mind. For example, suppose uniform national Medicaid eligibility and benefit criteria were established and it was desired that matching rates be designed to equalize the effective tax burden of the program across states. Then the cost to a typical taxpayer with state tax share $1/N$ would be:

$$\text{Cost} = \frac{BPR(1 - F)}{N} = tY \tag{1}$$

where B is the average real medical benefits per recipient, P is the price of medical services in the state, R is the number of recipients, F is the federal share of Medicaid costs, N is the number of taxpayers in the state, Y is the taxpayer's income, and t is the share of the taxpayer's income required to pay for the state share of the program costs.

The federal share (matching rate) that would result in an effective tax rate of t is obtained by solving equation 1 for the federal share, F. That is:

$$\text{Federal share} = 1 - \frac{tYN}{BPR} \tag{2}$$

Using the same value for t in every case, this formula would produce a matching rate for each state that would result in approximately the same tax burden on a typical taxpayer in every state. Of course, an individual's actual tax burden would depend on the state tax structure and the taxpayer's income. The variable t could be made a function of state income if a progressive rather than proportional tax across states were desired. Using this formula, the federal share would be inversely related to aggregate state taxpayer income, YN, and would be directly related to the number of poor persons who met the national eligibility criteria. The federal share would also increase with the cost of medical care in a state and with the real benefit level desired.

A limitation of these matching rates is that they do not necessarily provide enough incentive for states to provide benefits at the level of the specified national standards. Such an incentive could be provided by making the tax share, t, sufficiently small (and the federal subsidy sufficiently large) to ensure that every state desires at least the federally specified level of benefits. This leaves open the possibility that some states would want to provide benefits beyond the national standards without additional federal assistance.

119

Matching rate formulas could also be designed to equalize Medicaid benefits or promote other policy objectives. But whatever formula is used in the future, it should be chosen with an awareness of the incentives it would produce and of the redistribution and equity effects that would result.

General Principles

In light of the above analysis, a set of general principles, or guidelines, can be formulated that may steer future health programs away from some of the problems encountered by Medicaid. Consider the following set of objectives for a national health insurance program for low-income people:

- *Limited Burden for Basic Coverage.* All persons would be able to obtain basic medical-care benefits by spending no more than X percent of their income (or assets) on a health insurance plan.
- *Cost Consciousness.* Either providers or recipients or both would have an incentive to limit care of low marginal value relative to costs.
- *Progressive Taxpayer Equity.* Tax liability for the program will be approximately the same for taxpayers of equal incomes and will increase with income according to a progressive scale.
- *Self Support.* Where it does not result in too heavy a burden as defined in the first objective, persons pay the cost for their own health insurance either through premiums or copayments or indirectly through taxes.

Each of these objectives has been suggested in some way by the previous analysis in this paper. The first principle, limited burden for basic coverage, is one possible version of horizontal equity. But it will be shown that it is compatible with the basic elements of voter demand as well. Rather than imposing a requirement that all persons have identical insurance, it only requires that access to basic medical services not be impeded by low income. Adherence to such a condition would ensure that no one would be required to pay more than, say, 10 percent of income ($X = 0.10$) to obtain basic medical services. The figure X percent could be made a function of income to build some progressivity into the system if desired.

Cost consciousness is the second general principle. Medicaid's failure in this area has contributed to discontent with the program and has discouraged states from extending benefits to more recipients. Estimates indicate that a 20 percent reduction in costs per recipient would produce about a 6 percent increase in the number of recipients to whom voters are willing to provide care. This effect is small but significant; savings not channeled into increased recipients could be used in other areas.

The third criterion, progressive taxpayer equity, deals with the haphazard distribution of the tax burden that has been a characteristic of Medicaid. More equitable distribution of the cost of medical-care programs could be a factor in encouraging public support for such programs. A progressive financing system, either employing or paralleling the federal income tax structure, would be preferable to the current system.

The fourth guideline, self support, reflects the above analysis of taxpayer preferences. It recognizes that taxpayers are more willing to pay for medical care where recipient needs are greater. The condition implies that eligibility for publicly subsidized medical care will depend on recipient needs as measured by income and medical-care prices. Self support is a pragmatic guideline. It is not directly related to the principles of equity and efficiency, as are the other three criteria. If voters were willing to pay for publicly financed medical care for all, there would be no need for this guideline. But given the nature of voter preferences, a national health insurance plan without a self support feature is likely to be too expensive to be acceptable. Recipient cost sharing, where it does not produce too heavy a burden, can reduce the cost per recipient and permit scarce public resources to be directed where the need is greatest.

As a group, the four guidelines would promote both equity and efficiency in a national health insurance program. The guidelines reflect the interests of taxpayers as well as the needs of the low-income population and would provide for the common goal of insuring access to basic medical services for all.

Plans for Reform

The general principles of limited burden for basic coverage, cost consciousness, taxpayer equity, and self support could be applied through a number of administrative mechanisms. These include a federal-state program, a federalized program for the poor, or a universal national health insurance plan. The purpose of this section is to indicate how the four principles could be followed within each of the three types of administrative mechanisms. In addition, current legislative proposals from each of the three administrative categories will be examined to determine how well they meet the objectives of the four principles and to identify areas for potential improvement. But before proceeding we should consider a simple scheme for implementing the four principles.

A Basic Voucher Plan. Under any of the three administrative alternatives the four principles could be implemented through a voucher system similar to that of Enthoven's Consumer Choice Health Plan. As an example, suppose it was decided to establish a program that would limit to 10 percent ($X = 0.10$) the share of income any individual or family would have to spend to obtain basic health insurance coverage. Suppose also that in state A the actuarial cost of basic coverage is $300 a year for an individual adult and $900 a year for a family of four. The assumed coverage could allow for small copayments. In state A, a person with no income would receive a voucher for $300, which could be applied to an insurance policy or HMO plan of the individual's choice. The voucher value would decline to zero for persons with an annual income of $3,000 or for a family of four with an income of $9,000. A family of four with an income of $4,500 would receive a voucher worth $450. They could then purchase the basic benefit plan for an additional $450, or 10 percent of their income. Suppose in state B, the cost of the same basic coverage is $400 per person and $1,200 for a family. Not only would the typical voucher value be higher than in state A, but the subsidy would apply to higher income persons as well. A family of four would receive some benefits with an income of up to $12,000. For these higher income eligible families, the subsidy could be provided through a tax credit rather than a voucher.

Under this plan, persons with identical nominal incomes could be treated differently in different states but only in the interest of equalizing the burden of obtaining basic medical services. The plan would thus satisfy taxpayer demand for less restrictive eligibility requirements where high medical-care costs impede access to care.

Because higher income eligible families would receive vouchers or tax credits of relatively small value, they could choose to use the voucher to purchase inexpensive catastrophic coverage and use their own resources to cover more routine medical expenses. The self-support condition would be served by the income-sensitive subsidy, and persons would contribute to the cost of their own medical care to the extent their income permitted. The public contribution to medical insurance expense would thus be tapered with income to avoid the prominent differences in benefits between eligibles and not-quite-eligibles that currently exist in the Medicaid program. For eligible persons the marginal tax rate, X, would be low, so work disincentives would be small.

The plan would also have built-in cost consciousness. At the margin, the recipient would bear the full cost of additional insurance coverage so there would be an incentive to buy insurance with copayment provisions or to use an HMO to save costs.

The plan is sufficiently flexible to accommodate various policy concerns. Program costs could be predicted with greater accuracy since the government would provide fixed-value vouchers rather than open-ended reimbursement commitments. Budgeted funds not spent, due to unredeemed vouchers, could be used to finance an automatic minimum coverage program for low-income persons who neglect to redeem their vouchers for a private-sector plan. Because X could be set at any level, the plan could be consistent with any proposed budget for the program. It could also be made consistent with any desired degree of progressivity in income redistribution effects by making X a function of income.

Federal-State Plans. One means of implementing these proposals is to modify the existing federal-state system. There are several reasons why it may be desirable to maintain a state role in medical insurance programs for the poor. Perhaps the most important is that states have an incentive to help control costs when they have a financial stake in the program. Additionally, states may want to experiment with innovative forms of medical-care delivery or financing that may be particularly suited to the state. California's experience with HMOs is an example. For this purpose, state policy makers may be better aware of local needs and conditions than federal administrators. The Canadian system is based on several provincial programs; even within provinces decentralization is being pursued as a means of controlling costs. The effectiveness of these attempts is not yet clear, however.[8]

The above analysis provides some clues as to how a reformed federal-state program might be designed. With the proposed voucher system, benefit levels and eligibility criteria could be established at the national level, taking account of variation in medical-care prices. Then, as shown above, it would be possible to find matching rates that would both ensure that the state had adequate incentive to implement the program and equalize the burden on taxpayers across states. This would involve using equation (2) above to compute matching rates, making t, the effective state tax rate, a function of Y if a progressive tax were desired. The value of t would have to be small enough to ensure that all states would demand at least the federally specified level of benefits. Even if the voucher plan is not adopted, changes in the matching rates can be used to more nearly equalize the benefits and burden of costs across states. Much improvement is possible even within the current federal-state system.

A modified federal-state plan is the approach taken with the

---

[8] Eugene Vayda, Robert Evans, and William Mindell, "Universal Health Insurance in Canada: History, Problems, and Trends," *Journal of Community Health* (Spring 1979).

pending Child Health Assurance Program (CHAP). This plan would eliminate many of Medicaid's categorical eligibility criteria, and is designed to provide care to needy children regardless of their family status. The plan also would establish a uniform national income eligibility standard for children and pregnant women.

When measured against the criteria developed above, CHAP has a number of shortcomings. First, the income eligibility standard would not be related to medical-care costs in an area. This may not be a serious problem, however, because states would be permitted to set limits higher than the federal standard and presumably some states with high incomes and high costs would do so. Second, CHAP would not taper benefits with income. It therefore would preserve Medicaid's notch and would exclude completely low-income persons just above the income cutoff level.

A third problem is that, although it would provide additional federal funds through higher matching rates, CHAP would actually produce a less equitable distribution of program costs. As the program has been proposed, high-income states would receive greater increases in matching rates than low-income states. Low-income states would be required to finance greater percentage increases in state costs, while many high-income states would have lower state expenditures under CHAP than currently under Medicaid.[9] As a result, low-income states would be required to contribute a greater share of taxpayer income to the program than would high-income states. For example, state costs as a fraction of taxpayer income in Mississippi would be four to six times that in Connecticut.[10] In other words, this program, presumably intended to aid low-income persons, would actually be financed with a highly regressive tax. Because it fails to provide for an equitable distribution of program costs across states, CHAP needlessly faces opposition from low-income states that could benefit most from the program.

A Federalized Program. A federalized program could also be consistent with the goals outlined above. In a purely national program,

---

[9] U.S. Congress, House of Representatives, Committee on Interstate and Foreign Commerce, *Child Health Assurance Act of 1978*, Washington, D.C., August 11, 1978.

[10] Consider a program that provided $300 in medical benefits to every child in families with income below 75 percent of the federal poverty level. Using 1975 data and proposed CHAP matching rates, this would require 0.0218 percent of income in Connecticut and 0.0865 percent of taxpayer income in Mississippi. Using the Senate version of matching rates, Connecticut would still pay 0.0218 percent, but the effective tax rate for the state share of the program would be 0.137 percent—over six times as high—in Mississippi.

it is important to take account of regional variation in medical-care prices in determining both benefits and eligibility. The voucher system, which satisfies the limited burden for basic coverage criterion, would do this explicitly; other well-defined goals could be used as well. But in the absence of a carefully specified policy goal it is not clear that a federal plan would do better than individual state plans in adjusting for variations in prices and income from state to state. The Medicaid program has at least led to less restrictive eligibility requirements in high-cost areas where the need of the poor is greater. On the other hand, a point in favor of federalization is that there may be some cost saving from consolidating the administrative functions of small states.[11]

In one of several bills under consideration by the Senate Finance Committee, Senator Russell Long has included a federalized program for the poor along with a plan for universal catastrophic coverage. This bill (S.760) would eliminate Medicaid's categorical eligibility requirements and make benefits available to all low-income persons regardless of family status. The plan provides incentives for cost consciousness through copayments on physician visits. It would also discourage excessive stays in hospitals and nursing homes by requiring income-related copayments for persons institutionalized more than sixty days.

The Long plan would limit the burden of health expenses to a specific deductible amount (such as $3,500) for individuals covered by an employer or "individual coverage" catastrophic plan. A person with an income of less than $3,000 or a family of four with income less than $5,400 would qualify for full medical benefits, but the near-poor could only receive benefits by spending down to the low-income eligibility level. Under the spend-down provision, a family of four with an income of $8,900 would derive no additional benefits from the catastrophic plan with a $3,500 deductible, because after spending that much it would qualify for benefits as a low-income family. This hypothetical family could then potentially spend 39 percent of its income before becoming eligible for any benefits. This problem would be even more serious if the income eligibility level were set below $5,400. Although this plan would effectively limit the burden of health expenses for the poor and for higher income groups, it would do little for the near-poor.

New expenditures under the Long bill would come mostly out of federal funds, but states would contribute to a trust fund an amount based on historical state Medicaid expenditures. To the extent that new costs were paid for out of federal taxes, this portion of the financing would meet the criterion of progressive taxpayer equity. But the distribution of total cost of care for the poor would depend on the

---

[11] Grannemann, "Demand for Publicly Financed Medical Care," pp. 137–147.

extent to which states supplemented the federal program and on what federal subsidies would be available for this purpose. As a model for a federalized program for the poor, Senator Long's bill S.760 receives a mixed rating.

Universal National Health Insurance. Reforms of health care programs for the poor could also be incorporated into a universal national health insurance plan. A universal plan would still have to deal with the problems of financing care for the poor that result from interregional variations in income and prices. If the program is to gain public acceptance, it must also be designed to satisfy voter preferences for medical insurance for the poor. A universal program might confront additional problems because, depending on how it is financed, it could adversely affect low-income persons through its impact on the labor market.

In September 1979, two major national health insurance proposals were introduced in Congress. One is President Carter's National Health Plan Act, introduced as S.1812 and H.R.5400. The other is Senator Edward Kennedy's Health Care for All Americans Act, introduced as S.1720 and H.R.5191. Both of these universal plans provide for publicly financed health insurance for the poor and can be evaluated in terms of the four general guidelines developed above.

The first criterion is limited burden for basic coverage. Both plans would eliminate Medicaid's categorical eligibility criteria and assist persons without regard to their family status. The Kennedy plan would be financed through taxes and employer-employee contributions; care would be provided to the nonworking poor at no cost. The burden of financing care for the poor would fall on taxpayers and, with a progressive scale for employee contributions, high-wage workers would subsidize insurance for lower wage workers. The Kennedy plan would thus satisfy the limited burden criterion by shifting the cost of care for all to higher income groups.

Under the Carter plan, the burden for a low-income family would depend on its income relative to the program eligibility standards. A person with an income below 55 percent of the federal poverty level would be eligible for care with no out-of-pocket cost. But, unless a state program were available, other low-income persons would have to spend down to this level to be eligible for benefits. As with the Long bill, this requirement could result in a fairly high burden on low-income families with incomes just above the eligibility standard. These families would derive little benefit from the voluntary insurance plan with a high deductible and could face very burdensome medical expenses. Some families below the poverty level would be required to spend up to 40 percent of their income on medical care before becoming eligible for program benefits.

Another criterion is cost consciousness. With the Carter plan, persons participating in the voluntary governmental insurance plan would have an incentive to keep expenses to a minimum unless their expenses exceeded the $2,500 deductible. Similarly, government-approved private plans could provide for a deductible to encourage cost consciousness. The Kennedy plan, on the other hand, mandates full coverage for all and would provide no incentive for users to limit their own use of low-value services. To control costs, the Kennedy plan would rely on limits on provider reimbursement, implemented through negotiated fee schedules and budget constraints. Services would then be rationed through provider decisions rather than a market mechanism.

Both the Carter and Kennedy plans permit the use of HMOs, but, because individuals would not retain any of the costs saved if an HMO plan were selected, neither plan would provide an incentive for participants to choose an HMO over a fee-for-service arrangement.

Concerning self support, the Carter plan would require persons with incomes above 55 percent of the poverty level to pay for their own care until income was spent down to the eligibility level or the deductible was exhausted on a governmental or private plan. As noted above, the self-support requirement could be excessive for low-income persons who do not qualify for a less restrictive state program. The Kennedy plan does not have any provision for self support by the poor, although employed low-income persons would make some employee contributions. As a result, taxpayers would bear nearly the full cost of providing care to low-income persons.

Although the burden on taxpayers would be high under the Kennedy plan, the financing of care for the poor through the federal tax system would meet the requirement of progressive taxpayer equity. The Carter plan would also make some improvements in Medicaid's inequitable financing mechanism. The Carter plan involves both federal and state financing. The federal government would pick up new costs required to provide a standard set of benefits to all persons below 55 percent of the poverty level. This arrangement would tend to benefit low-income states with less extensive Medicaid programs and would be preferable to the CHAP financing scheme. But the bulk of state payments would be based on historical Medicaid expenditures, and, with high-income states receiving federal subsidies for more generous state programs, there is no guarantee that the program costs would be distributed equitably.

A final concern is the effect universal national health insurance would have on the market for labor. Both the Carter and Kennedy plans would require employers to make contributions toward the health insurance costs of their workers. This would raise the cost of labor to employers and discourage employment. This effect would be particularly strong in the unskilled labor market where employment is typically at the minimum wage. Producers would have an incentive to substitute capital and skilled labor for the now more expensive unskilled labor. Employment of skilled workers would be less affected because they are more likely to have employer-provided insurance coverage already and because their wages are above the legal minimum, so they could accept a compensating reduction in cash wages in return for the insurance coverage. Workers who already have employer-provided health insurance—and this includes much of organized labor—would benefit from their improved competitive position compared with unskilled labor. Thus national health insurance financed with employer contributions would benefit high-income workers at the expense of low-income persons, who would face reduced employment opportunities.

Each of the legislative proposals we have discussed would improve medical care programs for the poor. At a minimum, they would all eliminate some of the arbitrary categorical eligibility requirements, which exclude many needy persons from the Medicaid program. Each of the proposals would channel more public funds into medical-care programs and could be expected to increase use of medical services among one or more groups within the low-income population.

Except for the much more costly Kennedy plan, however, each plan would follow the same basic approach to determining eligibility and benefits that is used with Medicaid. This approach provides a complete package of benefits to persons below a specified income level and requires any others to spend all income down to this level before becoming eligible for benefits on the basis of low income. This requirement can mean burdensome medical expenses for low-income persons above the eligibility level. It also means that persons with income near the eligibility level face an effective marginal tax rate of 100 percent if they incur significant medical expenses.

Income-related subsidies for health insurance would eliminate these problems and could provide an attractive means of meeting the health insurance needs of the poor and near-poor. The subsidies could be provided through either vouchers or tax credits and could be administered in a way that would promote the principles of limited burden, cost consciousness, self support, and progressive taxpayer equity. Such a program could greatly improve health insurance coverage for low-income persons without the high cost and other problems of comprehensive universal national health insurance.

Conclusion

This paper has pointed out some of the problems of financing medical care for the poor that must be dealt with by any national health program. The implications of the wide interstate variation in income and prices must be considered if future programs are to meet the needs of the poor and also be acceptable to voters. Medicaid has had only limited success in this area because federal incentives for state policy makers have not reflected an awareness of underlying economic conditions and the nature of public preferences for medical-care programs for the disadvantaged.

The reforms that I have suggested could be implemented through any of several possible administrative structures, including a revised federal-state program or a federalized Medicaid plan. Universal national health insurance is also a possibility, but is not the only way to effectively deal with the medical-care needs of low-income persons. In fact, when compared with pending legislation for universal national health insurance, a less extensive plan employing income-related vouchers compares favorably in terms of limiting the burden of medical expenses for all, promoting cost consciousness in utilization of medical resources, and distributing the costs of the program equitably.

By pursuing adequate care for the poor in a way that promotes efficient use of resources, directs benefits to where they are needed most, and distributes the cost of the program equitably, we can greatly improve medical care for the disadvantaged. We need not wait for universal national health insurance to have a more efficient and equitable health program for the poor.

Appendix: Regression Results

The empirical analysis supporting this study employs a mixed cross-section and time series sample of observations on state Medicaid expenditures. The sample includes data for the forty-nine states with Medicaid programs for fiscal years 1973 to 1977. Recipient data are only for fiscal years 1973 through 1976. Explanatory variables that are available on a yearly basis for calendar years are matched with the following fiscal year. These explanatory variables are then, in effect, lagged one-half year.

The variables are defined as follows:

Dependent Variables

M = aggregate real Medicaid benefits provided in state.
$OLDM, CHM, ADM$ = aggregate real Medicaid benefits for recipients

129

eligible as over 65, children, and adults in families with dependent children respectively.

OLDREC, CHREC, ADREC = number of old, child, and adult Medicaid recipients divided on basis of eligibility.

RECPOP = ratio of recipients to total population.

OBEN, OBEN, ABEN = real Medicaid benefits per old, child, and adult recipient respectively.

Economic Variables

MEDIDX = An index of state medical-care costs, consisting of a weighted average of (1) hospital cost per patient day (*COST*) and (2) reasonable and customary physician fees (*CPRFEE*).

NTAX = number of taxpayers in state.

PMT = effective price of Medicaid to taxpayer = $[(1 - CORTAX) \times 1 - SHARE) \times MEDIDX]/NTAX$ where *CORTAX* is the share of state taxes paid by corporations, and *SHARE* is the Medicaid matching rate.

YTAX = mean adjusted gross income of taxpayers minus federal income tax deflated by the consumer price index.

NPOOR = estimated number of persons below poverty level.

GINI = an index of income inequality.

Characteristics of the Poor

BLACK = percentage of poor who are black (1970).

PCTOLD = percentage of poor over age sixty-five.

PCTCH = percentage of poor age sixteen or less (1970).

PCTPOOR = percentage of state population below poverty level (1973).

PCTRUR = percentage of the poor located in rural areas.

Characteristics of State Population

METRO = percentage of state population living in metropolitan areas.

EDUC = percentage of state population completing high school.

NEAST, SOUTH, WEST = regional dummies.

Medical Care Market Characteristics

PHY = physicians per capita.

BEDS = hospital beds per capita.

Time Dummies

$T74 = 1$ for fiscal 1974.
$T75 = 1$ for fiscal 1975.
$T76 = 1$ for fiscal 1976.
$T77 = 1$ for fiscal 1977.

REGRESSIONS ON AGGREGATE MEDICAID BENEFITS BY TYPE OF RECIPIENT ELIGIBILITY

Variable	Over Age 65 LN(OLDM) Coef. = elast.	t	AFDC Children LN(CHM) Coef. = elast.	t	AFDC Adults LN(ADM) Coef. = elast.	t
PMT	−.88	−3.81	−.67	−3.28	−.57	−2.99
MEDIDX	.97	1.66	.99	1.94	.67	1.42
YTAX	.51	0.89	2.44	4.89	2.81	6.04
NPOOR	.21	0.99	.38	2.05	.44	2.55
BLACK	−.12	−2.56	−.09	−2.27	−.08	−2.20
PCTOLD	.48	1.28	1.70	5.13	1.49	4.81
PCTCH	.98	1.08	3.35	4.20	2.74	3.67
PCTRUR	−.30	−2.15	−.08	−0.64	.01	0.10
EDUC	.17	0.37	−.33	−0.84	−1.17	−3.14
METRO	−.01	−0.09	−.04	−0.32	.16	1.41
BEDS	.26	0.92	.54	2.24	.56	2.45
PHY	−.05	−0.21	.54	2.49	.43	2.11
NEAST	−.01	−0.81	−.16	−1.38	−.12	−1.06
SOUTH	−.16	−1.24	−.28	−2.49	−.50	−4.81
WEST	−.51	−2.78	.12	0.76	.28	1.91
T74	.15	1.80	.10	1.39	.06	0.94
T75	.35	3.50	.38	4.34	.34	4.13
T76	.45	3.42	.45	3.93	.45	4.23
T77	.53	3.14	.46	3.12	.48	3.43
C	−11.06	−1.37	−34.91	−4.95	−31.72	−4.82
R²	.90		.93		.93	
N	228		228		228	

REDUCED-FORM REGRESSIONS ON NUMBER OF MEDICAID RECIPIENTS BY TYPE OF RECIPIENT ELIGIBILITY

Variable	Over Age 65 LN(OLDREC) Coef.= elast.	t	AFDC Children LN(CHREC) Coef.= elast.	t	AFDC Adults LN(ADREC) Coef.= elast.	t
PMT	−.43	−1.92	−.30	−1.66	−.25	−1.34
MEDIDX	1.86	3.22	1.03	2.22	1.12	2.28
YTAX	−2.25	−4.08	2.17	4.92	2.32	4.93
NPOOR	.63	3.13	.67	4.14	.75	4.33
BLACK	−.05	−1.19	−.04	−1.11	−.09	−2.38
PCTOLD	−.06	−0.15	1.78	5.98	1.28	4.03
PCTCH	−1.14	−1.27	3.50	4.88	1.72	2.25
PCTRUR	−.25	−1.80	.12	1.07	.12	1.03
EDUC	−1.13	−2.57	−.46	−1.31	−1.62	−4.31
METRO	.03	0.03	.27	2.57	.31	2.73
BEDS	.79	2.95	.69	3.22	.80	3.48
PHY	.35	1.40	.31	1.55	.31	1.44
NEAST	−.25	−1.89	.06	0.56	.13	1.16
SOUTH	.73	0.59	−.19	−1.97	−.29	−2.78
WEST	−.10	−0.55	.44	3.13	.62	4.14
T74	.03	0.33	.04	0.59	.01	0.14
T75	−.11	−1.16	.18	2.50	.17	2.21
T76	−.23	−1.84	.24	2.40	.22	2.14
C	25.38	3.17	−35.99	−5.63	−26.04	−3.82
R²	.92		.95		.94	
N	188		188		188	

REDUCED-FORM REGRESSIONS ON MEDICAID BENEFIT LEVEL BY TYPE OF RECIPIENT ELIGIBILITY

Variable	Over Age 65 LN(*OBEN*)		AFDC Children LN(*OBEN*)		AFDC Adults LN(*ABEN*)	
	Coef. = elast.	*t*	Coef. = elast.	*t*	Coef. = elast.	*t*
PMT	−.47	−2.33	−.26	−1.90	−.29	−2.12
MEDIDX	−.65	−1.24	−.05	−0.13	−.23	−0.65
YTAX	2.42	4.82	.26	0.76	.61	1.77
NPOOR	−.44	−2.36	−.17	−1.38	−.27	−2.12
BLACK	−.06	−1.52	−.07	−2.58	.00	0.06
PCTOLD	.63	1.85	−.05	−0.20	.24	1.02
PCTCH	2.49	3.04	−.10	−0.18	.95	1.71
PCTRUR	−.06	−0.44	−.23	−2.66	−.11	−1.24
EDUC	1.54	3.82	.39	1.44	.56	2.02
METRO	−.01	−0.09	−.22	−2.70	−.15	−1.85
BEDS	−.60	−2.44	−.11	−0.65	−.13	−0.76
PHY	−.42	−1.87	.08	0.57	−.08	−0.52
NEAST	.20	1.67	−.20	−2.43	−.24	−2.87
SOUTH	−.26	−2.28	−.00	−0.05	−.13	−1.75
WEST	−.46	−2.84	−.35	−3.20	−.28	−2.54
T74	.13	1.84	.07	1.52	.05	1.17
T75	.43	5.12	.20	3.69	.17	3.02
T76	.62	5.49	.21	2.81	.22	2.92
C	−33.03	−4.52	3.44	0.70	−4.41	−0.89
R²	.63		.44		.39	
N	188		188		188	

REGRESSIONS ON NUMBER OF MEDICAID RECIPIENTS
AS A FRACTION OF STATE POPULATION

Variable	LN(*RECPOP*) Coef. = elast.	*t*	LN(*RECPOP*) Coef. = elast.	*t*	LN(*RECPOP*) Coef. = elast.	*t*
PMT	−.08	−2.58	−.07	−2.27	−.07	−2.29
MEDIDX	.69	3.35	1.10	5.19	.98	2.96
YTAX	−.79	−2.41	−.06	−0.17	.13	0.32
GINI	.09	0.17	.39	0.71	.41	0.75
BLACK	−.06	−1.86	−.04	−1.27	−.04	−1.30
PCTOLD	.45	1.92	1.31	4.82	1.31	4.61
PCTCH	1.25	2.15	2.64	4.34	2.64	4.23
PCTRUR	−.11	−1.43	.14	1.49	.13	1.22
EDUC	−.89	−3.30	−1.44	−4.62	−1.44	−4.58
METRO	−.08	0.74	.18	1.70	.18	1.75
BEDS	.28	1.90	.82	4.58	.86	4.64
PHY	.49	3.03	.32	1.96	.28	1.70
NEAST			.11	1.37	.14	1.50
SOUTH			−.06	−0.72	−.05	−0.53
WEST			.64	5.34	.67	5.34
T74					.05	0.77
T75					.09	1.31
T76					.09	1.02
T77					.07	0.61
C	2.92	.53	−10.21	−1.79	−11.35	−1.93
R^2	.52		.58		.59	
N	218		218		218	

Bibliography

Bartlett, Lawrence. "HMOs and the Poor: Problems and Possibilities." *Public Welfare*, Spring 1979, pp. 50–53.

Bergstrom, Theodore C., and Robert P. Goodman. "Private Demand for Public Goods." *American Economic Review*, June 1973, pp. 280–296.

Borcherding, T., and R. Deacon, "The Demand for Services of non-Federal Governments." *American Economic Review*, December 1972.

Davis, Karen. "Medicaid Payments and the Utilization of Medicaid Services by the Poor." *Inquiry*, June 1976.

Davis, Karen. *National Health Insurance: Benefits, Costs, and Consequences*. Washington, D.C.: The Brookings Institution, 1975.

Davis, Karen, and Roger Reynolds. "The Impact of Medicare and Medicaid on Access to Medical Care." In *The Role of Health Insurance in the Health Services Sector*, edited by R. Rosett. New York: National Bureau of Economic Research, 1976, pp. 391–435.

Davis, Karen, and Kathy Schoen. *Health and the War on Poverty*. Washington, D.C.: The Brookings Institution, 1978.

Deacon, Robert T. "A Demand Model for the Local Public Sector." *Review of Economics and Statistics*, May 1978, pp. 184–192.

Enthoven, Alain C. "Consumer Choice Health Plan." *The New England Journal of Medicine*, Vol. 298, No. 12 (March 23, 1978), pp. 650–658 and No. 13 (March 30, 1978), pp. 709–720.

Gayer, David. "The Effects of Medicaid on State and Local Government Finances." *National Tax Journal*, December 1972.

Giertz, J. Fred, and Dennis H. Sullivan. "Donor Optimization and the Food Stamp Program." *Public Choice* 32, Spring 1977, pp. 19–35.

Godwin, R. Kenneth, and W. Bruce Shepard. "Political Processes and Public Expenditures: A Re-examination Based on Theories of Representative Government." *American Political Science Review* 70 (1976): pp. 1127–1135.

Grannemann, Thomas W. "The Demand for Publicly Financed Medical Care: The Role of Interdependent Preferences." Ph.D. dissertation, Northwestern University, 1979.

Hall, Charles, et al. "Medicaid and Cash Welfare Recipients: An Empirical Study." *Inquiry*, March 1977, pp. 43–50.

Helms, J., J. P. Newhouse, and C. E. Phelps. "Copayments and Demand for Medical Care: The California Medicaid Experience." *Bell Journal of Economics*, Spring 1978, pp. 192–208.

Hester, James, and Elliott Sussman. "Medicaid Prepayment: Concept and Implementation." *The Milbank Memorial Fund Quarterly*, Vol. 54, No. 4 (Fall 1974), pp. 415–444.

Holahan, John. *Financing Health Care for the Poor: The Medicaid Experience*. Lexington, Mass.: Lexington Books, 1975.

Holahan, John. "Foundations for Medical Care: An Empirical Investigation of the Delivery of Health Services to a Medicaid Population." *Inquiry*, December 1977, pp. 352–368.

Holahan, John, William Scanlon, and Bruce Spitz. *Restructuring Federal Medicaid Controls and Incentives*. Washington, D.C.: The Urban Institute, 1977.

Holahan, John, and Bruce Stuart. *Controlling Medicaid Utilization Patterns*. Washington, D.C.: The Urban Institute, 1977.

Holahan, John, et al. *Altering Medicaid Provider Reimbursement Methods*. Washington, D.C.: The Urban Institute, 1977.

Institute for Medicaid Management, DHEW, HCFA, Medicaid Bureau. *Data on the Medicaid Program: Eligibility, Services, Expenditures, Fiscal Years 1966–1978.* Washington, D.C., 1978.

Orr, Larry L. "Income Transfers as a Public Good: An Application to AFDC." *American Economic Review,* June 1976.

Orr, Larry L. "Income Transfers as a Public Good: Reply." *American Economic Review,* December 1978, pp. 990–994.

Pauly, Mark. "Efficiency in the Provision of Consumption Subsidies." *Kyklos,* 1970.

Pauly, Mark. "Income Redistribution as a Local Public Good." *Journal of Public Economics,* 1973, pp. 35–58.

Pauly, Mark. *Medical Care at Public Expense.* New York: Praeger Publishers, 1971.

Pauly, Mark. *The Role of the Private Sector in National Health Insurance.* Washington, D.C.: Health Insurance Institute, 1979.

Sloan, Frank, Janet Mitchell, and Jerry Cromwell. "Physician Participation in State Medicaid Programs." *Journal of Human Resources,* Supplement 1978, pp. 211–245.

Spiegel, Allen D., ed. *The Medicaid Experience.* Germantown, Maryland: Aspen Systems Corporation, 1979.

Spitz, Bruce, and John Holahan. *Modifying Medicaid Eligibility and Benefits.* Washington, D.C.: The Urban Institute, 1977.

Stevens, Robert B., and Rosemary Stevens. *Welfare Medicine in America: A Case Study of Medicaid.* New York: Free Press, 1974.

Stuart, Bruce. "Equity and Medicaid." *Journal of Human Resources,* Spring 1972, pp. 162–178.

Vayda, Eugene, Robert Evans, and William K. Mindell. "Universal Health Insurance in Canada: History, Problems and Trends." *Journal of Community Health,* Spring 1979.

Vogel, Ronald J., and John R. Morall, III. "The Impact of Medicaid on State and Local Health and Hospital Expenditures with Special Reference to Blacks." *Journal of Human Resources,* Spring 1973.

Preventive Care, Care for Children, and National Health Insurance

Gilbert R. Ghez and Michael Grossman

The numerous plans for national health insurance (NHI) introduced during the 1970s have emphasized the extension of coverage to two types of services where private health insurance benefits are thought to be lacking or inadequate: medical care services associated with catastrophic illness and medical care services with a large preventive component. Included in the latter category are prenatal care, pediatric care (care rendered by all physicians to children and adolescents), preventive checkups, and dental care.

Although some bills introduced in Congress during the Nixon-Ford administration focused solely on catastrophic illness, most of them, including those supported by the administration, contained benefits for preventive care. For example, the Mills-Schneebeli-Packwood Bill, introduced in 1974 and endorsed by the Nixon administration, provided benefits subject to a deductible of $150 per person and a coinsurance rate of 25 percent for prenatal and maternity care, well-child care to age six, dental care to age thirteen, and vision and eye examinations to age thirteen.[1] Preventive checkups for adults were excluded from the basic benefits, but the provisions of the bill to stimulate enrollment in prepaid group health plans (health maintenance organizations) would have resulted in an increase in the percentage of the population insured for this service.

Other bills, most notably those associated with Senator Kennedy, were even more liberal with respect to the coverage of preventive medi-

NOTE: We are grateful for the comments received from Edward F. X. Hughes, M.D., at the AEI conference on national health insurance. We also thank Ann Colle for excellent assistance. Grossman's research for this paper was supported by a grant from the Robert Wood Johnson Foundation to the National Bureau of Economic Research. This paper has not undergone the review accorded official National Bureau of Economic Research publications; in particular, it has not yet been submitted for approval by the Board of Directors.

[1] Saul Waldman, *National Health Insurance Proposals: Provisions of Bills Introduced in the 93rd Congress as of February 1974*, U.S. Department of Health, Education and Welfare, Social Security Administration, Office of Research and Statistics, 1974.

137

cal care. Although phase one of President Carter's recent national health insurance plan focuses on catastrophic illness, pregnant women and infants up to the age of one would be guaranteed free care regardless of family income.[2] Presumably, coverage would be extended to other types of preventive care after the initial phase-in period. Governor Jerry Brown has recently advocated an all-out emphasis on prevention.

The purpose of this paper is to examine issues related to the coverage of preventive care under national health insurance. In particular we try to answer two basic questions: Should preventive services be covered? If so, what would the best plan be like? As part of the second question, we investigate whether coverage should be universal or limited to certain groups in the population and certain preventive services.

To deal with these two basic issues, several other issues must be addressed. To shed light on the extent of "underinsurance," we first discuss the extent of present third-party (private and public) coverage of preventive medical care services. In the next section we review the literature on the effects of preventive medical care on health outcomes. This review is relevant, because one of the goals of coverage of preventive care under NHI is to improve the health of the population. In the third section we review the literature on the determinants of use of preventive medical care services. Here our focus is on the effects of variables that are under the purview of public policy (price, income, and health manpower) and on variables whose effects government policy might try to offset (socioeconomic and family characteristics). Implications for an optimal plan are treated in the final section.

Before turning to the main issues in the paper, we should discuss several conceptual issues. These revolve around the definition of preventive care, the types of medical services included under the rubric of preventive care, and the appropriateness of insuring this care.

We define preventive-care activities as activities that may improve health by reducing the probability of an illness or an accident or that reduce the seriousness of an illness or an injury given the occurrence of an unhealthy state. Preventive care is *efficacious* if there exists a course of action that can be taken after detection of an adverse symptom that will reduce the need or extent of later treatment. Whether preventive care is efficacious or not is a medical question. Preventive care is said to be *effective* if a unit of preventive activity by an individual improves his later health. For preventive care to be effective, the physician must adequately identify the symptoms, the care must be efficacious, and

---

[2] U.S. Congress, H.R. 5400, September 25, 1979; and "Comparison of Health Proposals," *New York Times*, June 14, 1979.

the patient must comply with the prescribed course of action. Hence effectiveness is a stricter requirement than efficaciousness.

Preventive activities are *not* limited to medical care. Indeed, much evidence suggests that preventive nonmedical activities have more impact on health than medical care. Studies have linked good health to such factors as proper diet, exercise and recreation, refraining from smoking cigarettes, avoiding alcohol abuse, and years of formal schooling completed.[3] By and large, we deal with preventive medical care in this paper, but the reader should not lose sight of the important role of nonmedical factors in health outcomes.[4]

We include four specific kinds of medical care services under the rubric of preventive care:

- prenatal care
- pediatric care (preventive and curative physicians' services delivered to children and adolescents)
- preventive physicians' services delivered to adults under the age of sixty-five, including physical examinations, multiphasic screening, and associated X-rays and laboratory tests
- dental care delivered to children, adolescents, and adults under the age of sixty-five.

To keep the paper manageable, we do not consider preventive care for persons age sixty-five and over and therefore do not discuss issues related to the Medicare program. We focus on the medical services just listed because they are all thought to have an important preventive component. This is obvious in the case of preventive physicians'

---

[3] See, for example, L. Breslow and B. Klein, "Health and Race in California," *American Journal of Public Health*, vol. 61, no. 4 (April 1971), pp. 763–775; Victor R. Fuchs, "Some Economic Aspects of Mortality in Developed Countries," in *The Economics of Health and Medical Care*, edited by Mark Perlman (London: MacMillan, 1974); Victor R. Fuchs, *Who Shall Live? Health, Economics and Social Choice* (New York: Basic Books, Inc., 1974); Michael Grossman, "The Correlation Between Health and Schooling," in *Household Production and Consumption*, edited by Nestor E. Terleckyj (New York: Columbia University Press for the National Bureau of Economic Research, 1975); Lawrence Manheim, "Health, Health Practices, and Socioeconomic Status: The Role of Education," Ph.D. dissertation, University of California at Berkeley, 1975; Linda N. Edwards and Michael Grossman, "Adolescent Health, Family Background, and Preventive Medical Care," *Annual Series of Research in Human Capital and Development*, vol. 3, edited by Ismail Sirageldin and David Salkever (Greenwich, Connecticut: JAI Press, forthcoming); and Linda N. Edwards and Michael Grossman, "Children's Health and the Family," *Annual Series of Research in Health Economics*, vol. 2, edited by Richard M. Scheffler (Greenwich, Connecticut: JAI Press, 1980).

[4] In the final section of this paper, we consider the implications, for an optimal health insurance plan, of the possible existence of complementarities between preventive medical care and preventive nonmedical care.

services for adults. In the case of children and adolescents, both preventive and curative services delivered early in life can have important long-run effects on health in adulthood. Moreover, the appropriate treatment of problems revealed by an annual checkup is an integral component of preventive care. The importance of prevention is underscored by making periodic checkups required in schools, in the armed forces, and sometimes at the place of work.

The alleged importance of the early period of life in health outcomes has led several researchers to propose that national health insurance should be limited at first to complete coverage of prenatal care, pediatric care, dental care for children, and in some instances catastrophic illness.[5] Bills limiting national health insurance solely to mothers, infants, and children were introduced in Congress in 1976 by Senator Javits and Congressman Scheuer. The content of our paper reflects the legislative and policy interest in preventive care for children; the paper contains a selective, rather than a comprehensive, discussion of preventive care for adults.[6] To keep the paper manageable and because of the key role of the physician in the medical care market, we do not deal with hospital care for children. Also to keep the paper manageable, we do not treat in any detail the preventive component of adult remedial care delivered in the early stages of illness, although we recognize that the benefits of prevention and intervention are perhaps greatest at this stage.

At first glance, it might seem anomalous to consider the coverage of preventive care under national health insurance. After all, the purpose of private insurance is to protect against uncertainty. That is, risk-averse consumers have an incentive to purchase health insurance to finance medical outlays associated with illness and injury. In this context, preventive care is a substitute for market insurance; it is a form of self-insurance or self-protection, to use the terminology introduced by

---

[5] Eli H. Newberger, Carolyn Moore Newberger, and Julius B. Richmond, "Child Health in America: Toward a Rational Public Policy," *Milbank Memorial Fund Quarterly*, vol. 54 (Summer 1976), pp. 249–298; Kenneth Keniston and the Carnegie Council on Children, *All Our Children: The American Family Under Pressure* (New York: Harcourt Brace Jovanovich, 1977); Theodore R. Marmor, "Children and National Health Insurance," in *Developing a Better Health Care System for Children*, volume III of the report of the Harvard Child Health Project Task Force (Cambridge, Mass.: Ballinger Publishing Company, 1977); and Theodore R. Marmor, "Rethinking National Health Insurance," *The Public Interest*, no. 45 (Winter 1977), pp. 73–95.

[6] Our focus on children is due in part to Phelps's excellent recent paper on insurance of preventive care for adults. See Charles E. Phelps, "Illness Prevention and Medical Insurance," *Journal of Human Resources*, vol. 13, Supplement (1978), pp. 183–207.

Ehrlich and Becker.[7] Put differently, there is a good deal of uncertainty with respect to the scope and size of remedial medical care outlays but no such uncertainty with respect to preventive medical care outlays.

If the sole purpose of national health insurance were to provide protection against uncertainty and if the insurance scheme satisfied several conditions mentioned later in the paper, there would be no justification for covering preventive care. The key point to realize, however, is that national health insurance has other goals in addition to reducing risk. If its goals include improvements in the health of certain segments of the population or correcting suboptimal private decisions due to externalities, NHI itself and coverage of preventive care could be justified even if there were no uncertainty.[8] We discuss theoretical justifications for coverage of preventive care under NHI and optimal intervention strategies in more detail in the final section.

Extent of Coverage

Private Health Insurance Coverage. Panel A of Table 1 shows the percentage of the civilian population of the United States under age sixty-five with private insurance for three types of medical services in 1970 and in 1976. The three services are (1) doctor office and home visits, (2) X-rays and laboratory exams, and (3) dental care.

Panel B shows the percentage of private expenditures for each service paid by health insurance. The percentage of expenditures covered is smaller than the percentage of persons covered because most health insurance policies contain deductibles; coinsurance rates; upper limits; and restrictions on, for example, the type of doctor office visits covered. The most notable trend in the table is the rapid increase in the percentage of the population with dental insurance—from 6.6 percent in 1970 to 24.0 percent in 1976.

Preventive physicians' services delivered to children and adults take the form of vaccinations and immunizations, checkups, detailed physical examinations, and multiphasic screening. Although these services are associated with doctor office visits, X-rays, and laboratory tests, the coverage figures in Table 1 cannot be extrapolated to these preventive services. This is because most health insurance plans do not

---

[7] Isaac Ehrlich and Gary S. Becker, "Market Insurance, Self-Insurance and Self-Protection," *Journal of Political Economy*, vol. 80 (July/August 1972), pp. 623–648.

[8] For a similar discussion, see Mark V. Pauly, *Medical Care at Public Expense: A Study in Applied Welfare Economics* (New York: Praeger Publishers, 1971).

TABLE 1

Private Health Insurance Coverage

Service Covered	1970	1976
A. *Percent Under 65 with Private Health Insurance Coverage by Type of Service*		
Doctor office and home visits	48.0[a]	62.2[b]
X-ray and laboratory examinations	73.8[a]	75.0[b]
Dentist's services	6.6[a]	24.0[b]
B. *Percent of Private Expenditures Paid by Private Health Insurance by Type of Service*		
Doctor office and home visits for people under 65 years of age (includes X-rays and laboratory tests associated with office visits)	22.1[c]	28.6[d]
Dentist's services	3.8[c]	14.9[e]

[a] SOURCE: Marjorie Smith Mueller, "Private Health Insurance in 1970: Population Coverage, Enrollment, and Financial Experience," *Social Security Bulletin*, vol. 35 (February 1972).

[b] SOURCE: Marjorie Smith Carroll, "Private Health Insurance Plans in 1976: An Evaluation," *Social Security Bulletin*, vol. 41 (September 1978).

[c] SOURCE: Ronald Andersen, Joanna Lion, and Odin W. Anderson, *Two Decades of Health Services: Social Survey Trends in Use and Expenditure* (Cambridge, Mass.: Ballinger Publishing Company, 1976).

[d] Computed as follows:

K_{70}, K_{76} = percentages paid by insurance in 1970 and 1976, respectively.

I_{70}, I_{76} = percentages of population with private health insurance coverage in 1970 and 1976, respectively.

Assume $\dfrac{K_{76}}{I_{76}} = \dfrac{K_{70}}{I_{70}}$, then $K_{76} = \dfrac{I_{76}}{I_{70}} \times K_{70}$.

[e] SOURCE: Robert M. Gibson and Charles R. Fisher, "National Health Expenditures, Fiscal Year 1977," *Social Security Bulletin*, vol. 41 (July 1978).

cover preventive care.[9] On the other hand, health maintenance organizations (HMOs) do cover preventive physicians' services. In 1976 approximately 4 percent of persons with private doctor office visit insurance were members of HMOs.[10]

---

[9] The percentage of the population with X-ray and laboratory examination insurance exceeds the percentage with doctor office visits insurance in Table 1 because sometimes the former type of insurance is limited to X-rays and tests performed in a hospital.

[10] Marjorie Smith Carroll, "Private Health Insurance Plans in 1976: An Evaluation," *Social Security Bulletin*, vol. 41, no. 9 (September 1978), pp. 3–16.

Fraud by physicians and patients can make insurance companies' exclusion from coverage of preventive services difficult to enforce. That is, in filling out an insurance claim, a physician can report that he delivered curative services when in fact he delivered preventive services. Although the extent of such fraud is not known, our own casual empiricism suggests it is important. Our own casual empiricism also suggests that dental insurance, especially the newer plans, do cover preventive checkups subject to deductibles, coinsurance, and specified maximum payments.[11]

According to the health survey conducted by the National Opinion Research Center and the Center for Health Administration Studies of the University of Chicago (the NORC survey), 51 percent of children between birth and age five, and 53 percent of children between the ages of six and seventeen, had insurance covering doctor office visits in 1970.[12] This insurance covered 13.6 percent of the private outlays on doctor office visits on behalf of the younger children and 20.7 percent of the private outlays on behalf of the older children. There is evidence that the NORC estimates of the percentage of children with doctor office visit insurance are too large. Unpublished data from the National Center for Health Statistics indicate that approximately one-third of all children had such coverage in 1972.[13]

In 1970, 74 percent of all live births to women not eligible for Medicaid or other public funds were covered by private health insurance.[14] This insurance financed 49 percent of total private expenditures per live birth and 46 percent of obstetrical services delivered by physicians. Obstetricians typically charge pregnant women a flat fee for prenatal visits and the delivery of the child, rather than a fee for each prenatal visit. Therefore, the figures just cited give a good indication of the extent of coverage for all physicians' services associated with births. Data on prenatal insurance coverage are not available for years

---

[11] For a detailed discussion of this point, see Phelps, "Illness Prevention," pp. 183–207.

[12] Ronald Andersen, Joanna Lion, and Odin W. Anderson, *Two Decades of Health Services: Social Survey Trends in Use and Expenditure* (Cambridge, Mass.: Ballinger Publishing Company, 1976).

[13] Harvard Child Health Project, *Toward a Primary Medical Care System Responsive to Children's Needs*, vol. 1 of the report of the Harvard Child Health Project Task Force (Cambridge, Mass.: Ballinger Publishing Company, 1977). This estimate agrees with the one reported by Colle and Grossman based on their research with children between the ages of one and five in the NORC survey. See Ann D. Colle and Michael Grossman, "Determinants of Pediatric Care Utilization," *Journal of Human Resources*, vol. 13, Supplement (1978), pp. 115–158.

[14] Andersen, Lion, and Anderson, *Two Decades*.

after 1970, but Andersen, Lion, and Anderson report that such insurance increased over time between 1963 and 1970.[15]

To summarize, preventive physicians' services for children and adults are not usually covered by private health insurance except in the case of HMOs. Between one-third and one-half of all children have doctor office visit insurance, most of which finances curative (remedial) medical care services. The percentages of the population with prenatal and dental insurance have risen substantially over time.[16]

Public Coverage. The main public sources of coverage for the medical care services considered in this paper are Medicaid, the maternal and child health program, and the neighborhood health center program.[17] All of these programs are aimed primarily at low-income families. Of the three programs, Medicaid is by far the largest. In 1976, it accounted for approximately 95 percent of total public expenditures on the three programs combined.[18]

The Medicaid program was enacted in 1965 as Title XIX of the Social Security Act. It is a joint federal-state program designed to finance the medical care services of specified groups of needy persons. Medicaid eligibility is linked to welfare eligibility. States that elect to participate in the program (all states except Arizona have elected to do so) must cover all families covered by the aid to families with dependent children (AFDC) program.[19]

States may also provide Medicaid coverage to the medically needy. These are persons whose incomes net of medical expenses are 133⅓ percent or less of the AFDC eligibility income level in each state.

---

[15] Andersen, Lion, and Anderson, *Two Decades.*

[16] Prenatal care, pediatric care, preventive physicians' services for adults, and dental care all are eligible for the medical expense deduction under the federal income tax. Due, however, to the sizable deductible that must be satisfied (3 percent of adjusted gross income), this cannot be an important source of "insurance" of preventive care for most taxpayers.

[17] Our discussion is based on Anne-Marie Foltz, "Uncertainties of Federal Child Health Policies: Impact in Two States," U.S. Department of Health, Education, and Welfare, Public Health Service, National Center for Health Services Research, 1978; Anne-Marie Foltz and Donna Brown, "State Response to Federal Policy: Children, EPSDT, and the Medicaid Muddle," *Medical Care,* vol. 13 (August 1975), pp. 630–642; Anne-Marie Foltz, "The Development of Ambiguous Federal Policy: Early and Periodic Screening, Diagnosis and Treatment (EPSDT)," *Milbank Memorial Fund Quarterly,* vol. 53 (Winter 1975), pp. 35–64; and Karen Davis and Cathy Schoen, *Health and the War on Poverty* (Washington, D.C.: The Brookings Institution, 1978).

[18] Robert M. Gibson and Charles R. Fisher, "National Health Expenditures, Fiscal Year 1977," *Social Security Bulletin,* vol. 41 (July 1978), pp. 3–20.

[19] We do not discuss persons covered under Medicaid because they are aged, blind, or disabled recipients of supplemental security income (SSI).

Twenty-eight states provide coverage for the medically needy. In twenty-six states AFDC is restricted to families without a father present in the home. Twenty-four states extend AFDC and Medicaid coverage to families with unemployed fathers who do not receive unemployment compensation. Seventeen states cover all children under the age of twenty-one in families with incomes below the AFDC eligibility level, regardless of the employment status of the parents or the family composition.

It is well known that AFDC income eligibility levels vary considerably among states. This factor, together with the factors mentioned above, causes a considerable percentage of low-income persons to be ineligible for Medicaid. Davis and Schoen estimate that in 1970 45 percent of the poverty population of children under age twenty-one and 39 percent of the poverty population of adults between the ages of twenty-one and sixty-four did not receive Medicaid benefits.[20] Comparable figures are not available for later years, but the percentage of the poverty population who did not receive Medicaid benefits declined from 41 percent in 1970 to 35 percent in 1974.[21]

In some states, Medicaid recipients are eligible for benefits for all four medical care services discussed in this paper: prenatal and obstetrical care, pediatric care, preventive physicians' services for adults, and dental care. All states must cover physicians' services. Coverage of dentists' services is optional, and in 1974 only 16 percent of all white persons covered by Medicaid and 15 percent of all non-white persons covered saw a dentist.[22]

Although Medicaid has no deductibles or coinsurance, states can in a number of ways restrict the kind and amount of physicians' services covered. In twenty states, single women pregnant with their first child are ineligible for prenatal and obstetrical care because the AFDC programs of these states do not cover "unborn children." Some states limit the number of physician office visits per person to a specified number per month or per year. Some states exclude routine physical examinations and screening for adults.[23] Moreover, Medicaid does not cover the indirect costs of obtaining medical care: outlays on trans-

---

[20] Davis and Schoen, *War on Poverty*.

[21] Karen Davis and Roger Reynolds, "The Impact of Medicare and Medicaid on Access to Medical Care," in *The Role of Health Insurance in the Health Services Sector*, edited by Richard Rosett (New York: Neale Watson Academic Publications, 1976); and Davis and Schoen, *War on Poverty*.

[22] Davis and Schoen, *War on Poverty*.

[23] For a detailed outline of the benefits provided in each state, see Health Care Financing Administration, *Data on the Medicaid Program: Eligibility, Services, Expenditures: Fiscal Years 1966–78* (Washington, D.C.: The Institute for Medicaid Management, 1978).

portation and the value of the time spent in traveling, waiting, and obtaining information about alternative sources of care.[24]

In 1967 an early and periodic screening, diagnosis, and treatment (EPSDT) program was created under Medicaid. By July 1, 1969, all states were *mandated* to provide EPSDT services to children under the age of twenty-one who were eligible under the state's Medicaid program. The enactment of this program changed the nature of Medicaid from simply a payment mechanism for financing services to an active deliverer of services to poor children. States were required to seek out such children, advise them or their families of the availability of benefits, and ensure that they receive them.

The emphasis of the EPSDT program has been on screening. The screening examination must include a physical examination, appropriate immunizations, vision and hearing tests, laboratory tests, and a dental examination for children three years of age and older.

In fiscal 1977, 2 million children of an estimated Medicaid population of 11 million children received screening services. This increased the number of children with up-to-date assessments to 3 million.[25] The failure of Medicaid to cover all pregnant women and children in the poverty population and the failure of the EPSDT program to screen all children eligible for Medicaid has led the Carter administration to propose the Child Health Assurance Program (CHAP). A bill to amend Title XIX of the Social Security Act to create CHAP was introduced in Congress in 1978 (H.R. 13611) and modified and reintroduced in 1979 (H.R. 4053). To date, the legislation has not been enacted.

Under CHAP, national income standards would be established for determining the eligibility of pregnant women and children for Medicaid. For pregnant women, the standard is $3,000, increased by $600 for each additional family member.[26] For children, the standard is $2,400 for an individual (relevant for older children who do not live with their parents), $3,000 for a family of two, and an additional $600 for each additional family member. These uniform national standards would add to the Medicaid rolls 100,000 pregnant women and approximately 2 million children. States would be required to finance

---

[24] The effects of indirect costs on utilization are discussed in the third section of this paper, "Determinants of Utilization."

[25] These data are from an unpublished memorandum supplied to us by Malcolm Curtis, Human Resources Division, Congressional Budget Office. For a careful review of EPSDT see Edward F. X. Hughes and his associates, *An Assessment of the Validity of the Results of HCFA's Demonstration and Evaluation Program for the Early and Periodic Screening, Diagnosis and Treatment Program: A Metaevaluation*, Center for Health Services and Policy Research, Northwestern University, June 1979.

[26] Note that under this standard, women pregnant with their first child would be eligible for Medicaid in all states.

prenatal care for pregnant women and routine dental care for children.[27]

Funds are authorized to publicize the availability of these services. CHAP would increase the cost of Medicaid by roughly $400 million; this should be compared with total federal and state expenditures on Medicaid of $14 billion in fiscal 1976.

With the exception of the EPSDT program, Medicaid is a mechanism for financing the medical care services of poor people rather than a mechanism for delivering these services. On the other hand, the maternal and child health program (MCH) and the neighborhood health center program (NHC) focus both on delivery and on financing of services to poor people. The MCH program was created by Title V of the Social Security Act of 1935. In 1963 Title V was amended to include special grants for maternity and infant care projects designed to provide adequate prenatal care. In 1965 Title V was further amended to include children and youth projects. These supply comprehensive medical care services in poverty areas.

In 1965 the program to create and fund neighborhood health centers was started by the Office of Economic Opportunity as part of the War on Poverty. By 1973 overall control of the centers had been shifted to the Bureau of Community Health Services of the U.S. Department of Health, Education, and Welfare. These centers provide ambulatory care services to all age groups in the population. Children and adults not eligible for Medicare are the main recipients of services delivered by NHCs.[28]

In both the MCH and NHC programs, funds are allocated directly to suppliers: state and local health departments; special clinics and centers for the medical care of pregnant women, infants, children, and youths; and neighborhood health centers. Note that suppliers are not physicians or dentists in private practice. Taken together, the MCH and NHC programs cover prenatal care, pediatric care, preventive physicians' services for adults, and dental care. But these programs are very small relative to Medicaid: In fiscal 1976, Medicaid outlays were nineteen times as large as outlays on the MCH and NHC programs.[29]

To summarize, a network of public programs exists to finance prenatal care, pediatric care, preventive physicians' services for adults, and dental care for the poverty population and to deliver these services to this population. This network has been criticized because it fails to

---

[27] Currently, EPSDT covers the cost of a dental examination and treatment of problems uncovered by the examination. States have the option of covering or not covering routine dental care for children that is not associated with the EPSDT assessment.

[28] Davis and Schoen, *War on Poverty*.

[29] Gibson and Fisher, "National Health Expenditures," pp. 3–20.

cover a significant proportion of the poverty population and because it emphasizes financing rather than delivery. Nevertheless its existence should be kept in mind, particularly since we argue in the final section that a convincing case can be made for limiting preventive care under national health insurance to low- and moderate-income families.

Effects of Preventive Medical Care on Health Outcomes

In this section we discuss the effects of preventive medical care on health outcomes. We do not argue that in those instances where care is more effective it necessarily provides greater benefits than where care is less effective. After all, benefits depend not only on the health outcome but also on the value of a unit of improved health in the form of reduction in income loss or relief from pain and suffering. By concentrating on health outcomes rather than on measures of full benefit from care, we bypass the difficult issues of monetary valuation. Our aim is to distinguish those forms of care that are effective from those that are not. Our review of the literature on this subject is selective rather than comprehensive. Studies are cited to illustrate our main points.

Prenatal Care. There is a growing consensus that prenatal care is effective in terms of infant health outcomes, although its relative importance remains an open issue. Lewit reports that prenatal care, measured by the number of prenatal visits to physicians, is an important determinant of birth weight and neonatal mortality in the 1970 New York City birth and death cohort.[30] He also reports that birth weight has a strong negative effect on postneonatal mortality, so that prenatal care has an indirect impact on postneonatal mortality. Williams finds that the mortality rate is inversely related to the number of board-certified obstetrician-gynecologists per birth.[31]

Other evidence suggests that selective public intervention strategies are effective. With various socioeconomic variables held constant, Williams shows that the infant mortality rate is negatively related to expenditures per birth under maternal and infant care (M and I) projects in a subsample of states of the United States in 1966 and 1967.[32] Davis and Schoen summarize studies that point to dramatic

---

[30] Eugene M. Lewit, "Experience with Pregnancy, the Demand for Prenatal Care, and the Production of Surviving Infants," Ph.D. dissertation, City University of New York Graduate School, 1977.

[31] Ronald L. Williams, "Outcome-Based Measurements of Medical Care Output: The Case of Maternal and Infant Health," Ph.D. dissertation, University of California at Santa Barbara, 1974.

[32] Williams, "Outcome-Based Measurements."

148

declines in infant mortality rates over time in the late 1960s and early 1970s in areas served by M and I projects.[33] These declines exceeded those experienced by similar residents of the same city or county who were not served by the M and I project in their area. Davis and Schoen also point out that the infant mortality rate of blacks in Lee County, Mississippi, was cut in half between 1970 and 1974. This large decline followed the opening of a neighborhood health center in the county in 1970. Currently, the black infant mortality rate in Lee County is below the state average, "a remarkable achievement considering that the county has the lowest educational level of any county in the state and one of the highest poverty rates."[34]

Because birth weight rises with prenatal care, the benefits of appropriate care are not limited to infant mortality outcomes. Birth weight has strong positive effects on intellectual development in samples of school-age children.[35] Moreover, Shakotko, Edwards, and Grossman find that health in adolescence is positively associated with intellectual development in childhood in a longitudinal sample.[36] Because they control for health in childhood, the finding implies causality from IQ to health. It means that birth weight has favorable impacts on health throughout the life cycle.

Recent trends in infant mortality in the United States provide suggestive, although not definitive, evidence of the importance of prenatal care. From 1964 to 1974, the infant mortality rate declined by 3.9 percent per year. This was an extremely rapid rate compared to the comparable figure of 0.6 percent per year from 1955 to 1964.[37] The latter period witnessed the introduction of Medicaid, maternal and infant care projects, and the neighborhood health center program. Rogers and Blendon associate the trend in infant mortality with these developments, although they are careful to emphasize that there is no evidence of a cause-and-effect relationship.[38] Fuchs is somewhat more cautious

---

[33] Davis and Schoen, *War on Poverty*, p. 176.

[34] Ibid.

[35] For example, Linda N. Edwards and Michael Grossman, "The Relationship between Children's Health and Intellectual Development," in *Health: What is it Worth?*, edited by Selma Mushkin and David Dunlop (Elmsford, N.Y.: Pergamon Press, Inc., 1979).

[36] Robert A. Shakotko, Linda N. Edwards, and Michael Grossman, "The Dynamics of Health and Cognitive Development in Adolescence," paper presented at the fifty-fourth annual conference of the Western Economic Association, Las Vegas, Nevada, June 1979.

[37] Victor R. Fuchs, "The Great Infant Mortality Mystery, or What Caused the Slump? " mimeographed, 1978.

[38] David E. Rogers and Robert J. Blendon, "Feeling Fine," *New York Times*, June 27, 1977.

because the period in question also witnessed the legalization of abortions and the widespread adoption of oral contraceptive techniques.[39] Nevertheless, Fuchs does not deny the effectiveness of adequate medical care during pregnancy and delivery, especially for high-risk pregnancies.

Pediatric Care. Even such an enthusiastic supporter of national health insurance for children as Marmor realizes that pediatric care makes small contributions at best to favorable child outcomes.[40] To be sure, immunizations against rubella, measles, diphtheria, tetanus, pertussis, polio, and the mumps are extremely efficacious. Sharp declines in the reported number of cases of each disease occurred in the years immediately following the general availability of an immunization against it.[41] But routine pediatric care has small and often statistically insignificant effects on the health of children and adolescents in a number of recent studies.

Edwards and Grossman study the prevalence of obesity, abnormal corrected distance vision, and anemia (reflected by low hematocrit levels) among white adolescents who were members of Cycle III of the U.S. Health Examination Survey.[42] Youths who saw a doctor for a preventive checkup within the past year (approximately 60 percent of the sample) have one-half percentage point smaller probabilities of being obese or of having abnormal corrected distance vision than other youths, and a one-fifth percentage point *higher* probability of having anemia. None of these three differentials is statistically significant.

Kaplan, Lave, and Leinhardt measure medical care input by enrollment in a comprehensive health care clinic and measure health output by number of days absent from school in a sample of elementary school children from low-income families in Pittsburgh, Pa.[43] With race and sex of the child held constant, enrollment in the clinic has a small negative effect on number of days absent from school. Unfortunately, the

---

[39] Fuchs, "Infant Mortality Mystery"; and Fuchs, *Who Shall Live?* In research in progress, Jacobowitz and Grossman are studying the effects of Medicaid, M and I projects, the legalization of abortion, the use of oral contraceptive techniques, and other factors on variations in infant mortality rates among counties of the U.S. See Steven Jacobowitz and Michael Grossman, "Determinants of Variations in Infant Mortality Rates Among Counties of the United States," in progress.

[40] Marmor, "Children and National Health Insurance."

[41] National Center for Health Statistics and the National Center for Health Services Research, *Health: United States, 1978*, U.S. Department of Health, Education, and Welfare, Public Health Service, 1978.

[42] Edwards and Grossman, "Adolescent Health."

[43] Robert S. Kaplan, Lester B. Lave, and Samuel Leinhardt, "The Efficacy of a Comprehensive Health Care Project: An Empirical Analysis," *American Journal of Public Health*, vol. 62 (July 1972), pp. 924–930.

authors could not control for parents' education, which has been shown to be an extremely important factor in child health outcomes.[44]

Hu measures medical care by the dollar value of Medicaid benefits and by the receipt of a regular checkup in a sample of first-grade children in a coal mining county in Pennsylvania, mainly from low-income families.[45] Medicaid benefits have a positive and statistically significant effect on hearing correction[46] but have no effect on vision correction. The receipt of a regular checkup has no impact on either health measure.

Kessner studies the prevalence of middle ear infection and hearing loss, vision defects, and anemia in a sample of black children between the ages of six months and eleven years in Washington, D.C.[47] He focuses on the relationship between these three health problems and the usual source of pediatric care (physicians in private solo practice, prepaid group practice, hospital pediatric outpatient departments, hospital emergency rooms, and public clinics). Kessner finds that source of care has no effect on prevalence of the three health conditions with socioeconomic status held constant. Using more sophisticated statistical techniques, Dutton and Silber have reexamined Kessner's basic result.[48] They report higher than average illness probabilities in solo practice and lower than average probabilities in prepaid group practice and in the hospital outpatient departments. These differences are small, however, and are not always statistically significant. Dutton also indicates that the frequency of a preventive health checkup has no significant impact (at the 5 percent level) on the presence of anemia in the Kessner sample.[49]

Inman estimates child health production functions in which preventive pediatric visits and curative pediatric visits appear as separate

[44] For example, Edwards and Grossman, "Adolescent Health"; Edwards and Grossman, "Children's Health and the Family"; and Shakotko, Edwards, and Grossman, "Dynamics of Health."

[45] Teh-Wei Hu, "Effectiveness of Child Health and Welfare Programs: A Simultaneous Equations Approach," *Socio-Economic Planning Sciences*, vol. 7, no. 6 (December 1973), pp. 705–721.

[46] A problem arises in interpreting Hu's result for hearing correction because of the way in which he coded this variable: zero if the child had normal hearing, one if the child had hearing defects corrected, and minus one if the child had uncorrected defects. This coding scheme gives children with a corrected defect more "health" according to this index than children with no defect.

[47] David M. Kessner, *Assessment of Medical Care for Children* (Washington, D.C.: Institute of Medicine, 1974).

[48] Diana B. Dutton and Ralph S. Silber, "Children's Health Outcomes in Six Different Ambulatory Care Delivery Systems," mimeographed, March 1979.

[49] Diana B. Dutton, "Hematocrit Levels and Race: An Argument Against the Adoption of Separate Standards in Screening for Anemia." Paper presented at the American Public Health Association Meetings in Los Angeles, October 18, 1978.

inputs.[50] His data sample is the one analyzed by Kessner, and his health measures are absence of ear, nose, and throat infections and absence of ear infection. The two pediatric care inputs tend to have positive effects on health, but their regression coefficients are small and rarely statistically significant.

In a sense it is not surprising that pediatric care has little impact on children's health. Many of their health problems are either self-limiting, such as morbidity from acute conditions, or irreversible, such as congenital abnormalities of the neurological system. But the studies reviewed above indicate that this lack of potency extends to health problems that are capable of being affected by pediatric care and by family decisions concerning diet and other forms of at-home health care, as modified by the advice of physicians.

Dental Care. Although appropriate pediatric care has little impact on children's physical health outcomes, appropriate dental care is extremely important in their dental (oral) health outcomes. This is illustrated strikingly by multivariate analyses of the number of decayed teeth and the periodontal index (a negative correlate of good oral health)[51] of white adolescents who were members of Cycle III of the U.S. Health Examination Survey. Edwards and Grossman[52] find that there are large significant impacts of the receipt of a preventive dental visit in the past year on both the periodontal index and the decay index. In particular, adolescents who did not have a preventive dental checkup within the past year (approximately 30 percent of the sample) have periodontal indexes and decay scores that are each about 30 percent of a standard deviation worse than adolescents who received a checkup.

Edwards and Grossman also provide strong results pertaining to the efficacy of a publicly provided form of preventive dental care— water fluoridation. Youths exposed to fluoridated water have signifi-

---

[50] Robert P. Inman, "The Family Provision of Children's Health: An Economic Analysis," in *The Role of Health Insurance in the Health Services Sector*, edited by Richard Rosett (New York: Neale Watson Academic Publications, 1976).

[51] Kelly and Sanchez describe the periodontal index as follows:
Every tooth in the mouth . . . is scored according to the presence or absence of manifest signs of periodontal disease. When a portion of the free gingiva is inflamed, a score of 1 is recorded. When completely circumscribed by inflammation, teeth are scored 2. Teeth with frank periodontal pockets are scored 6 when their masticatory function is unimpaired and 8 when it is impaired. The arithmetic average of all scores is the individual's [periodontal index]. . . .
See James E. Kelly and Marcus J. Sanchez, *Periodontal Disease and Oral Hygiene Among Children*, National Center for Health Statistics, U.S. Department of Health, Education, and Welfare, Public Health Service, 1972, pp. 1–2.

[52] Edwards and Grossman, "Adolescent Health."

cantly better oral health than other youths at conventional levels of confidence. The fluoridation differentials are smaller, however, than the corresponding preventive dental care differentials in oral health.

Nevertheless, given that the per-child cost of fluoridation is also substantially below the cost of a preventive dental visit,[53] this still remains a cost-effective method of improving dental health. Moreover, in 1975 approximately 50 percent of the population of the U.S. resided in communities that had water supplies with less than optimal fluoride levels.[54]

Research by Newhouse and Friedlander questions the effectiveness of dental care in adult health outcomes.[55] Using adults in Cycle I of the U.S. Health Examination Survey, they report an insignificant positive effect of the number of dentists per capita in the county of residence on the periodontal index. They do not explicitly recognize, however, the common-sense proposition that an increase in a community's dental manpower will not improve oral health outcomes unless it encourages more use of dental services. Despite the findings by Newhouse and Friedlander, there is a consensus that the receipt of appropriate dental care in childhood and in adulthood contributes to better oral health at all stages in the life cycle.[56]

Preventive Physicians' Services for Adults. There is little evidence that annual physical checkups and mass screening programs for adults lead to improvements in health. Spark and Phelps summarize a number of studies that contain evidence that screening and checkups are economically wasteful and only occasionally detect conditions that are aided by early treatment.[57] These authors and others conclude that preventive physicians' services for adults can raise medical-care costs without significantly raising the level of health.

To be sure, there are selected health problems for which preventive care may be efficacious. The best documented cases are for glaucoma, breast cancer, cervical cancer, hypertension, and syphillis. For such major illnesses as angina and stomach cancer, however, the efficacious-

---

[53] "Fluoridation: The Cancer Scare," *Consumer Reports*, vol. 43 (July 1978), pp. 392–396.

[54] National Center for Health Statistics and the National Center for Health Services Research, *Health: United States, 1978.*

[55] Joseph P. Newhouse and Lindy J. Friedlander, *The Relationship Between Medical Resources and Measures of Health: Some Additional Evidence* (Santa Monica, Calif.: The Rand Corporation, May 1977).

[56] National Center for Health Statistics and the National Center for Health Services Research, *Health: United States, 1978.*

[57] Richard Spark, "The Case Against Regular Physicals," *The New York Times*, July 25, 1976, sec. 6, p. 10; and Phelps, "Illness Prevention," pp. 183–207.

ness of secondary prevention is uncertain.[58] Moreover, even when diagnosis and treatment are possible, there are problems associated with false positives; low prevalence rates; adverse side effects of, for example, frequent mamographies to detect breast cancer; and poor follow-up compliance.

The above conclusions are highlighted by a longitudinal study of members of the Kaiser-Permanente Health Plan by Collen and his associates.[59] In 1964 approximately 10,000 members of the plan between the ages of thirty-five and fifty-four were randomly assigned to two groups comparable in socioeconomic status. The study group was urged to come in for frequent periodic physical exams; the control group was not. By mid-1975, 41 percent of the control group had not received a checkup, while only 16 percent of the study group had not received a checkup. Yet between 1965 and 1975, the overall mortality experience of the two groups was very similar. By 1975, 6.9 percent of the study group and 7.1 percent of the control group had died, a difference which is not statistically significant. The control group did, however, have higher death rates from two illnesses that offer substantial potential for postponement or prevention: colorectal cancer and hypertension complications. But even these findings where efficacy of prevention is established cannot be interpreted as evidence in favor of the effectiveness of selective, as opposed to mass, screening. The cost of detecting one case of colorectal cancer is extremely high. Only fifty-five cases were detected by protoscopic exams administered to 47,207 patients in a Mayo Clinic study.[60] The detection of one case of hypertension is relatively cheap and a standard course of treatment exists to reduce blood pressure to normal. Despite this, the hypertension mortality differential in the Collen sample is not statistically significant.

It is universally recognized that lowering blood pressure in cases of extreme hypertension reduces both mortality and other severe complications.[61] There is also some evidence that reducing blood pressure in

---

[58] For example, Donald Louria et al., "Primary and Secondary Prevention among Adults: An Analysis with Comments on Screening and Health Education," *Preventive Medicine*, vol. 5 (1976), pp. 549–572.

[59] Morris F. Collen, ed., *Multiphasic Health Testing Services* (New York: John Wiley and Sons, 1978); and Loring G. Dales, Gary D. Friedman, and Morris F. Collen, "Evaluating Periodic Multiphasic Health Checkups: A Controlled Trial," *Journal of Chronic Disease*, vol. 32, no. 5 (1979), pp. 385–404.

[60] Spark, "Regular Physicals."

[61] For example, M. Sokolow and D. Perloff, "Five-Year Survival of Consecutive Patients with Malignant Hypertension Treated with Antihypertensive Agents," *American Journal of Cardiology*, vol. 6 (November 1960), pp. 858–863; E. R. Mohler and E. D. Freis, "Five-Year Survival of Patients with Malignant Hypertension Treated with Antihypertensive Agents," *American Heart Journal*, vol. 60

patients with moderately severe or with mild hypertension also reduces mortality and morbidity. The recognition of the role of hypertension in heart disease and stroke has contributed in part to the rapid reduction in deaths from these causes since 1968.[62] For these reasons, it is worth considering the case of hypertension screening in more detail.

The Veterans Administration Cooperative Study Group examined a group of 143 male hypertensive patients with diastolic blood pressures between 115 and 126 mm Hg randomly assigned to active or placebo treatment.[63] In the placebo group there were twenty-seven cases of severe complications, while there were only two in the treated group. Four sudden deaths occurred in the control group and none in the treated group. The Veterans Administration Study Group also studied 380 male hypertensives with diastolic blood pressures between 90 and 114 mm Hg.[64] Treatment was estimated to reduce morbidity from 55 percent to 18 percent over a five-year period: terminating morbid events occurred in thirty-five patients in the control group and only nine patients in the treated group. There was no reduction in myocardial infarction or sudden death. This study was confined to a small group of men and had very strict criteria. Hence it is difficult to generalize these results to the population at large.

Although hypertension is easy to detect and treatment is efficacious, in the sense that there is a known course of treatment, screening for hypertension seems to have limited value. Lauridsen and Gyntelberg report on a study of male employees in public and private companies in Copenhagen.[65] A sample of 5,249 males aged forty to fifty-nine was initially examined in 1970–1971. Of these, 196 had previously undetected severe or moderately high hypertension. Although some dropped

(September 1960), pp. 329–335; and S. Bjork et al., "The Effect of Active Drug Treatment in Severe Hypertensive Disease," *Acta Medica Scandinavica*, vol. 169 (June 1961), pp. 673–689.

[62] Surgeon General of the United States, *Healthy People: The Surgeon General's Report on Health Promotion and Disease Prevention*, U.S. Department of Health, Education, and Welfare, Public Health Service, Publication no. 79-55071, 1979.

[63] Veterans Administration Cooperative Study Group on Antihypertensive Agents, "Effects of Treatment on Morbidity in Hypertension, II. Results in Patients with Diastolic Blood Pressures Averaging 115 Through 129 mm Hg," *Journal of the American Medical Association*, vol. 202, no. 11 (December 11, 1967), pp. 1028–1034.

[64] Veterans Administrative Cooperative Study Group on Antihypertensive Agents, "Effects of Treatment on Morbidity in Hypertension, I. Results in Patients with Diastolic Blood Pressures Averaging 90 Through 114 mm Hg," *Journal of the American Medical Association*, vol. 213, no. 7 (August 17, 1970), pp. 1143–1152.

[65] Lone Lauridsen and Finn Gyntelberg, "A Clinical Follow-Up Five Years After Screening for Hypertension in Copenhagen, Males Aged 40–59," *International Journal of Epidemiology*, vol. 8 (March 1979), pp. 11–14.

out of the program, 150 were examined in an outpatient clinic, treated if judged necessary, and then referred to their own personal physician for further treatment. A five year follow-up was undertaken on the 150 men. At follow-up, their mortality was twice as high and their prevalence of major cardiovascular complications (nonfatal myocardial infarction and stroke) was three times as high as the expected rate for Danish middle-aged men. This relatively poor prognosis may be the result of inadequate compliance: Only 31 percent of these 150 men were well controlled on antihypertensive medication at the time of follow-up.

Other studies have also shown the low efficiency of public screening for hypertension.[66] Finnerty and his colleagues have reported that by screening in supermarkets they were able to reach 61 percent of an adult urban, largely stable population, but that despite all efforts only 30 percent of those identified as having high blood pressure were available for treatment.[67]

The failure of mass screening in a best possible case (high prevalence, easy detection, known course of treatment) raises the question of the effectiveness of preventive care for adults. Future research may shed light on the effectiveness of preventive care in areas where current evidence is insufficient or not conclusive.[68] Until such time, however, we believe that the burden of proof should fall on the advocates of effectiveness.

Proponents of health maintenance organizations, which provide preventive care at no charge to their members, cite the lower rates of hospitalization of HMO members compared to the general population as evidence in favor of the effectiveness of these delivery systems and of preventive care. On the other hand, Pauly argues convincingly that

---

[66] For example, Milton Weinstein and William Statson, *Hypertension—A Policy Perspective* (Cambridge, Mass.: Harvard University Press, 1976); M. F. D'Souza, A. V. Swan, and D. J. Shannon, "A Long-Term Controlled Trial of Screening for Hypertension in General Practice," *Lancet*, vol. 1 (June 5, 1976), pp. 1228–1231; W. E. Miall and S. Chinn, "Screening for Hypertension: Some Epidemiological Observations," *British Medical Journal*, vol. 3 (September 1974), pp. 595–600; and R. Stamler et al., "Adherence and Blood Pressure Response to Hypertension Treatment," *Lancet*, vol. 2 (December 20, 1975), pp. 1227–1230.

[67] F. A. Finnerty, Jr., L. W. Shaw, and C. K. Himmelsbach, "Hypertension in the Inner City, Part 2: Detection and Follow-Up," *Circulation*, vol. 47 (January 1973), pp. 76–78.

[68] See Mark V. Pauly, "Efficiency, Incentives and Reimbursement for Health Care," *Inquiry*, vol. 7 (March 1970), pp. 114–131. For careful empirical evaluations of HMOs, see Harold S. Luft, "How Do Health Maintenance Organizations Achieve Their 'Savings'?: Rhetoric and Evidence," *New England Journal of Medicine*, vol. 298 (June 15, 1978), pp. 1336–1343; and Harold S. Luft, "Why Do HMOs Seem to Provide More Health Maintenance Services?" *Milbank Memorial Fund Quarterly*, vol. 56 (Spring 1978), pp. 144–168.

these lower hospitalization rates can arise from the differential reimbursement schemes in HMOs compared to other delivery systems.[68] In particular, physicians in private practice are paid on a fee-for-service basis, while reimbursement in an HMO setting takes the form of capitation payments. Because an HMO's cost is increased when a patient is hospitalized while its revenue is not altered, it has an incentive not to hospitalize patients if possible. In light of this factor and the results of the Collen study, it is unlikely that the lower hospitalization rates of HMO enrollees implies that their health is better than that of other groups in the population.

To summarize, prenatal care and dental care are effective but pediatric care (other than immunizations) and preventive physicians' services for adults are not.

Many government health policies are directed at blacks and other low-income children and adults. Therefore, it is useful to point out that in general there is a correspondence between health measures for which care is effective and health measures for which race and income differences are observed. Black babies weigh less at birth than white babies and are more likely to die within the first year of life. Similar conclusions emerge when babies from low-income families are compared to those from high-income families.[69] Data from the Center for Disease Control reveal higher prevalence rates of measles and rubella among black children than among white children and among children who reside in poverty areas than among children who do not.[70] Edwards and Grossman show that the oral health of children is better if they are from high-income families or if they are white.[71] Newhouse and Friedlander reach similar conclusions with respect to the oral health of adults.[72] Edwards and Grossman report that the physical health of children is not related to race or parents' income, with parents' schooling and other

---

[69] For example, Brian MacMahon, Mary Grace Kovar, and Jacob J. Feldman, *Infant Mortality Rates: Socioeconomic Factors*, U.S. Department of Health, Education, and Welfare, Public Health Service and Mental Health Administration, 1972; Fuchs, "Mortality in Developed Countries"; Fuchs, *Who Shall Live?*; Steven L. Gortmaker, *Poverty, Race, and Infant Mortality in the United States*, Institute for Research on Poverty Discussion Paper No. 404-77, University of Wisconsin, 1977; Lewit, "Experience with Pregnancy"; and Selma Taffel, *Prenatal Care in the United States, 1969–1975*, U.S. Department of Health, Education, and Welfare, Public Health Service, National Center for Health Statistics, Vital and Health Statistics, series 21, no. 33 (September 1978).

[70] Center for Disease Control, "United States Immunization Survey, 1976," U.S. Department of Health, Education, and Welfare, Public Health Service, 1977.

[71] Edwards and Grossman, "Adolescent Health"; and Edwards and Grossman, "Children's Health and the Family."

[72] Newhouse and Friedlander, *Medical Resources and Measures of Health*.

factors held constant.[73] Mortality and morbidity rates of white adults are *positively* related to income in a number of studies, although black adults have higher mortality rates than whites.[74]

The above suggests that there are income- and race-related differences in health to offset in some cases but not in others.[75] These differences could be offset by lowering the price of preventive care for the poor via national health insurance, but they could also be offset by income transfers and other policies. We consider the choices among alternative policy options in more detail in the next two sections.

Determinants of Utilization of Preventive Medical Care Services

In this section we discuss the determinants of utilization of preventive medical care services. The coverage of preventive care under national health insurance would presumably lower the price of care. Yet the effects of other variables on utilization as well as price are also discussed in this section to identify variables whose effects government policy might try to offset. These variables include race, income, and other socioeconomic and family characteristics. Another reason for considering other variables is to compare a program of price cuts under national health insurance with programs to alter other variables in the purview of public policy—income and health manpower.

For these reasons and because there are few multivariate studies of prenatal care and preventive doctor care for adults, the section is organized around the effects of sets of determinants rather than on the determinants of the four kinds of care. The sets of determinants are as follows: (1) income, race, and Medicaid; (2) money and time prices; and (3) socioeconomic and family characteristics represented by school-

---

[73] Linda N. Edwards and Michael Grossman, "Income and Race Differences in Children's Health," National Bureau of Economic Research Working Paper No. 308, 1979; Edwards and Grossman, "Adolescent Health"; and Edwards and Grossman, "Children's Health and the Family."

[74] For example, Richard D. Auster, Irving Leveson, and Deborah Sarachek, "The Production of Health: An Exploratory Study," *Journal of Human Resources*, vol. 4 (Fall 1969), pp. 411–436; Michael Grossman, *The Demand for Health: A Theoretical and Empirical Investigation* (New York: Columbia University for the National Bureau of Economic Research, 1972); Grossman, "Health and Schooling"; Fuchs, "Mortality in Developed Countries"; and Fuchs, *Who Shall Live?* These studies control for reverse causality from poor health to low income in a variety of ways.

[75] In general, conclusions reached with respect to the existence or nonexistence of income and race differences are valid whether or not medical care is held constant. When care is efficacious, sensitive to income, and not held constant, the gross difference exceeds the net (medical care-constant) difference. This pertains to infant health and oral health. In the case of prevalence of infectious diseases, net differences do not seem to exist.

ing and family size. Income, race, and Medicaid are treated together because proverty is more prevalent among blacks than among whites and because Medicaid is aimed at low-income groups.

Income, Race, and Medicaid. Data on the utilization of the medical care services between 1963 and 1976 reveal two facts with regard to race and income differences in utilization.

First, cross-sectional surveys in selected years reveal that whites and high-income families made more use of almost all these services. Second, trend data on utilization of the same service reveal that income and race differences declined over time. To a large extent, these declines can be traced to Medicaid, which reduces the net or out-of-pocket price of medical care to zero from the point of view of the consumer.[76] In the case of pediatric care, one of the declines has been substantial: income differences in the average number of physician visits by children disappeared in 1975.[77] Nevertheless, income and race differences in most measures of utilization still are large.

Taffel reports that in 1969 72.4 percent of all white mothers but only 42.7 percent of all black mothers started prenatal care in the first trimester of pregnancy.[78] In 1975 the comparable figures were 75.9 percent for whites and 55.8 percent for blacks. Hence the difference between the probability that a white mother would obtain care within the first trimester and the probability that a black mother would do so fell by ten percentage points over a five-year period. But the 1975 differential of twenty percentage points is sizable. A similar differential emerges when high-income mothers are compared to low-income mothers. In 1972, 71.2 percent of pregnant women whose family income was $15,000 or over saw a doctor within the first trimester of pregnancy. The corresponding figure for women whose family income was under $5,000 was 47.2 percent.[79]

In 1976, white children and children from nonpoverty areas were more likely to have been immunized against measles, rubella, polio, mumps, and DPT (diphtheria, whooping cough, and tetanus) than black

---

[76] For example, Davis and Reynolds, "Access to Medical Care"; Colle and Grossman, "Pediatric Care," pp. 115–158; and Davis and Schoen, *War on Poverty*.

[77] National Center for Health Statistics, *Physician Visits: Volume and Interval Since Last Visit, 1975*, U.S. Department of Health, Education, and Welfare, Public Health Service, Vital and Health Statistics, series 10, no. 128 (April 1979).

[78] Taffel, *Prenatal Care*.

[79] National Center for Health Statistics, *Use of Selected Medical Procedures Associated with Preventive Care, 1973*, U.S. Department of Health, Education, and Welfare, Public Health Service, Vital and Health Statistics, series 10, no. 110 (March 1977).

children and children from poverty areas.[80] The percentage of all children between the ages of one and four immunized against polio declined from 88 percent in 1964 to 75 percent in 1975.[81] This trend and the variations in immunization rates by race and income have been responsible in part for the EPSDT program under Medicaid and for the proposed CHAP program.

We have already indicated that the income difference in physician visits by children vanished by 1975. Based on a multiple regression analysis of physician visits in the 1969 U.S. Health Interview Survey, Davis and Reynolds show that this result can be attributed almost entirely to Medicaid.[82] In particular, children from families with an income of under $5,000 who were eligible for welfare made approximately one more visit in 1969 than children from families with an income of under $5,000 who were not eligible for welfare. Note that a substantial fraction of children from low-income families are not eligible for Medicaid.[83] Therefore income differences in visits remain for these children compared to children from high-income families.[84] Moreover, visits rise with income in the 1975 data if the lowest income category is not considered.[85] Note finally that black-white differences in visits have not been eliminated. Black children made approximately one fewer visit than white children in 1975.[86]

Gross income or race differences in other dimensions of pediatric care utilization have not been altered as much by Medicaid as the per-capita number of visits. In 1973, 18.7 percent of poor children below the age of seventeen but only 11.9 percent of nonpoor children had not seen a physician in the past two years.[87] The race difference is almost

---

[80] Center for Disease Control, "United States Immunization Survey, 1975," U.S. Department of Health, Education, and Welfare, Public Health Service, DHEW (CDC) 76-8221, 1976.

[81] Center for Disease Control, "United States Immunization Survey, 1971," U.S. Department of Health, Education, and Welfare, Public Health Service, DHEW (HSM) 72-8094, 1971; and Center for Disease Control, "Immunization Survey, 1975."

[82] Davis and Reynolds, "Access to Medical Care."

[83] As indicated above, this figure was 45 percent in 1970.

[84] In 1975 children from families with an income of under $5,000 made exactly the same number of visits on average as children from families with an income of $15,000 or over. This means that children who received Medicaid benefits made *more* visits than their counterparts in the $15,000 or over family income class.

[85] National Center for Health Statistics, *Physician Visits.*

[86] National Center for Health Statistics, *Physician Visits.*

[87] Ronald W. Wilson and Elijah L. White, "Changes in Morbidity, Disability, and Utilization Differentials between the Poor and Nonpoor: Data from the Health Interview Survey: 1964 and 1973," *Medical Care*, vol. 15 (August 1977), pp. 636–646.

identical to the income difference: 19 percent of black children and 12 percent of white children had not seen a doctor within the past two years.[88] With respect to routine physical exams, in 1973 8.9 percent of white children under the age of seventeen, 14.8 percent of nonwhite children, 20.3 percent of children from families with an income under $3,000, and 44 percent of children from families with an income of $15,000 or more received exams.[89]

Among children with at least one physician contact in a given year, white children and nonpoverty children are more likely to see private-practice physicians in their offices. Black children and poverty children are more likely to see physicians in hospital outpatient departments and public clinics not associated with hospitals.[90] Among children with positive visits to physicians in private practice in a given year, parents' income is positively related to the number of visits. Colle and Grossman estimate an income elasticity of visits of 0.4 in 1970,[91] a figure that is much larger than the income elasticity of visits for adults.[92] In addition, in a sample of users of physicians in private practice, parents' income is positively related to the probability that the usual source of care is a board-certified or nonboard-certified pediatrician as opposed to a general practitioner.[93] In addition, in such a sample black children and Medicaid recipients are more likely to see general practitioners and the latter group makes fewer visits than non-Medicaid recipients.[94]

The last two findings indicate that families on the Medicaid rolls encounter substantial barriers when they try to take their children to specialists or to make a relatively large number of visits to physicians in private practice. In particular, the findings reflect the reluctance of some physicians in private practice to accept Medicaid recipients as their patients because of uncertainties and rigidities associated with

---

[88] Wilson and White present data that reveal a downward trend in these differentials between 1964 and 1973. See Wilson and White, "Changes in Morbidity," pp. 636–646.

[89] National Center for Health Statistics, *Preventive Care*.

[90] Colle and Grossman, "Pediatric Care"; and National Center for Health Statistics and the National Center for Health Services Research, *Health: United States, 1978*.

[91] Colle and Grossman, "Pediatric Care," pp. 115–158.

[92] For example, Charles E. Phelps, "Effects of Insurance on Demand for Medical Care," in *Equity in Health Services*, edited by Ronald Andersen, Joanna Kravits and Odin W. Anderson (Cambridge, Mass.: Ballinger Publishing Company, 1975).

[93] Colle and Grossman, "Pediatric Care," pp. 115–158; and Fred Goldman and Michael Grossman, "The Demand for Pediatric Care: An Hedonic Approach," *Journal of Political Economy*, vol. 86 (April 1978), pp. 259–280.

[94] Colle and Grossman, "Pediatric Care."

Medicaid reimbursement schedules, some of which fail to recognize physician specialties.[95]

Interactions and relationships among parents' income, race, and Medicaid in pediatric care utilization are highlighted in a study by Colle and Grossman with the 1970 NORC health survey.[96] They performed a multivariate analysis of the probability in 1970 that a child between the ages of one and five had a preventive physical examination—that is, an examination for reasons other than illness or because it was required. For whites the observed probability is 34.6 percent and for blacks it is 28.7 percent. This gross difference of 6 percentage points is reduced to 1.9 percentage points when several variables are held constant. The latter differential is not statistically significant.

Put differently, differences in characteristics other than race between black and white families fully explain the preventive care differential. Black children would have the same probability of receiving an examination as whites if they had the same mean values of these characteristics.

In the multiple regression analysis, the probability of having an exam rises with income and is higher for those who receive welfare than for those who do not. Of course, blacks have lower income than whites, but they are more likely to be on welfare. Colle and Grossman show that black children would be more likely, by 2.7 percentage points, to have a preventive exam if they had the same mean family income as whites. On the other hand, blacks would have a 2.4 percentage point lower probability of having an exam if the proportion of blacks on welfare equaled the proportion of whites.

In other words, the welfare program, of which Medicaid is an integral part, is an effective policy tool for eliminating income-related differences in the utilization of preventive care. Blacks and whites would have the same observed probabilities if all their characteristics except for income and welfare eligibility were the same.[97]

Dental care is an optional service under Medicaid. Therefore, income and race differences in use of dental care by children and adults have not declined over time by nearly as much as the corresponding

---

[95] For example, Davis and Schoen, *War on Poverty*; and Frank Sloan, Janet Mitchell, and Jerry Cromwell, "Physician Participation in State Medicaid Programs," *Journal of Human Resources*, vol. 13, Supplement (1978), pp. 211–245.

[96] Colle and Grossman, "Pediatric Care," pp. 115–158.

[97] The sources of the observed differences in the probability of receipt of preventive care are discussed in the section, "Determinants of Utilization of Preventive Medical Care Services." Colle and Grossman perform a similar analysis of the probability that a child had at least one physician contact in 1970. They reach a similar conclusion: the income-related difference in the probability of use between blacks and whites is entirely offset by the welfare program.

differences in use of pediatric care. Wilson and White report substantial differences for both children and adults in 1973.[98] Data for that year indicate that 58.3 percent of poor children under the age of seventeen had not seen a dentist in the past two years. The corresponding figure for nonpoor children was 37.2 percent. The differential in the probability of use grew smaller between 1964 and 1973, but the difference in the mean number of dental visits by the two groups of children remained constant. A similar picture emerges when the utilization rates for poor and nonpoor adults are examined, except that there was a slight reduction in the gap between the mean number of visits by the two groups.

In a multivariate context Edwards and Grossman find that family income has a positive and statistically significant effect on the probability that a white youth obtained a preventive dental checkup in the past year in Cycle III of the U.S. Health Examination Survey.[99] The computed income elacticity of this probability equals 0.15. Manning and Phelps estimate a somewhat higher income elasticity of 0.51 for white children of all ages in the NORC survey.[100] They also report income elasticities of 0.64 for white adult females and 0.73 for white adult males. Manning and Phelps also compute income elasticities of demand for dental visits by the three groups of whites. These equal 0.55 for adult females, 0.61 for adult males, and 0.87 for children.

With regard to the use of preventive physician services by adults, the U.S. Health Interview Survey for 1975 shows a mild positive correlation between number of physician visits per person for general checkups and family income up to $15,000 (rising from 0.37 to 0.39 visits) and a strong positive correlation at higher levels of income (0.49 visits for incomes between $15,000 and $25,000 and 0.55 visits for incomes in excess of $25,000).[101] Preventive care as measured by general checkups increases also relative to other forms of care: they constitute less than 5 percent of all visits when family income is less than $3,000 and approximately 10 percent when family income is at least $15,000.

Gross comparisons over time reveal that the percentage of persons with family incomes less than $5,000 who had a general checkup during the year rose from 28 percent in 1971 to 37 percent in 1975, with little change in the fraction of the population in income brackets above

[98] Wilson and White, "Changes in Morbidity," pp. 636–646.
[99] Edwards and Grossman, "Adolescent Health."
[100] Willard B. Manning, Jr., and Charles E. Phelps, *Dental Care Demand: Point Estimates and Implications for National Health Insurance* (Santa Monica, Calif.: The Rand Corporation, 1978).
[101] National Center for Health Statistics, *Physician Visits.*

$5,000 who had general checkups.[102] This remarkable increase in utilization at the lower end of the income scale occurred during the time when Medicaid was expanded. It may be tentatively interpreted as a direct result of the fall in cost, especially since over the period 1971 to 1975 aggregate real income did not change much.

The 1963 and 1970 NORC data reveal similar patterns.[103] For both years the percentage of the population who had never had a physical examination is negatively related to income; it was, however, lower in 1970 than in 1963. Moreover, the interval of time between checkups is shorter the higher is family income, and the mean intervals by income class seem to be more similar in 1970 than in 1963. The proportion of the population having never had a physical exam is higher for nonwhites than it is for whites, but the frequency of exams within a year is about the same for both races.

The NORC data distinguish between physical examinations elicited by the occurrence of self-assessed symptoms; those that are required for a job, school, insurance, armed forces, or similar circumstances; and those that are preventive.[104] Preventive exams are positively related to income in both 1963 and 1970. This positive income effect on prevention is consistent with the evidence from the U.S. Health Interview Survey reported above. By contrast, the fraction of exams that are required is highest for the middle-income groups, and the fraction of visits elicited by symptoms falls with family income. These patterns are consistent with the higher prevalence rates of disease at the lower end of the income distribution.[105]

The fraction of physical exams that are preventive rose from 29 percent in 1963 to 37 percent in 1970. The fraction of such exams was lower for nonwhites than for whites in 1963, although by 1970 the difference was eliminated.

More detail on preventive care is available from the 1973 U.S.

---

[102] National Center for Health Statistics, *Physician Visits*. These figures assume that persons will have only one general checkup within a year. Comparable figures cannot be obtained prior to 1971 because general checkups were recorded under a more narrow definition starting in 1971.

[103] Andersen, Lion, and Anderson, *Two Decades of Health Service*.

[104] The NORC questionnaire specifies "there was nothing particularly wrong and the examination wasn't required—it was just time for a checkup or physical examination." The NCHS definition of general checkup is less inclusive than the NORC definition of physical examination because it excludes those checkups occasioned by a specific condition. On the other hand it is more inclusive than the NORC definition of preventive physical examination because it includes those exams that are required.

[105] The above statement is not inconsistent with our proposition at the end of the second section, that morbidity and mortality rates of white adults rise with income. The latter proposition refers to studies that control for schooling and also for reverse causality from poor health to low income.

Health Interview Survey. It gives information on the utilization of selected preventive services by specific population groups. These services include electrocardiograms, chest X-rays, glaucoma tests, eye examinations, pap smears, and breast examinations. In general, high-income persons were more likely to have received these services than low-income persons.[106] These patterns are, however, not always clear-cut. For chest X-rays, glaucoma tests, pap smears and breast examinations, the fraction of persons ever having had an exam rises monotonically with income, but for electrocardiograms this fraction rises only when family income exceeds $15,000.

Moreover, intervals since last visits for these specific tests are shorter uniformly by income group only for pap smears and breast exams. For electrocardiograms and chest X-rays, intervals are shortest at the low and the high end of the income distribution; for glaucoma tests, intervals shorten only when family income reaches $15,000.

Whites are more likely to have had any one of these tests than blacks, except for chest X-rays where the likelihoods are the same. For all tests, however, except glaucoma, the percentage having had a test in less than a year is higher for nonwhites than it is for whites.

Our survey of the impacts of income and Medicaid on utilization reveals that pediatric care and preventive physicians' services for adults are sensitive to these variables, although the effectiveness of pediatric care and checkups is questionable. One explanation of these results is that people want to verify that they are healthy,[107] and the demand for this information is sensitive to income and price (Medicaid). A second explanation is that, although preventive care may not be effective for the average individual, it may have impacts on certain individuals. Such differential impact effects are probably subject to a considerable amount of uncertainty.

Money and Time Prices. The coverage of preventive care under national health insurance would lower the net or out-of-pocket price of care from the point of view of the consumer. Therefore, estimates of the price elasticity of demand for care play a central role in predictions about the effects of NHI on the utilization of these services. We have just discussed price effects related to Medicaid; now our focus turns to price variations associated with private health insurance and other factors.

Because the consumer's time is required to produce health and obtain medical care, the relevant price in the demand function for care contains a money price component and a time price component.

---

[106] National Center for Health Statistics, *Preventive Care.*
[107] For example, Phelps, "Illness Prevention," pp. 183–207.

In the case of a visit to a physician or a dentist, the money price pertains to the direct payment to the provider net of insurance payments. The time price pertains to the sum of the time spent traveling to reach the provider and return home and waiting to see him at the source of care multiplied by the opportunity cost of time.[108] For pediatric care or dental care for children, since the mother typically is responsible for the child, the opportunity cost of time is evaluated by her actual or potential hourly wage rate in studies by Inman, Colle and Grossman, and Goldman and Grossman.[109]

The existence of a time price component implies that the money price elasticity of demand for care should fall in absolute value as income rises. This is because the value of time rises with income. Therefore, a 1 percent reduction in money price is associated with a smaller percentage reduction in total price for the rich.[110]

The possibility of differential price elasticities by income is relevant if price cuts under national health insurance are directed at low-income families and if coverage of time costs is excluded. Empirical evidence with respect to income-related differences in price elasticities and with respect to the effects of both money price and time price is reviewed below.

To our knowledge there are no studies of the effects of money or time price on the receipt of prenatal care. Information on the effects of these variables on the receipt of preventive doctor care by adults also is very limited. Luft reports that the greater use of preventive services by HMO enrollees is due to their better financial coverage rather than to incentives of HMOs to supply such services.[111] In particular, he finds that differences in the use of preventive services disappear when HMO enrollees are compared to persons with private health insurance that covers preventive care, or to persons with Medicaid.

Estimates of money price elasticities of demand for physician visits by children in studies by Inman, Colle and Grossman, and Goldman and Grossman are presented in Table 2.[112] The elasticities are

---

[108] If the trip to the source of care is made by a mode of transportation other than walking, the direct cost of the trip would be included in the total price of a visit.

[109] Inman, "Family Provision of Children's Health"; Colle and Grossman, "Pediatric Care," pp. 115–158; and Goldman and Grossman, "Demand for Pediatric Care," pp. 259–280.

[110] For a rigorous derivation of the above proposition and some exceptions to it, see Michael Grossman and Elizabeth H. Rand, "Consumer Incentives for Health Services in Chronic Illness," in Consumer Incentives for Health Care, edited by Selma J. Mushkin (New York: Prodist, 1974).

[111] Luft, "Health Maintenance Services," pp. 144–168.

[112] Inman, "Family Provision of Children's Health"; Colle and Grossman, "Pediatric Care," pp. 115–158; and Goldman and Grossman, "Demand for Pediatric Care," pp. 259–280.

TABLE 2

ESTIMATES OF INCOME AND PRICE ELASTICITIES OF PEDIATRIC VISITS

	Colle and Grossman (1978)	Goldman and Grossman (1978)	Inman[a] (1976)
Average income in sample	$10,000	$6,500	$8,700
Estimate of income elasticity	0.38	1.32	0.23
Estimate of price elasticity	−0.11	−0.06	−0.09
Sample and year	NORC 1970	Bronx, New York, residents 1965–66	Kessner 1970

[a] Inman fits separate functions for preventive and curative visits. His estimates of income and price elasticities of each service are very similar. We show simple averages in the table.

fairly similar; they range in absolute value from 0.06 to 0.11. None of the studies explicitly investigates whether there are income-related differences in the price elasticity. Yet the results in the table shed some light on this issue because the mean level of family income varies among the samples analyzed. There is no evidence that the price elasticity falls in absolute value as income rises; if anything the reverse is true.

The table also shows that in each study the income elasticity exceeds the price elasticity by a substantial amount. This suggests that it might be more efficient to increase physician visits by means of income transfers to low-income families rather than by means of national health insurance.

Another aspect of the impact of money price on pediatric care services involves its effect on the choice of a specialist or a general practitioner as the usual source of care. Colle and Grossman and Goldman and Grossman find that parents who face lower money prices are more likely to select board-certified pediatricians. This can be explained by the presence of the time price component in the total price of care. Consider two families, one of which has health insurance for doctor visits with a 25 percent coinsurance rate. If time prices do not vary by source of care, the health insurance policy will lower the total price of a visit to a pediatrician relative to a general practitioner because pediatricians charge higher fees than do general practitioners.

Hence a national health insurance plan that either pays a fixed percentage of the fee of a visit or reduces money price to zero would increase the demand for specialists relative to general practitioners. This might be desirable if visits to pediatricians contributed to favorable child health outcomes. As we earlier pointed out, however, there is no evidence in support of this proposition.

Both Inman and Goldman and Grossman report that the number of visits falls as the time cost of a visit rises. The elasticities are —0.15 in the Inman study[113] and —0.12 in the Goldman-Grossman study. Colle and Grossman do not find evidence of a negative time cost coefficient in their demand curve for visits. They do indicate, however, that the time cost of a visit has a negative and statistically significant effect on the probability that a child obtained a preventive physical examination within the past year. If the time cost of a visit goes up by one dollar, the probability of obtaining preventive care goes down by 1.2 percentage points.

Colle and Grossman also report that children who walk to the doctor's office are more likely than others to have seen a physician within the past year and to have made more visits. This variable serves as a negative correlate of direct transportation costs.

In summary, all three studies show that time and transportation costs are significant rationing mechanisms in the pediatric care market. Consequently, even some Medicaid families may act as if the price of care is substantial.

Manning and Phelps provide price elasticities of demand for dental care for white children, white adult males, and white adult females.[114] Price elasticities of the probability of a dental checkup in the past year are —0.59 for children, —0.03 for adult males, and —0.56 for adult females. Price elasticities of the number of dental visits are —1.40 for children, —0.65 for adult males, and —0.78 for adult females.

Manning and Phelps allow for an interaction between income and price in their demand functions and obtain the result that price elasticities increase in absolute value rather than decrease as income rises.[115] They also show that the demand for dental visits would be dramatically altered if dental care were covered under national health insurance. "Demand appears roughly to double for adults and triple for children, when they pay nothing for dental care, rather than the full price."[116]

---

[113] This estimate pertains to the time cost elasticity of curative visits. Preventive visits are insensitive to time costs.

[114] Manning and Phelps, *Dental Care Demand*.

[115] The price elasticities reported in the text were computed by Manning and Phelps at sample means.

[116] Manning and Phelps, *Dental Care Demand*, p. 23.

Holtmann and Olsen study the effects of waiting time and travel time on the number of dental visits per family who resided in New York and Pennsylvania in the period 1971–1972.[117] Waiting time has a negative effect on the number of visits, but travel time has a positive effect. Their results should be interpreted with caution because they aggregate visits by children and adults in the same family. On the other hand, Manning and Phelps report significant differences between the coefficients of demand functions for care by adults and demand functions for care by children.[118] Additional evidence on the role of time costs in the demand for dental care is contained in a study by Edwards and Grossman.[119] They find that the probability that a youth had a preventive dental checkup within the past year is smaller if his mother works full time in the labor market. Presumably, such mothers place a bigger value on their time than mothers who do not work.

Time prices are difficult to estimate. It is not surprising that their effects are so variable across studies. Another way of looking at time prices is to estimate their effect indirectly, namely through the effects of health manpower availability on utilization.

Recently enacted federal legislation is designed to increase the availability of physicians and dentists in medically underserved areas to expand the use of preventive care in such areas. The Emergency Health Personnel Act of 1970 (PL 91-623) created the National Health Service Corps, whose members are assigned to areas with shortages of health manpower. The Health Professions Assistance Act of 1976 (PL 94-484) encourages new graduates of medical and dental schools to locate in urban ghettos and rural regions by forgiving their medical education loan obligations. Further, the Health Maintenance Organization Act of 1974 (PL 93-222) gives priority for developmental funding of HMOs in medically deprived areas.

In general, research on the determinants of preventive care utilization shows that the receipt of care is sensitive to the availability of medical care inputs. Using data from the 1973 U.S. Health Interview Survey, Kleinman and Wilson show that the proportion of births to mothers who began prenatal care in the first trimester of pregnancy was lower in areas designated by the Secretary of Health, Education, and Welfare as medically underserved areas (MUAs) than in other areas.[120]

---

[117] A. G. Holtmann and E. Odgers Olsen, Jr., "The Demand for Dental Care: A Study of Consumption and Household Production," *Journal of Human Resources*, vol. 11 (Fall 1976), pp. 546–560.

[118] Manning and Phelps, *Dental Care Demand*.

[119] Edwards and Grossman, "Adolescent Health."

[120] Joel C. Kleinman and Ronald W. Wilson, "Are 'Medically Underserved Areas' Medically Underserved?" *Health Services Research*, vol. 12 (Summer 1977), pp. 147–162.

They also indicate that persons below the age of seventeen were more likely not to have had a routine physical examination during the past two years in MUAs. Finally, based on the indicators of preventive physicians' services for adults mentioned previously (such as chest X-rays and pap smears), adults in MUAs were less likely to receive preventive care.

In multivariate analyses, Colle and Grossman, Manning and Phelps, and Edwards and Grossman find that health manpower has large and statistically significant effects on the likelihood that a family has obtained preventive dental and doctor care for its children.[121] For example, an increase of one dentist per thousand population in the county of residence increases the probability that youths visited the dentist for preventive care by approximately 17 percentage points both in Cycle III of the Health Examination Survey and in the NORC survey.[122]

These results are unlikely to reflect demand manipulation by physicians or dentists. The concept of demand manipulation refers to the ability of health personnel to shift the demand curve for their services, with all direct and indirect costs of these services held constant. In his extensive treatment of this phenomenon, Pauly shows that the demand manipulation effect should be larger in a sample of consumers with positive utilization than in a sample of all consumers. Moreover, his model gives no basis for expecting a demand manipulation effect in an equation that explains the probability of a checkup.[123]

Based on the above considerations, it is appropriate to interpret the role of physicians or dentists in the preventive care demand function as a reflection of information, entry, travel, waiting, and direct costs in the parents' decision to obtain care for their offspring. In the study by Edwards and Grossman, all factors are at work because they have no measure of the money price of dental care or pediatric care and only a crude proxy for time price. Manning and Phelps control for money price but not for time price. Colle and Grossman control for both prices so that their findings indicate the importance of information, inconvenience, and other kinds of entry costs.

As a prelude to our analysis of optimal health insurance in the final section, it is useful to review Edwards and Grossman's estimates of the impacts of three government programs to improve the oral health of

---

[121] Colle and Grossman, "Pediatric Care," pp. 115–158; Manning and Phelps, *Dental Care Demand*; and Edwards and Grossman, "Adolescent Health."

[122] Manning and Phelps, *Dental Care Demand*; and Edwards and Grossman, "Adolescent Health."

[123] Mark V. Pauly, *Doctors and Their Workshops* (Chicago, Ill.: University of Chicago Press for the National Bureau of Economic Research, forthcoming).

youths.[124] First, they consider a $1,000 income transfer to low-income families. This transfer would lower the periodontal index of youths from these families by 0.01 points and would lower their decay index by 0.02 points. (Such a program would also have other beneficial effects on children and their families.) These estimates take account of the direct favorable impact of income on oral health with preventive dental care held constant, and they also take account of the indirect favorable impact of income. In particular, an increase in income increases preventive dental care, which increases oral health.[125]

Next Edwards and Grossman consider a program to reduce or eliminate regional differences in the number of dentists per thousand population. Dentists are more numerous in urban areas than in rural areas. To take two sites in the Health Examination Survey, in 1968 there were 1.1 dentists per thousand population in San Francisco, California, while there were 0.2 dentists per thousand population in San Benito, Texas. Suppose that this difference were eliminated by raising the number of dentists in San Benito by one per thousand population. Then the periodontal index of youths in San Benito would fall by 0.04 points, and their decay index would fall by 0.05 points. Here the mechanism is an indirect effect alone; the number of dentists per capita is positively related to the receipt of a preventive dental exam, and the latter improves oral health.

Finally, they consider an 80 percent reduction in the price of a dental checkup due to the enactment of a national health insurance plan for dental care with a 20 percent coinsurance rate. Based on research by Manning and Phelps on the impact of price on the propensity to obtain preventive dental care for children and youths, Edwards and Grossman estimate that such a policy would raise the probability of obtaining care by 16 percentage points.[126] This would improve both the periodontal and the decay scores by 0.04 points.

Edwards and Grossman view their computations as illustrative rather than definitive. To choose among the three programs, information on the cost of each program and on the number of youths affected clearly is required. Moreover, Edwards and Grossman indicate that definitive computations of impact effects should take account of the supply elasticity of dental care and the exact nature of the relationship between dental manpower and the indirect costs (costs other than money price) of obtaining dental care.

---

[124] Edwards and Grossman, "Adolescent Health."

[125] Technically, Edwards and Grossman estimate the impact of each program from the solved reduced form of an oral health production and preventive care demand model.

[126] Manning and Phelps, *Dental Care Demand*.

We would add one further point. A health manpower program differs much more in form than in substance from a program to cover preventive care under national health insurance. After all, both programs seek to reduce the *total* price of preventive care. NHI cuts the money price component of care, while manpower programs cut both the money price and the indirect price components. If indirect costs are an important determinant of utilization, as our review indicates, NHI will be much more successful if policy makers recognize these costs and try to deal with them than if they ignore them. Put differently, health manpower programs and programs to develop delivery systems that lower indirect costs should not be ignored when NHI policies are being formulated.

Schooling and Family Size. With race, income, and price held constant, parents' schooling and family size are extremely important determinants of the receipt of preventive care. After controlling for husband's education (a proxy for income), Lewit finds that more-educated women are more likely to see a physician within the first trimester of pregnancy and to make a greater number of prenatal visits than less-educated women.[127] Similarly, pregnant women with few living children receive more prenatal care than those with many living children.

Colle and Grossman report that mother's schooling is a positive correlate of the probabilities that a child had a physician contact and a physical examination within the past year.[128] The number of children in the family is a negative correlate of these two probabilities. Edwards and Grossman indicate similar effects of mother's schooling and family size on the probability that a youth received a preventive dental examination within the past year.[129] More-educated adults have higher probabilities of receiving preventive care services such as chest X-rays and pap smears.[130]

The importance of mother's schooling and family size in preventive care utilization are underscored by Colle and Grossman's analysis of differences between black and white children in the probability of an ambulatory contact and the probability of a preventive physical examination within the past year.[131] They show that the welfare program, including Medicaid, almost completely eliminates income-related differences in these two indexes of pediatric care between black and white children.

---

[127] Lewit, "Experience with Pregnancy."

[128] Colle and Grossman, "Pediatric Care," pp. 115–158.

[129] Edwards and Grossman, "Adolescent Health."

[130] National Center for Health Statistics, *Preventive Care*.

[131] Colle and Grossman, "Pediatric Care," pp. 115–158.

Black-white differences in these measures persist primarily because black mothers have less education than white mothers and because black mothers have more children than white mothers. One can speculate that income-related differences in these measures and others persist over time for similar reasons. In particular, high-income mothers have more education and fewer children than low-income mothers. Although researchers have not examined the latter issue explicitly, Edwards and Grossman show that income-related differences in several measures of the health of white children are due primarily to differences in mother's schooling and to a lesser extent family size.[132]

The implications of these findings are at the same time disheartening and heartening. They are disheartening because they imply that policies to reduce differences in utilization through NHI and policies to reduce differences in health through income transfers and NHI may not succeed. This is because the key differences are in schooling and family size. These differences are extremely costly to reduce and will not be altered, at least in the short run, by NHI and income transfers.[133]

At the same time, the findings are heartening because black-white differences in schooling have narrowed over time, particularly since 1970. In 1960, the difference between the median school years completed by white females and the median school years completed by black females stood at 2.6 years. This difference declined to 2.0 years in 1970 and to 1.0 years in 1977.[134] Recall that the infant mortality rate, which historically has been higher for blacks than for whites, declined rapidly from 1964 to 1974. Is there a hint in these trends that a future policy of laissez faire may be the best one?

Implications for Optimal National Health Insurance

In this concluding section we consider whether preventive care should be covered under NHI and the nature of the optimal plan. Our purpose here is to pull together the conclusions we made earlier about the effects and determinants of preventive care after first considering theoretical justifications for government subsidization of preventive care.

Our intention is neither to design an optimal plan nor to estimate the costs of alternative plans. Rather our intention is to underscore relevant factors that should be kept in mind when decisions are made about

---

[132] Edwards and Grossman, "Children's Health and the Family."

[133] In the long run, NHI might result in a reduction in family size by making contraceptive information and abortion more readily available. Also in the long run, income transfers could narrow schooling differentials by making it easier for low-income families to finance a college education for their children.

[134] Bureau of the Census, *Statistical Abstract of the United States, 1978* (Washington, D.C., 1978).

preventive care under NHI. We do not have all the answers, but we want to raise some relevant questions.

The main justification for government interference with the decisions of its citizens about preventive medical care is the existence of externalities. Two basic types of health-related externalities have been identified. Production externalities refer to situations in which the health of some persons depends on the health or preventive medical care utilization of others. Consumption externalities refer to situations in which the utility, rather than the health, of some persons depends on the health or preventive medical care consumption of others.[135]

In either situation, it is easy to show that free-rider problems will lead at least some persons to choose levels of health or preventive medical care that are less than optimal from society's point of view. When there is a one-to-one correspondence between health and preventive medical care, it makes little difference whether the externality is specified in terms of health or in terms of care.

This is likely to be true for immunizations against infectious diseases. But in the more common case there is a multivariate health production function, where medical care can substitute for other inputs. Here it makes a difference whether a consumption externality is specified in terms of health or in terms of the input of preventive medical care. It also makes a difference whether a production externality is specified in terms of preventive medical care or in terms of all preventive activities including preventive nonmedical activities, such as careful driving. We discuss some implications of this distinction below.

The other justification that we wish to consider for government attemtps to modify the preventive care decisions of its citizens is the existence of moral hazard. We refer to situations in which an individual pays a fixed premium for the purchase of a health insurance policy that covers remedial (curative) medical care services associated with illness or accidents. That is, the premium does not reflect the individual's probability of becoming ill, a probability that is negatively related to preventive care.

Pauly shows that moral hazard results in overinsurance of remedial care and too little preventive care.[136] Put differently, it results in a substitution toward remedial care and away from preventive care.[137]

---

[135] For an excellent treatment of health-related externalities with a focus on consumption externalities, see Pauly, *Medical Care at Public Expense.*

[136] Mark V. Pauly, "Overinsurance and Public Provision of Insurance: The Role of Moral Hazard and Adverse Selection," *The Quarterly Journal of Economics*, vol. 88 (February 1974), pp. 44–62.

[137] For a similar conclusion see Ehrlich and Becker, "Market Insurance." Zeckhauser, Pauly, Phelps, and others have constructed models in which moral hazard is present even in the absence of preventive care. Here the concept refers to a

Clearly, there is a close correspondence between a theoretical argument to cover preventive care under NHI to combat moral hazard and a practical argument to cover preventive care in order to contain the cost of NHI.[138]

Armed with the above justifications for government intervention in the preventive care market and with our detailed treatment of the extent of third-party coverage of care and the effects and determinants of care, we offer the following theoretical and empirical implications with respect to preventive care and NHI.

1. When production and consumption externalities are specified in terms of preventive medical care, the optimal way to deal with these externalities is to subsidize the full (money and indirect) price of care.

This justifies covering preventive care under NHI to lower the money price. But as demonstrated by Pauly, the optimal price cut should not be the same for everyone. Because the private demand for preventive care rises with income, the optimal price reduction should fall with income. Beyond some income, no price reduction is required. Moreover, the optimal insurance plan does not and should not eliminate income-related differences in utilization. Instead, it should reduce such differences.

2. The size of the optimal price cut depends on the price elasticity of demand for care at each income level.

For example, if more refined estimates suggest that the price elasticity

---

substitution of remedial medical care for other consumption goods in general due to insurance-related reductions in the price of care. Because preventive and remedial care are likely to be good substitutes, it seems more natural to use the concept developed in the text. See Richard Zeckhauser, "Medical Insurance: A Case Study of the Tradeoff Between Risk Spreading and Appropriate Incentives," *Journal of Economic Theory*, vol. 2 (March 1970), pp. 10–26; Pauly, *Medical Care at Public Expense*; and Charles E. Phelps, "Demand for Reimbursement Insurance," in *The Role of Health Insurance in the Health Services Sector*, edited by Richard Rosett (New York: Neale Watson Academic Publications, 1976).

[138] Another reason for the government to modify the preventive care decisions of its citizens is that they may have imperfect information about the effects of care. A special case of imperfect information, which is particularly relevant to children's health and closely related to externalities, arises because parents' health affects the health of their offspring. Parents may ignore or may not be aware of these effects when they decide how much to invest in their health. (For an interesting model along these lines, see Edward Lazear, "Intergenerational Externalities," National Bureau of Economic Research Working Paper No. 145, 1976). We do not deal with imperfect information because it will almost always be more desirable for the government to deal with the problem directly than to subsidize the price of care. In the case of parent-child externalities, since these pertain to a small number of people in the same family, they are likely to be small and to be internalized by the family in a number of ways. Moreover, the issue of imperfect information most frequently is raised not in the context of the effects of preventive care but in the context of the quality of physicians (for example, Pauly, *Medical Care at Public Expense*).

of demand for care goes up as the level of income goes down, a relatively small price cut would achieve substantial effects. It follows that the optimal price cut need not be monotonically related to income if price elasticities of demand for care fall sufficiently rapidly as income increases.[139] This points to the need to obtain precise estimates of response to price changes in order to formulate an actual price structure that is in any way near optimal.

3. The indirect costs of travel, waiting, entry, and information are important determinants of utilization.

From an administrative point of view, these costs probably would be difficult to measure and allocate under NHI. For this reason, health manpower programs and programs to develop delivery systems that lower indirect costs should not be ignored when NHI policies are being formulated.

4. When production and consumption externalities are specified in terms of health and the health production function has a multivariate form, the optimal policy involves reductions in the prices of all inputs that contribute to favorable health outcomes.

Because practical difficulties might preclude this approach, an income transfer program might be a second best solution.[140] Such a program could be accompanied by reductions in the prices of easily identified inputs, especially inputs whose shares in health costs are large. This alternative solution is why income transfers should not be

---

[139] If ΔM_i denotes the change in medical expenditures of the ith income group required to achieve optimality, and if income groups are listed starting from lowest, then optimality requires:

$$\Delta M_1 > \Delta M_2 > \Delta M_3 \geqq 0$$

Hence optimality requires:

$$S_1 \, \Delta P_1 > S_2 \, \Delta P_2 > S_3 \, \Delta P_3 \geqq 0$$

where S_i stands for the effect on medical care of the ith group resulting from a unit change in the price of care (with all S_i negative), and ΔP_i is the reduction in the price of medical care for the ith group. Therefore, the pattern of ΔP depends on the size and pattern of the S_i. In particular, if

$$|S_1| > |S_2| > |S_3|$$

the optimal price cuts need not be inversely related to income throughout the whole range of incomes. Quite conceivably the optimal price cut could be greater for those with modest incomes than for the very poor.

[140] It is well known that, unless total consumption of some persons (say, the poor) enters the utility functions of others, price reductions of specific goods are preferable to income transfers. Indeed, price reductions may be preferable even if the good in question is total present and future consumption of poor children rather than consumption of all poor persons. Poor parents would receive income transfers directed at their children and might spend them on their own consumption. To avoid this, the rich might prefer to subsidize health and schooling investments of poor children, which would raise their earnings prospects and hence their future consumption.

ignored when NHI is being considered. Both approaches would accomplish the same goal.

Regardless of the nature of the optimal program, if the private demand for health rises with income,[141] the optimal transfer or price reductions should fall with income. Income-related differences in health or differences due to factors correlated with income such as race or schooling are reduced but not eliminated by the optimal plan.[142]

5. The application of a common coinsurance rate (possibly zero) to preventive medical care and curative medical care under NHI might or might not reduce moral hazard.

The price of the former relative to the latter is unaffected by NHI only if the time price components and the gross money prices of each are the same, or if the ratio of time price to total price is the same for each type of care. This is unlikely because the money price of curative care in the event of serious illness undoubtedly exceeds the money price of preventive care, while the time price of the former is smaller than that of the latter. Even if the relative price ratio is not affected, undesirable substitutions away from other goods, including preventive nonmedical care, and toward curative care might occur.[143]

6. Prenatal care and dental care are effective, but pediatric care (except for immunizations) and preventive doctor care for adults are not. Moreover, health outcomes in which care is effective correspond to outcomes in which income differences in health are observed. These empirical results and the theory of health as a consumption item suggest that the optimal NHI plan should have benefits that fall as income rises.

In addition, the plan should be selective rather than general with respect to the types of services covered. For instance, instead of providing complete coverage for preventive physicians' services to persons of all ages under NHI, the government should direct its attention to prenatal care and physicians' services during the first year of life.[144]

Similarly, the effectiveness of dental care throughout the life cycle

---

[141] The properties of the private demand functions for health and the differences between this demand function and the demand function for medical care are analyzed in detail by Grossman. See Grossman, *The Demand for Health.*

[142] The above statement pertains to gross schooling or race differences in health. Net (income-constant) differences would be unaffected unless the price reduction or income transfer depended on race or schooling as well as on income. Undoubtedly, the transactions costs of a program whose benefits depended on many characteristics of consumers would be prohibitive.

[143] Phelps, "Illness Prevention," pp. 183–207.

[144] If future research provides definitive evidence on the efficacy of screening for certain adult diseases, possibly in subsets of the population, coverage could be expanded to include the administration of these tests to groups with high prevalence rates.

suggests that the payoffs to the coverage of dental care from the age it is first received until age eighteen or beyond are substantial.[145] It should be kept in mind, however, that a cost-effective alternative to preventive dental care exists in the form of water fluoridation and that half of the population of the United States resides in communities with less than optimal fluoride levels. So perhaps the optimal policy might be to attach significant coinsurance rates to dental care under NHI and simultaneously to encourage communities to adjust the fluoride content of their water supply systems.

7. We do not know the income levels at which benefits for prenatal and dental services should end. We do know that there is little theoretical justification for providing benefits to persons from all income levels.

Moreover, trends in the private health insurance market indicate that benefits might cease at a fairly moderate income level. We refer to the rapid increases in the percentages of the population with obstetrical care and dental care insurance in the recent past. The reductions in net price associated with these increases in coverage imply that the private demand of many families for effective services may be substantial.[146]

8. Any discussion of preventive NHI cannot ignore the network of public programs that already exists to finance and deliver preventive services to the poverty population.

This network consists of Medicaid, the maternal and child health program, and the neighborhood health center program. It constitutes a preventive NHI system for many poor persons. Despite valid criticisms, this system has made at least some improvements in the health of the poor. We can see no reason to scrap it.

Rather, what is called for is a more uniform set of eligibility standards and some modifications in the way services are delivered and providers are reimbursed. In particular, less fragmentation of the health care delivery system would be desirable. Indeed it has been

---

[145] To the extent that smaller dollar weights are placed on improvements in oral health relative to physical health, the above statement would have to be qualified. Nevertheless, if the impact of preventive doctor care on physical health is nil, coverage cannot be justified regardless of the size of the dollar weights.

[146] Fuchs interprets these trends as a form of "pre-commitment." See Victor R. Fuchs, "Economics, Health, and Post-Industrial Society," *Milbank Memorial Fund Quarterly*, vol. 57 (Spring 1979), pp. 153–182. Phelps develops a model that explains them in terms of situations in which consumers and insurance companies share the gains of preventive care activities by consumers. Another factor is that employers' contributions to fringe benefits are excluded from employees' taxable income. Therefore, the price of preventive care is reduced if it is financed through a work-related health insurance plan. As income and hence marginal tax rates rise over time, the incentive to finance preventive care in this manner increases. See Phelps, "Illness Prevention," pp. 183–207.

shown that this fragmentation is a major source of delay and non-compliance to treatment of recognized illness as well as for follow-ups to early detection.[147]

9. We will not discuss Medicaid reform in any detail because that topic is the subject of another paper in this volume. We will comment, however, on two aspects of the proposed reforms.

First, our lack of enthusiasm for coverage of preventive physicians' services delivered to persons beyond the age of one under NHI does not imply that we think that existing Medicaid coverage of these services should be cut back. Instead, we are not enthusiastic about future expansions in this area.

Second, some persons view the declining trend in the percentage of children immunized against polio with alarm. They use this trend as evidence in favor of the CHAP expansion of the EPSDT program under Medicaid. Yet the trend may simply reflect a reduction in the benefits associated with immunization in a period during which the incidence of polio has been practically eliminated. Similar comments apply to arguments marshaled in support of CHAP based on income-related differences in rates of immunization against other infectious diseases. In the United States today, externalities associated with these diseases are of little importance.

To the extent that higher income parents "demand" a lower probability that their children contract these diseases, income-related differences should persist in equilibrium. This is not to say that the present differentials are the optimal ones dictated by a consumption-externality model. But we would like to suggest that, in a climate of "tight" federal and state budgets, the prenatal care initiatives in CHAP should be given a much higher priority than the other parts of the program.

10. Even in cases in which preventive care is effective, the provision of more care to blacks or low-income persons will not and should not eliminate differences in health.

Moreover, income transfers will not eliminate these differences because health varies among individuals with income and preventive care held constant. In particular, the studies we have reviewed point to mother's schooling as a key "preventive nonmedical determinant" of infant health and oral health outcomes. Race and income-related differences in mother's schooling are extremely costly to offset. Further, mother's schooling and preventive care may be complements. It is known that more educated mothers make more use of prenatal care and

---

[147] See Howard Greenwald, Selwyn Becker, and Michael Nevitt, "Delay and Noncompliance in Cancer Detection—A Behavioral Perspective for Health Planners," *Milbank Memorial Fund Quarterly*, vol. 56 (Spring 1978), pp. 212–230.

dental care; and it is plausible that the impact of care on certain health outcomes rises as schooling rises.[148]

Another example of complementarity may be compliance with the treatment prescribed as a result of a screening examination. For instance, in the case of hypertension, more-educated consumers may be more likely to modify their diets and take the appropriate medication.

Lest the reader be disheartened, he should recall the dramatic decline in the difference between black female and white female schooling levels since 1970. This decline may narrow race- and income-related differences in health in the future and curtail the amount of preventive medical care that the government should finance on the grounds of consumption externalities.

11. Finally, it is worth repeating that our arguments in favor of national health insurance rest on externalities. Yet there is a market for private contributions for medical care through several nonprofit institutions. It is an open question to what extent production and consumption externalities are already internalized through private giving and voluntary transfers.

Our answers to the three questions posed by this conference are as follows:

> *Preventive NHI: What Now?*   Medicaid reform with an emphasis on prenatal care; mandatory dental coverage for Medicaid children.
> *Preventive NHI: What Later?*   A preventive NHI program for moderate-income families with an emphasis on prenatal care and dental care; mandatory dental coverage for Medicaid adults.
> *Preventive NHI: What Never?*   Complete coverage of all preventive medical care services for all groups in the population.

These answers appear to be at variance with the widespread support for comprehensive and universal NHI expressed in the media and in public opinion polls. Are we simply "bucking" an inevitable trend? We think not. Although most people say they favor NHI, a recent survey by the Health Insurance Institute shows that this percentage falls dramatically when it is pointed out that the enactment of NHI is likely to be accompanied by higher taxes.[149] Thus, when people are asked "to put their money where their mouths are," there is much less enthusiasm for comprehensive NHI.

---

[148] Inman is the only researcher who has tested this proposition. His results are inconclusive. This is not surprising since they pertain to pediatric care which is not efficacious. See Inman, "Family Provision of Children's Health."

[149] Health Insurance Institute, *Health and Health Insurance: The Public's View* (Washington, D.C.: The Health Insurance Institute, 1979).

Commentaries

Paul B. Ginsburg

Professor Friedman concludes that there is no significant market failure in the private provision of health insurance, including catastrophic health insurance (CHI), but that federally sponsored CHI may nevertheless be desirable.

To argue that there is no market failure, Friedman makes the following points:

- Coverage for catastrophic illness is both widely available and extensively purchased.
- Adverse selection is not important in the market for health insurance policies.
- Opportunities for free care make it rational for many not to buy CHI.

He then offers a number of arguments in favor of federal sponsorship of CHI. A federal program would avoid the undesirable redistributions inherent in the current system of privately provided free care. Such a reduction in the provision of free care would also end the competitive advantages that Blue Cross plans enjoy through their discount, which is used to promote first-dollar coverage. Friedman also suggests that a federal CHI program might be a useful replacement for Medicaid, and might reduce opposition by organized labor to proposals to reduce tax subsidies to the purchase of health insurance.

Friedman's paper makes two important contributions to the debate about the federal role in providing CHI. First, the data presented on the extensiveness of private CHI show that there is more coverage for high-cost illness than many people believe. Clearly, the magnitude of the problem of absence of catastrophic coverage for those people with some insurance coverage is smaller today than it was in the early 1970s when the idea of federal sponsorship of CHI emerged. Second, Friedman stresses the role of free care. Opportunities for free care may be an important explanation for the absence of almost universal private CHI

181

coverage. More important from a policy perspective is the existence of an extensive cross-subsidy system resulting in substantial redistributions from the insured sick to the uninsured sick.

The following remarks will focus on my own perspectives on the issues treated by Professor Friedman.

Market Failure

I agree with Friedman that private CHI is extensive today. It is probably more extensive than many think, since it has grown so rapidly in recent years. The Congressional Budget Office is currently studying depth of coverage in employment-related health insurance. The data base for this study is a 1977 Bureau of Labor Statistics survey of provisions of employment-related health benefit plans. Some preliminary results have become available. For a hypothetical $10,000 claim, the average health plan would cover about 92 percent of charges. I would interpret this result as supporting Friedman's contention that for those with insurance coverage, the coverage tends to be deep.

Free Care

Free care is potentially important but has had very little study. I am skeptical, though, that its availability explains much of people's not insuring for catastrophic expenses. For one thing, people may be poorly informed about such opportunities at the time they are making decisions on insurance purchases. Also, there are more compelling reasons for not purchasing CHI that I discuss below. Nevertheless, the reduction in free care that would result from a federal CHI program is a major effect, and must be analyzed carefully.

Adverse Selection

Friedman dismisses this too easily as an explanation for the absence of coverage by some. He points out that the uninsured, on average, have the same rate of medical care utilization as those with individual insurance.

But averages are averages. The uninsured group is likely to be heterogeneous—composed of those expecting to be low utilizers and those rejected by insurers on the basis of expected high utilization. Thus, the finding of similar utilization rates between these two groups does not reject a hypothesis of adverse selection.

The fact that HMOs have long offered enrollment only to employed groups implies that they fear adverse selection. With marketing considered to be a major problem area for HMOs, restricting enrollment offerings to groups implies that concerns with adverse selection are indeed serious ones.

Irrational Behavior

I feel that the single most important explanation for people's not having CHI is their difficulties in making decisions when small probabilities of large losses are involved. How much would you pay to reduce the risk of a loss equal to a year's income from 0.2 percent to 0.1 percent? Laboratory experiments by economists and psychologists consistently reveal "irrational" behavior when individuals are faced with similar quandaries.[1]

A decision with strong similarities to the one concerned with the purchase of CHI is insurance against property damage from earthquakes and floods. The probability of loss is low, but the losses are large. Federal aid is often available to those incurring major losses (the analog of free care). Apparently, few purchase this insurance (the case with CHI before the late 1960s).

Howard Kunreuther has performed field studies and conducted laboratory experiments on earthquake and flood insurance.[2] From interviewing homeowners who had not purchased insurance, he finds that a significant number of homeowners in flood and earthquake prone areas either knew nothing about the availability and terms of insurance, or had inaccurate information. The survey also revealed that many residents had little idea of the probability or potential damage from a future disaster. Furthermore, the insurance decisions of persons who did have firm notions of expected losses, premium costs, and so on were often inconsistent with what would have been predicted by the expected utility model.

One of the most surprising results was ' the large number of uninsured homeowners who expected no federal aid at all in the aftermath of a major disaster. This indicated that neglect of insurance could not be attributed to expectations of generous government relief.

In laboratory experiments, Kunreuther found that people preferred to insure against relatively highly probable, low-loss hazards and reject insurance in situations where there are small chances of large losses. People were generally disinclined to worry about low-probability

---

[1] For a review of this literature, see P. Slovic et al., "Cognitive Processes and Societal Risk Taking," in John S. Carroll and John W. Payne, eds., *Cognition and Social Behavior* (New York: Halstead Press, 1976).

[2] Howard Kunreuther, *Recovery from Natural Disasters: Insurance or Federal Aid?* (Washington, D.C.: American Enterprise Institute, 1973).

hazards. This is understandable given the large number of such hazards that people face.[3]

Such "irrational" behavior in the face of low-probability hazards is likely a major reason for the failure (until recently) of many to purchase CHI.

Recent Growth in CHI

The preceding discussion of "irrational" behavior gives a useful perspective on the recent growth in CHI. I suspect that in the late 1960s people's perceptions about the probabilities of large losses changed. Part of this was undoubtedly the publicity about catastrophic expenses. Some hard facts may also have been behind this adjustment in perceptions. According to Trapnell, catastrophically expensive illnesses are accounting for a growing share of medical expenses.[4] As the perceived probability of a catastrophic expense rises, "irrational" behavior leads to greater CHI purchases growing much faster than the perceptions of risks.

Long-Term Care

This is a frequently ignored area of catastrophic medical expenses. There is virtually no private coverage here. Existing private coverage tends to be restricted to limited periods of recuperation from acute hospital stays. Such stays are a very small proportion of long-term care use. Nevertheless, the expenses are often catastrophic, as many long-term care stays are very long.

This may be a classic case of market failure. If private insurance for long-term care expenses were sold, adverse selection would probably be extreme. Only those elderly with poor health would seek to purchase it. To avoid this adverse selection, insurers would have to offer a very long-term contract. Perhaps you would buy a policy at age fifty to protect against nursing home expenses that might occur at age seventy-five. The problems with market provision of such a contract are apparent.

Desirability of Federal CHI

The Congressional Budget Office does not make recommendations concerning legislation before the Congress, so I will not state a position

---

[3] Kunreuther, *Recovery from Natural Disasters.*

[4] Gordon R. Trapnell, "The Increasing Cost of Catastrophic Insurance." Paper presented at the American Public Health Association Convention, Miami, Florida, October 19, 1976.

on whether or not federal sponsorship of CHI is desirable. There are a number of comments that I can make that are relevant to this issue, however.

1. It is naive to think of a federal CHI plan as a replacement for Medicaid. For CHI to serve such a role, it would have to be a very expensive plan, with a deductible that varied with income. Most plans currently under discussion do not have such a provision. Although such provisions might be a good idea, they would cause practical problems, which I shall discuss momentarily.

2. Fears that federal CHI would skew the medical-care system towards tertiary care have been overstated. Although we do not have any information on the demand elasticities in this range of expenses, we do know that current coverage for catastrophic illness is extensive. Whatever skewing that might be caused by CHI should already be well under way. Making CHI universal should not add appreciably to these tendencies.

3. In contemplating what type of federal CHI (if any) to enact, Congress might consider an income-related deductible or stop-loss. A single dollar stop-loss cannot provide protection against catastrophes to everyone—unless it is so small that the policy is comprehensive rather than catastrophic. A $2,500 medical bill would be unpleasant to a family with an income of $30,000 per year, but a catastrophe to a family with an $8,000 income.

But income-related deductibles are probably not practical in private insurance. A person's income would have to be measured both at premium-setting time and at the time of claim. Verification by the insurers would be impossible under existing statutes to protect privacy. This would rule out an employer mandate of such private coverage.

Government provision of insurance would probably be required to achieve a program of income-related deductibles. But Congress may be unwilling to sanction a major displacement of private health insurance by public insurance because it would eliminate a major industry and would dramatically increase federal outlays.

To make coverage with an income-related deductible feasible, we would have to maintain most private insurance but supplement it with publicly provided catastrophic insurance. The trick here would be to prevent private insurers from setting limits on benefits that would approximate the income-related deductible. One proposal under discussion in Congress would require that private policies not have such limits; in return, Congress would continue the exclusion from income taxes of employer contributions to such plans. Another plan would mandate that employers provide plans with a uniform out-of-pocket maximum. Those employees with an income-related deductible lower than the uniform deductible would get federal benefits until the latter were reached.

Research Agenda

Unfortunately, there has been little research on many of the issues important for analyzing federal support of CHI. A particularly important area is the temporal pattern of catastrophic expense. To what extent does a calendar year stop-loss protect people against catastrophes? This depends on the proportion of catastrophic expense accounted for by acute versus chronic episodes.

CBO is looking into this issue with claims data from the federal employees health benefit program. We are also looking into illness types and procedure types that involve catastrophic expense, and the relationships between individual and family expense patterns. A report on these analyses is due in the fall of 1980.

Karen Davis

The Grannemann paper is an important contribution to our knowledge about lessons to be learned from the Medicaid programs. It is a thoughtful review of the net financial redistribution of the program and of the wide variation in benefits and coverage of the poor among states. Exploration of the many facets of Medicaid experience is extremely important now, as policy makers consider a major expansion of the financial access for the poor as part of a national health plan.

The major findings of the Grannemann paper include the following:

• There is no net financial redistribution between low-income and high-income states as a result of Medicaid.

• There appears to be substantial net financial redistribution in favor of the Northeast at the expense of other regions.

• There is an inverse relationship between the number of individuals covered and the average level of benefits provided per beneficiary.

• There is a direct relationship between the federal matching rate and the level of Medicaid expenditures.

• The Medicaid program results in disproportionately lower expenditures for children—perhaps because, Grannemann concludes, greater federal matching is available for the aged in combined Medicare-Medicaid coverage or because children are relatively greater users of preventive and primary care services whose reimbursement rates are controlled by the states.

These findings are not generally known about the Medicaid program, and they provide useful insights into how the program works and how it might respond to changes in the current legislation.

Grannemann's chapter builds upon a theoretical model of voter choice to explain state government behavior. The chapter does not make a case for why the state is an appropriate level of government for the reflection of voter preferences, yet most of the policy options examined retain state government roles. It might be argued that the federal government is a more appropriate level for making decisions about financing health care for the poor. Voters may take more time to learn about stands on issues and voting records in congressional races than in elections for state representatives. If so, political actions at the national level may be more responsive to voter choices than to special interest groups that provide campaign support for relatively more obscure candidates for state office. Further, voters may be concerned about the poor generally rather than the poor in a specific state. If so, statewide decisions would not adequately reflect the preferences of all citizens regarding the level of care received by the poor in that particular state. Some examination of the rationale for political decision making would greatly strengthen Grannemann's chapter.

The interpretations and conclusions reached from the empirical analysis are in many cases unjustified. Several illustrations make the point:

• Grannemann argues that when medical care prices are higher, voters are more willing to cover the poor under Medicaid because high prices deter access of the poor to care. Yet, on the other hand, he argues that when there are few hospital beds (and physical access to care by the poor is curtailed) voters are less willing to cover the poor for fear that the poor will take away needed hospital beds from voters. This would appear almost logically inconsistent—either voters are more benevolent when they sense the poor are being denied care or they are not. Rather than trying to force this somewhat complicated interpretation on the empirical results, a simpler explanation is more convincing. What the regression shows is that Medicaid expenditures are higher when medical prices are higher, and that is to be expected because of the definitional relationship between expenditures and prices. Further, expenditures could be expected to be higher in states with greater hospital bed capacity, because utilization would be expected to be higher in such states.

• Grannemann concludes that the absence of coinsurance leads to too much use of medical services, yet there is no analysis on which to base this conclusion. No attempt is made to compare the utilization

187

patterns of Medicaid recipients with other persons, or to analyze the benefits or types of care received by Medicaid recipients.

• Grannemann concludes that hospital cost containment would lead to a reduction in hospital beds, which would lead voters to urge their elected state representatives to curtail the number of poor enrolled in Medicaid. The opposite would seem to be the experience of state cost commissions. In states where cost containment programs have curtailed the price of services to Medicaid, states have been more generous. In the absence of effective cost containment, fiscal pressures on states have generally led to cutbacks in program coverage and benefits.

He favors the Consumer Choice Health Plan approach to coverage for the poor. Part of the rationale given for this is that benefits can be tapered off gradually as income rises—but this is equally true for other approaches, where spend-downs can be designed on a two-for-one, a four-for-one, or any desired rate. Grannemann does not really deal with the problems generated with a Consumer Choice type of plan, such as:

• What evidence is there that individual buying of insurance is more economical than group purchasing?

• Is it expected that individuals or insurance companies could be more successful at obtaining favorable reimbursement rates from providers than are state governments or the federal government purchasing these services on behalf of the poor?

• How would adverse risk selection be avoided? Would not any effort to prevent insurance companies from acting in their own economic self-interest entail detailed regulation of the insurance industry?

• How would underutilization be avoided if the poor were required or given strong incentives to be financially at risk for health care services?

Edward F. X. Hughes, M.D., M.P.H.

It is both a pleasure and a predicament to be able to comment on this important paper by Ghez and Grossman, "Preventive Care, Care for Children, and National Health Insurance."[1] It is a pleasure because I essentially concur in their principal policy recommendation, namely, that

NOTE: I am grateful for the thoughtful comments on this commentary of Tryfon Beazoglou, Bernard Friedman, Martin Gaynor, James Horney, Susan Hughes, Stephen LaTour, Lawrence Lawson, Andrew Melczer, Janet Reis, and William Shadish and for the assistance of Sandra Sherman, Edythe Seltzer, and Carl Goad in its preparation.

[1] The research for this commentary is supported in part by a grant from the Robert Wood Johnson Foundation.

an optimal national health insurance plan should stress price reductions that fall with income and should be targeted at specific social health needs for which efficacious care exists. The paper is important, particularly to me as a physician, because it summarizes evidence that medical care, specifically prenatal care, can have a positive impact on the health of individuals.[2]

The predicament about the paper, however, arises when it moves beyond prenatal care to the question of the benefits of both preventive and curative care for children (with the exception of immunizations) and preventive care for adults. In addressing these topics, the authors give evidence of an implicit bias against medical care that fosters an uncharacteristic lack of rigor in their interpretation of the studies presented. This lack of rigor entails confusion as to (1) the appropriate definition of a number of the concepts underlying the assessment of medical care, (2) which of the concepts is being evaluated in each study and when validly so, and (3) what inferences may be appropriately drawn therein. This confusion leads the authors to draw a number of inferences that are not supported by the data presented or that are subject to rival competing hypotheses. In addition, a selectivity, albeit an acknowledged one, in the studies chosen by the authors for citation reinforces one's concern that a bias permeates the paper. There is also a disturbing ambiguity in the authors' inclusive equating of pediatric preventive and nonhospital curative care, which further undermines the paper. I would first like to address these concerns and then discuss briefly a number of additional significant points raised by the paper, especially as they relate to the need to develop new knowledge to better understand this important area of medical care.

An understanding of six of the many concepts underlying the assessment of medical care is requisite for an appropriate evaluation of this paper. These concepts are efficacy, effectiveness, process, compliance, outcome, and efficiency. "Efficacy" refers to whether a therapy (for example, a drug or a procedure) technically produces a desired physiologic response. Efficacy is most often measured in rigorous laboratory situations or in controlled clinical trials. In such situations, great stress is placed on ensuring both that all of the components of the therapy are appropriately delivered (for example, correct dose and frequency) and that the patient performs all of the tasks required of him for the therapy

---

[2] This evidence shows a positive association between prenatal care and increased infant birth weight, between increased infant birth weight and intellectual development, and hence between prenatal care and improved health throughout the life cycle. The implications of this work, much of it generated by Grossman and his co-workers, are especially important when one realizes that it was not many years ago that distinguished health economists were alleging that medical care, including prenatal care, had virtually no impact on the health of people.

to produce its desired effect (for example, he takes the pills prescribed for him at appropriate intervals). The various components or steps in the delivery of a therapy (or medical care in general) are referred to as the "process" of medical care, and the extent to which a patient fulfills the above-mentioned tasks required of him in receiving that care is referred to as "compliance." The net change in the patient's health status as a result of a therapy (or medical care in general) is referred to as the "outcome" of care. "Efficiency" refers to the resources consumed per unit of efficacious care delivered.

The critical task in evaluating the efficacy of care is to eliminate, or reduce as much as possible, provider-specific or patient-specific variance that might mask or mimic a valid physiologic response. This task requires as controlled a clinical setting as possible.[3] When a positive outcome is demonstrated in such a controlled setting, it is valid to infer that it could be obtained in any situation where similar clinical indications, process, and compliance prevail.

The term "effectiveness" refers to the extent to which the desired outcome of an efficacious therapy is obtained in a "real world" setting. Accordingly, effectiveness is a more complex concept than efficacy and is highly dependent on the behavior of the particular providers and consumers in each setting. Thus, it is inappropriate to generalize about the effectiveness of a therapy from the results in one setting without first assessing the process and compliance involved in that setting and demonstrating that they are generalizable qualities of the therapy and not situationally specific.

Although in the current version of the paper, Ghez and Grossman provide appropriate definitions of efficacy and effectiveness, they often use the words in an ambiguous, if not an inappropriate, context in the text.[4] They also tend to cite, and generalize from, findings of poor effec-

---

[3] For a vivid example of the effort investigators expend to achieve such a controlled setting, see Veterans Administration Cooperative Study Group on Antihypertensive Agents, "Effects of Treatment on Morbidity in Hypertension, I. Results in Patients with Diastolic Blood Pressures Averaging 115 Through 129 mm Hg," *Journal of the American Medical Association*, vol. 202 (December 11, 1967); and Veterans Administration Cooperative Study Group on Antihypertensive Agents, "Effects of Treatment on Morbidity in Hypertension, I. Results in Patients with Diastolic Blood Pressure Averaging 90 Through 114 mm Hg," *Journal of the American Medical Association*, vol. 213 (August 17, 1970).

[4] For instance, in their discussion of "Prenatal Care," Ghez and Grossman state, "There is a growing consensus that prenatal care is effective in terms of infant health outcomes." The context and the following discussion would suggest that the authors mean to convey that there is a growing consensus that prenatal care is "efficacious." There is also a confusion of efficacy and effectiveness in their discussion of the meticulous Veterans Administration's antihypertensive therapy trials. Ghez and Grossman accurately present the results of these trials of reduced mortality from stroke but argue that it is difficult to extrapolate these results to

tiveness or efficiency of preventive care (as they inclusively define it) in specific field settings without addressing the issue of whether the process and the compliance achieved in these settings was conducive to enhanced outcomes. They subtly formulate these generalizations in such a way as to cast aspersions on the very efficacy of that care and thereby insinuate a bias against policies that might be directed at increasing the effectiveness and efficiency of preventive care or curative care. For instance, in their discussion of preventive care for adults, they cite the Lauridsen and Gyntelberg study in which 150 Danish men, found to have treatable hypertension, were referred to their own physicians for care. After five years, these men had both higher death rates and higher cardiovascular complication rates than would normally be expected for middle-aged men.[5] In addition, the authors cite a study by Collen and others as evidence of lack of a decreased hypertensive death rate in a population of men randomized into a group "urged to come in for frequent periodic physical exams" and a nonintervention control group.[6]

Critical to a valid interpretation of the results of these and similar studies is the question whether the process of medical care delivered in, or the compliance achieved in, either study was conducive to an improved outcome. Indeed, the recently published results of the Hypertension Detection and Follow-up Program have shown dramatically increased five-year survival rates in men and women hypertensives treated in a systematic antihypertensive treatment program as compared with controls referred to their usual source of care.[7] These recent findings suggest that the effectiveness of antihypertensive therapy can be significantly increased through appropriate attention to process and compliance and they contrast sharply with the impression Ghez and Grossman convey. In part, these results answer Ghez and Grossman's call for "future research [to] shed light on effectiveness of preventive care in areas where current evidence is insufficient or not conclusive." Most critically, however, these results argue against the bias in the paper

---

"the population at large." It is precisely because the studies were performed to evaluate efficacy that one would not envision extrapolating the results to the population at large.

[5] L. Lauridsen and F. Gyntelberg, "A Clinical Follow-Up Five Years after Screening for Hypertension in Copenhagen, Males Aged 40–59," *International Journal of Epidemiology*, vol. 8 (March 1978). In addition to the point to be made below, the comparison group in this study, that is, expected mortality experience of middle-aged men, may well be inappropriate.

[6] M. F. Collen, ed., *Multiphasic Health Testing Services* (New York: John Wiley and Sons, 1978).

[7] Hypertension Detection and Follow-up Program Cooperative Group, "Five Year Findings of the Hypertension Detection and Follow-up Program: I. Reduction in Mortality of Persons with High Blood Pressure, Including Mild Hypertension," *Journal of the American Medical Association,* vol. 242 (December 7, 1979).

against the effectiveness (and, implicitly, the efficacy) of preventive care ("the burden of proof should fall on the advocates of effectiveness") and argue forcefully for a substantial investment in mechanisms to increase the effectiveness of efficacious preventive care.

In addition to appearing to overlook the importance of process and compliance in generalizing about effectiveness of preventive care for adults, Ghez and Grossman seem to draw inferences as to the efficacy of "pediatric care" (even though they use the word, "effectiveness") from studies about which similar concerns as well as serious questions can be raised concerning the appropriateness of the outcome measures used. For instance, they cite the study of Edwards and Grossman, which found no statistically significant reduction in the prevalence of obesity, abnormal corrected distance vision, or anemia associated with a "preventive checkup within the past year."[8] They then proceed to cite a study by Kaplan, Lave, and Leinhardt that found only a small negative effect on the number of days absent from school associated with enrollment in a comprehensive health care clinic.[9]

We have no knowledge of the process of care in the preventive checkups in the Edwards and Grossman study. Even if the process had been directed at the outcome measures selected, two of the measures—prevalence of obesity and anemia—entail conditions whose resolution is heavily dependent on exogenous social factors, such as diet, exercise, and so forth. These factors are often beyond the purview of even "comprehensive care," especially in adolescence. The recalcitrance of these conditions, especially obesity, is such that even if the process had been relevant to them, the probability of an improved outcome resulting from one preventive checkup would, a priori, appear small. The appropriateness of the prevalence of abnormal corrected distance vision as an outcome measure for adolescents is also problematical insofar as the condition commonly begins during adolescence. Hence, it is quite possible that a valid negative finding on a preventive checkup could be followed by a valid positive finding a year later.[10]

The issue of which outcome measures are appropriate to evaluate "pediatric care" is further reinforced by the Kaplan, Lave, and Leinhardt study. This study used differential absentee rates from school to evaluate

---

[8] L. N. Edwards and Michael Grossman, "Adolescent Health Family Background and Preventive Medical Care," volume III of the *Annual Series of Research in Human Capital and Development*, eds. Ismail Sirageldin and David Salkever (Greenwich, Conn.: JAI Press, 1980).

[9] R. S. Kaplan, Lester B. Lave and S. Leinhardt, "The Efficacy of a Comprehensive Health Care Project: An Empirical Analysis," *American Journal of Public Health*, vol. 62, no. 7 (July 1972).

[10] Lawrence J. Lawson, M.D., Department of Ophthalmology, Northwestern University Medical School, personal communication.

the impact of comprehensive care versus regular care. It found a small positive effect on absenteeism associated with comprehensive care (parents' education not held constant).[11] This outcome measure (absentee rate) is again subject to any number of influences other than health care and, at very best, could be considered only slightly sensitive to many pediatric care interventions.[12] For instance, even if the preventive checkups in the Edwards and Grossman study had dramatic impact on the obesity, vision, and anemia status of the adolescents in that study, it is unlikely that any one of these improved health outcomes would translate into changes in school attendance rates.

Interestingly, T. W. Hu's study, cited as further evidence of the lack of efficacy of pediatric/preventive care, carries in its positive and statistically significant findings of an association between Medicaid benefits and hearing correction a suggestion of both the efficacy and effectiveness of acute care.[13] The findings suggested that low income children with otitis media—the most common cause of hearing loss—who are being treated for their acute condition under Medicaid are being referred for correction of residual hearing defects. Children not being treated under Medicaid, however, are receiving neither the acute nor the follow-up care, hence their poorer outcomes.[14] The lack of association between Medicaid benefits and vision correction reported in Hu's study is readily understandable. It results from the lack of a common, acute, and treatable eye problem analogous to otitis media to focus attention on, and thereby to contribute to, vision correction.

I have examined these studies in such detail to illustrate that reasonable rival hypotheses can be entertained to explain the apparent lack of effectiveness (or efficacy) of pediatric care alleged by Ghez and Grossman and to question the validity of their conclusion that "pediatric care has little impact on children's health." In developing evidence for that specific conclusion, Ghez and Grossman review the findings of six studies, three of which I have alluded to. W. Shadish of the Center for Health Services and Policy Research at Northwestern University has conducted

---

[11] It should be noted that the comparison here is between "comprehensive care and regular source of care," not between pediatric care and no care. Hence the use of the study by Ghez and Grossman to bolster their case that pediatric care has no impact on child health is inappropriate.

[12] Children's Defense Fund, "Children Out of School in America" (Washington, D.C.: Children's Defense Fund, 1974).

[13] T. W. Hu, "Effectiveness of Child Health and Welfare Programs: A Simultaneous Equations Approach," *Socio-Economic Planning Sciences*, vol. 7 (1973).

[14] An empirical test of this hypothesis might be possible. If Hu's data set identified the diagnosis for which care was rendered to the children for which benefits were paid, a higher frequency of treatment for otitis media would be expected among the children with corrected hearing defects than those without.

a literature review on the effectiveness of preventive health care.[15] Of the 147 articles and books abstracted by him, 38 were empirical studies with a control group of some kind. Each of these was reviewed in some detail with attention focused on the methodologic rigor of the study. Thirty-two of these studies dealt with nondental preventive care.[16] Shadish concludes:

> The bulk of the evidence suggests that [child health] prevention does have a beneficial effect on the dependent variables reported by the authors. Only four studies could reasonably be interpreted to suggest that it has no effect (Braren & Elinson, 1972; Gordis & Markowitz, 1971; Klein et al., 1973; Moore & Frank, 1973). On the other hand, at least [eleven] studies could be interpreted as suggesting that prevention has an unambiguous positive effect (Alpert et al., 1968; Beiner, 1975; Crawford, 1970; Department of Public Health, Portsmouth, Virginia, 1973; Gordis, 1973; Leodolter, 1978; MacCready, 1974; Perrin et al., 1974; Spencer, 1974; Vaughn, 1968; Webb et al., 1973). Positive effect is defined as unambiguous change on the only measure reported, or beneficial change on most or all measures reported. Admittedly, such attempts to classify magnitude of effects are crude and judgmental at best. However, the fact that the number of strong positive effects so greatly outnumber the no effect findings would suggest that were the judgments made by other people with other means, the results might still have favored positive conclusions.
>
> The remaining [seventeen] studies fall somewhere in between. At one extreme are studies like those by Yankauer and colleagues (1955, 1956, 1957, 1962) which suggest a very minimal benefit, if any. At the other extreme are studies which report quite a few benefits, but also fail to find benefits on a number of other variables (e.g., McKee, 1963; Mawson et al., 1968). What unifies the [seventeen] is that they all show at least some benefit. Every attempt was made to classify studies conservatively, not assigning a study to a category implying more benefit unless the reported evidence is strong. This conservative bias was deliberate so as to avoid the probability of finding a positive effect unless the evidence clearly supported it.

---

[15] W. Shadish, *Effectiveness of Preventive Child Health Care*, Working Paper #38, Center for Health Services and Policy Research, Northwestern University, March 1980.

[16] The quotation is presented deleting reference to the six dental studies reviewed by Shadish. Shadish and Ghez and Grossman strongly reinforce each other on the issue of dental care. Interestingly, only one of the thirty-two nondental articles analyzed by Shadish, that of Kaplan, Lave, and Leinhardt (1972), is included in the Ghez and Grossman paper.

A comprehensive review, conducted by the Canadian Task Force on the Periodic Health Examination, of the research on periodic health examinations across the human lifespan also supported the conclusions reached by Shadish for pediatric screening.[17] The Canadian Task Force also examined the quality of evidence supporting the efficacy, effectiveness, and efficiency of various preventive procedures. While the task force found that the quality of available evidence was generally poor, it concluded that the demonstrated effectiveness of a number of pediatric preventive screening procedures warranted their continuation.

Given the positive results reported by Shadish and the Canadian Task Force on the effectiveness of pediatric preventive care, why does the literature contain so many instances of ineffective or inefficient preventive programs (both for children and adults)?[18] A partial answer would appear to be that the seeking of preventive care involves an individual's making decisions both about the consumption of care in highly complex social situations and very often about the style of life he prefers, whose benefits may not be evident for years, if indeed they are ever palpably evident. We know very little about consumers' perception of the value of preventive medical care (or of all medical care for that matter) and very little about the preventive-care-seeking behavior of individuals, especially of parents for their children or of children for themselves. Accordingly, in view of the demonstrated efficacy of many elements of preventive care, for example, antihypertensive therapy, it would appear appropriate that attention in the health services research community be directed at developing a behavioral model of the preventive-care-seeking behavior of individuals so that we might more effectively market efficacious preventive care. The potential benefits of a more effective marketing of an efficacious preventive regimen such as antihypertensive therapy would appear to be substantial. Not only is hypertension a major contributor to the first and third most common causes of death—heart disease and diseases of the cerebro-vascular system—it is also one of the major precipitating conditions responsible for individuals' requiring lifelong maintenance dialysis in the End Stage Renal Disease program.

One of the major policy problems in preventive care is that pre-

---

[17] Task Force on the Periodic Health Examination, *Periodic (vs. annual) Health Examination* (Quebec: Department of National Health and Welfare, Health Services and Promotion Branch, November 1979).

[18] For instance, see F. A. Finnerty, Jr., et al., "Hypertension in the Inner City, Part 2: Detection and Follow-up," *Circulation*, vol. 47 (1973); and J. Reis et al., "An Assessment of the Validity of the Results of HCFA's Demonstration and Evaluation Program for the Early and Periodic Screening, Diagnosis, and Treatment Program (EPSDT): A Metaevaluation," Working Paper #29, Center for Health Services and Policy Research, Northwestern University, June 1979.

ventive care programs, including massive ones such as EPSDT (Early and Periodic Screening, Diagnosis, and Treatment Program), are often launched without adequate behavioral research to determine the most effective and efficient way to market and manage such programs. Moreover, such programs are often launched or managed by advocates of the program who are not persuaded of the need for such research. Also needed are rigorous studies of the efficacy of, and the cost effectiveness of, specific preventive techniques so that, in well-marketed programs, scarce resources can be concentrated on activities proven to be efficacious and possessing an acceptable cost-effectiveness ratio (however such a standard is set). The recent revision of its screening guidelines by the American Cancer Society is salutary evidence of an increased sensitivity to these important issues by an organization long known for its advocacy in this field.[19]

Within our HCFA Policy Center initiative at Northwestern, we are planning an investigation of the preventive-care-seeking behavior of families eligible for EPSDT in an attempt to understand why so many eligible individuals apparently decide not to participate in the program. In that regard, Ghez and Grossman's paper again reaffirms the singular importance of maternal education in preventive- and dental-care-seeking behavior. For years, this finding has been used to question the importance of medical care to health and has served to focus attention away from policies that might serve to increase the consumption of efficacious medical care. In reality, rather than viewing this finding as "disheartening," the health services research community should strive to identify the operational factor that, under the rubric of maternal education, is influencing the behavior of mothers to seek preventive and dental care. Maternal education is not an explanatory variable. Despite years of research on the topic, it remains a "black box." Somewhere within that black box is a mechanism that, if identified, would enable preventive care to be marketed with far less social cost and in far less time than would be required to reproduce the level of education found significant in these studies.[20] The potential benefits of the identification of this mechanism to the delivery of health services could be substantial.

Despite the problems in its handling of "pediatric care" and "adult preventive care," the paper is eloquent both in reviewing the association between the process of dental care and positive dental outcomes and in

---

[19] "Cancer Society Reports It Finds Some Detection Tests Unneeded," *New York Times*, March 21, 1980, p. 1.

[20] J. D. Finn, J. Reis and L. Dulberg, "Sex Differences in Educational Attainment: A Process Model," *Comparative Educational Review*, 1980 (in press). Implementing the level of education, if it could be accomplished, could be expected to entail benefits beyond those of the consumption of preventive and dental care, however.

evaluating various policy options to increase the consumption of dental care. In our metaevaluation of the fifteen demonstration and evaluation projects performed from 1972 to 1978 for the EPSDT program, dental pathology was a common finding among the children screened.[21] Sometimes, as many as 30 percent of the children screened in certain settings were found to have dental pathology. A critical question that has not been addressed to my knowledge, however, relates to the value to society of improving people's dental health. In addition to certain long-run health benefits, an individual's self-esteem, employment opportunity, and educational opportunity could be influenced by improved dental health, and therein benefits could accrue to society. In view of the size and scope of the problem, however, it would appear worthwhile to attempt to document and quantify the perceived benefits.

As stated at the outset of this discussion, the authors include "under the rubric of preventive care," "preventive and curative physicians' services delivered to children and adolescents" (outside of hospital), and lump the latter two items under the heading "pediatric care." Proceeding to argue as we have discussed, they conclude that "pediatric care has little impact on the health of children." Notwithstanding the errors in interpreting the results of the studies presented and the selectivity in the choosing of those studies, the very lumping of preventive and curative physicians' services into one category causes me some concerns that I feel should be explicated.

Ghez and Grossman are moved to merge the two because, "In the case of children and adolescents, both preventive and curative services delivered early in life can have important long-run effects on health in adulthood." This is unquestionably true as almost all efficacious curative services have some preventive payoff: the earlier in life those services are delivered, the greater the preventive return. The equating of the two here and the subsequent analysis does a disservice to "pediatric care," however, and clouds some important realities. As one who has had one child with florid scarlet fever and another with bronchiolitis and pneumonia (times two), under the age of six months, I can attest that the impact of pediatric care can be substantial. Similarly, ambulatory therapeutic intervention in conditions such as otitis media, infantile diarrhea, and now Wilm's tumor can be dramatic and, in the latter two cases, potentially lifesaving. Shadish's review suggested that preventive care is effective in impacting on child health, and it is my bias that curative care also has a positive impact on child health. In addition to its impact on child health, pediatric care, even when only ruling out the possibility of "dread disease," conveys a reassurance and psychic benefit possibly

---

[21] J. Reis et al., "An Assessment of the Validity of the Results of HCFA's Demonstration and Evaluation Program."

greater than any other area of medical care. It is critically important that the value of this component of pediatric care also be factored into any discussion of its benefits.

In view of Ghez and Grossman's analysis of the benefits of "pediatric care," it is somewhat surprising to see them suggest that, in developing a national health insurance plan, "the government should direct its attention to [among other things] physicians' services during the first year of life." Indeed, with the exception of the acknowledged value of immunizations, there is nothing in the paper to support the inclusion of such physicians' services in a publicly funded program.[22] Accordingly, one is tempted to speculate that this suggestion conveys some sensitivity on the authors' part to the potential efficacy of pediatric care.

The health services research and delivery community has made enormous strides in recent years in developing methodologies to assess care and to weed out nonefficacious therapy from the efficacious. The task remains to improve the effectiveness of the delivery of these services. In their discussion of the utilization of services, Ghez and Grossman report evidence of major strides in that area. Within this framework, it is appropriate that a critical component of our delivery system, pediatric care, receive its appropriate due.

---

[22] Interestingly, this suggestion is not explicitly mentioned in their three answers as to "Preventive NHI: What Now, What Later, What Never?" given at the end of the paper.

Part
Three

Solving the Problem of Overinsurance

Overinsurance: The Conceptual Issues

Mark V. Pauly

The primary cause of inflation in medical care expenditures has been the extent and form of medical insurance. With the exception of some of the poor and the near-poor, most people have too much insurance of the wrong kind.

In this paper I will try to explain what these strong statements mean, and what they imply about the appropriate form of national health insurance policy. I will show that, in the case of insurance against medical care, it is indeed possible to have (as Clark Havighurst has put it) "too much of a good thing." I will then discuss reasons why insurance is too extensive and of the wrong kind. Finally, I will indicate three types of solutions: (1) changes in the extent or amount of insurance, (2) changes in insurance markets, and (3) changes in the form of insurance. I will also discuss ways that these changes could be incorporated into a national health insurance policy.

Ideal Insurance

We begin by assuming that people are risk averse. By this we simply mean that, faced with a choice between sacrificing a particular dollar amount with certainty or running a risk of losing the same average or expected amount, a risk-averse person will prefer the certain loss to the risk.

If a person is, in fact, faced with a risk with a particular expected value, but can buy insurance at an actuarially fair premium (that is, a premium equal to the average or expected loss), it follows that the risk-averse person will prefer to insure—pay the certain premium— rather than run the risk. Against how much of the loss will he wish to insure? If he is risk averse, he gains by buying actuarially fair insurance against all risk. So he will insure the full amount of the loss, and he will buy insurance against all uncertain events. Thus, if the probability of an event occurring and the magnitude of the loss are both independent of the insured's behavior, and if insurance is available at a premium equal to its actuarial value, we conclude that a risk-averse person should (and will) buy full insurance coverage against any uncertain loss. Note that this proposition applies regardless of the amount of the loss: A $100 loss will be fully insured as well as a $100,000 loss.

What if insurance is not actuarially fair, as is almost certain to be the case? The insurer will need to ask for an amount in excess of the expected loss to cover administrative costs associated with transactions, including both the purchase of insurance and the payment of claims. He may also demand a payment to compensate himself for his own absorption of additional risk, even though his risk-aversion payment should be less than the value the insured would have placed on suffering the risk.

The form of optimal coverage depends on how this administrative cost or "loading" varies with premiums or losses. If this cost is just a flat percentage of the premium, then the optimal coverage will be full coverage above a deductible. If the cost is a function of the number of losses, but not of the amount of each loss, then optimal coverage will involve no payment for losses below a certain amount, but full coverage (without deductible) for large losses. Finally, if the insurer is risk averse, optimal coverage may involve sharing some of the risk with the insured in the form of copayments. These optimal copayments need not be proportional but (depending on the exact form of insurer and insured's attitudes toward risk) will probably tend to decrease as the size of the loss increases. In no case will there be a complete upper limit on the payment by the insurer.

These observations give us a qualitative picture of the coverage pattern that is likely to be optimal. How large the deductibles will be depends upon the magnitude of administrative costs. With average health insurance administrative cost at about 12 to 14 percent of premiums, the optimal deductible for insurance against the cost of medical care might not be very large. Given the large number of independent experiences pooled by a typical insurer, and given the ability of owners of insurance firms to further spread risks by holding a diversified portfolio of common stocks (insurance company or otherwise) and other securities, optimal copayments should probably be small. Determining how small is appropriate would require detailed information on the magnitude of risk aversion and on the distribution of losses.

However, there is an important difference between insurance against the cost of medical care and the ideal insurance against uncontrollable uncertain events that we have been discussing. That difference, to be discussed in the next section, is the "moral hazard" associated with consumer and producer behavior under medical insurance.

MARK V. PAULY

Moral Hazard and the Ideal Amount of Insurance

The typical form of medical insurance makes payments on the basis of events or facts over which the insured has at least partial control. The occurrence of illness itself can, through the use of preventive medicine or of lifestyle practices, be affected by actions or nonactions of the insured. In addition to medical care labeled "preventive," almost all of medicine is preventive in some sense, because it serves to stave off future and usually uncertain "complications."

More importantly, however, the patient and physician in combination are subject to few limits in determining the amount and type of medical care to be provided once illness has occurred. Because the insurance covers a large part, if not all, of the cost of each unit of medical care, the insured will desire increased consumption of medical care. Under most reimbursement arrangements, the provider will have no incentive to oppose this.

Some of this increased consumption will show up as increases in the kinds of units with which we usually measure the quantity of medical care—doctor visits, hospital admissions, and days of stay. But because the time cost per unit is usually higher for those measures of medical care we label "quantity" (such as doctor visits, hospital inpatient days) than for those we label "quality" (laboratory tests per patient day, physician board certification), much of this additional use will show up as higher quality, in the form of higher costs per unit, rather than as higher quantity.

In short, the insured person can affect the amount of medical care cost incurred on his behalf, possibly by merely acquiescing to his physician's suggestions. In this sense, insurance against the cost of medical care is subject to "moral hazard"; the insured experiences higher costs when there is insurance coverage than when it is absent.[1]

The empirical evidence for the existence of this effect is quite strong, though its precise magnitude is subject to dispute. For hospital care, Feldstein[2] has estimated a price elasticity of about 0.7, and Rosett and Huang[3] have provided even higher estimates. Newhouse and Phelps,[4] however, have obtained much smaller estimates for hospital

---

[1] Mark Pauly, "The Economics of Moral Hazard," *American Economic Review*, vol. 58 (June 1968), pp. 531–37.

[2] Martin S. Feldstein, "Hospital Cost Inflation: A Study in Nonprofit Price Dynamics," *American Economic Review*, vol. 61 (December 1971), pp. 853–72.

[3] Richard Rosett and L. F. Huang, "The Effect of Health Insurance on the Demand for Medical Care," *Journal of Political Economy*, vol. 81 (March 1973), pp. 281–305.

[4] Joseph Newhouse and Charles Phelps, "Estimate of the Price Elasticity of Demand for Medical Care," in Richard Rosett, ed., *The Role of Health Insurance in*

and physicians' services, in the neighborhood of 0.2. However, at high levels of coverage, relatively small additional reductions in price can have large predicted effects even if elasticity is "low," because such changes represent large proportional reductions in price. These estimates are of the response of *quantity* to insurance; the response of quality or of unit cost is likely to further increase the size of the change in total spending.

"Moral hazard" is, of course, just another way of looking at the much-discussed financial barriers to access. If the absence of insurance deters the use of medical care that one might (on some other grounds) regard as appropriate, it follows that the presence of insurance will encourage additional use. One cannot at the same time assert that (a) individuals do not respond to financial incentives in their consumption of medical care, and (b) that the absence of insurance provides a financial deterrent to use. If we were able to determine what "appropriate" use was, we would still have to design insurance to encourage only that use. An across-the-board increase in coverage as proposed by some national health insurance schemes will encourage *all* use, whether appropriate or not.

Why does the presence of moral hazard affect the amount of insurance that individuals ought to hold? The reason is that the extra medical care it encourages the individual to consume is worth less to him than it costs him in out-of-pocket payments and insurance premiums combined. The individual chooses to purchase medical care as long as its value to him exceeds the out-of-pocket price for an additional unit. Although his additional use raises his own premium, it is spread over so many other insureds that it is virtually ignored. But when all insureds engage in the same behavior, total premiums must rise to cover the extra cost. In a sense, there is an "insurance illusion" that tricks the individual into using care as if it were available at the low user price; in fact, either the user or someone else must eventually pay through substantially higher insurance premiums. This difference between apparent price and real cost leads to what economists call a welfare cost: an excess of the cost of medical care over its value to the consumer.

Additional insurance means additional stimulus to the use of medical care, which in turn means more welfare cost. When moral hazard is present, this welfare cost accompanies any increment in insurance, and it must be set against risk-reduction benefits. When moral hazard exists, it will not be optimal to fully insure any medical expense. Welfare cost increases as the level of insurance coverage

the Health Services Sector (New York: Neale Watson Academic Publications, Inc., 1977).

increases, but the benefits from risk reduction decrease. Insuring the last dollar of a risk provides only a small benefit to the insured, because his income was virtually free of risk anyway. But it carries a high welfare cost, because the value to the consumer of the additional units is virtually zero, while the cost is surely positive. With medical care, as with other goods, it is possible to have "too much of a good thing."

Why does moral hazard occur? In the most fundamental sense, it happens because the insurer is unable, or finds it too costly, to obtain some information that the insured possesses. Consider a simple situation in which the true loss depends upon the state of the person's health. For instance, the cost of medical care needed to restore a person to full health might be greater for a "serious" version of an illness than for a less serious one. If the insurer could observe the state of the person's health, and pay a fixed indemnity based on the level of that state, there would be no moral hazard. The person would simply receive a fixed sum, which would not vary with his medical care costs. He would then have no incentive to purchase medical care worth less than its cost, because every unit of medical care purchased would reduce his wealth by the price of one unit. Because the insurance would increase his financial (and real) wealth when he is sick, he might spend more than in comparison with the no-insurance care. But as long as the purchaser was appropriately informed and faced prices equal to cost, he would buy the "right" amount of medical care.

Except for certain "dread disease" policies and indemnities in accident insurance, medical insurance does not make payments that are contingent on the event of illness of a particular type—the state of the person's health. Instead, it makes payments that, in effect, depend upon the event of agreement by patient and provider to consume care, an event at least partly under the control of the insured. The reason for such an arrangement is obviously because it is costly or impossible to observe the state of the person's health. But although perfect indemnity insurance is not possible in all situations, I will argue below that a case can be made for a much broader use of indemnities than at present.

The spread of insurance will, therefore, be accompanied by an increase in medical care expenses. There is good reason to suppose that much of the explosion in the cost of medical care over the past fifteen years has been due to the substantial expansion in insurance coverage that followed the passage of Medicare and Medicaid in 1966, and the spread of private coverage for the rest of the population. Feldstein and Taylor,[5] for example, conclude that "the primary reason (for inflation)

---

[5] Martin S. Feldstein and Amy Taylor, *The Rapid Rise of Hospital Costs*, a report to the Council on Wage and Price Stability, Washington, D.C., 1977.

is that patients are much more willing to pay for expensive care (and doctors are willing to order it) because insurance finances a much larger share of those payments."

This expansion has taken several forms. There has been a modest increase in the number of units of medical care consumed, at least measured by visits per capita or hospital admissions per capita. But probably the most important consequence has been a change in what Feldstein has termed the "style" of care, with more resources per unit being demanded and provided by the medical care system. Insurance has even affected the rate and character of technical change, making possible the implementation of the imperative for high-cost technology.

In each case, the argument is not that resources have been expended to provide no benefit to patients. Evidence for this kind of "pure inefficiency" is at best anecdotal, and it is difficult in any case to believe that it has been increasing. Moreover, one person's inefficiency is another person's higher quality, as is evidenced by the debate between health planners and physicians over *CAT* scanners. Rather, the argument is that the positive benefit from additional care, or from changes in the style of care, is too small to justify the costs of these changes.

To say that the spread of insurance and the consequent increase in moral hazard is responsible for the increase in medical care costs is not to allege that there is necessarily anything undesirable about that rate of increase. Rising expenditures are not per se undesirable; what is desirable is the *proper* rate of change, one that reflects the benefits and costs to individuals. If rising expenditures accompany increases in insurance coverage that provide sufficient risk-reduction benefits to cover the increase in welfare cost, the increase in insurance and, of necessity, the rising costs that accompany it will not necessarily be undesirable. The situation will, of course, be less desirable than if moral hazard did not exist or could be avoided—that is, if the increase in expenses could somehow be prevented. But we may have to settle for a "second-best" situation in which more coverage can only be bought at the cost of more inflation.

There are two critical questions. One is whether this trade-off between insurance coverage and inflation has been correctly taken into account in decisions to purchase insurance in the United States. "Over-insurance" will be said to result if insurance has been obtained whose risk-reduction benefits are *less than* the marginal welfare cost generated by it. That is, overinsurance occurs if people purchase insurance whose benefit falls short of its cost. The second critical question is whether there are ways of preventing or at least reducing moral hazard that might make more extensive levels of coverage *not* constitute overinsurance. These two questions will be discussed in the remaining sections of this paper.

Causes of Overinsurance

Why would a person not make the proper trade-off between risk reduction and moral hazard? To answer this question, we first have to determine whether there exists an institutional arrangement under which the proper trade-off would be made; we can then suggest that deviations from that arrangement might lead to improper trade-offs.

One's intuition here (not yet confirmed by economic theory) is that if the insurance market is competitive, if adverse selection is not a problem, if there are no economies of scale in monitoring experience or loss-reducing or preventing activities of the insured, *and* if the insurer can always determine the total amount of insurance the individual has purchased, then an efficient arrangement will be achieved in "neutral" (neither taxed nor subsidized) markets.

The structure of insurance premiums will, one would suppose, come to reflect the effects of moral hazard. Insurers, in setting rates based on the experience of various types of policyholders, will notice that total expenditures are related to the level of insurance coverage. Individuals or groups with relatively incomplete coverage will tend to have lower total expenditures than those with relatively complete coverage. If coverage is doubled, claims will more than double, because total expenses will increase when coverage increases.

Individuals or groups will eventually face a schedule of prices for "units" of health insurance measured, say, by the number of percentage points of total expense covered, in which the price for each additional unit will increase as the total number of units purchased increases. The result will be that consumers will take into account, when contemplating the purchase of additional insurance, both the benefit from risk reduction and the cost of the additional medical care use they will generate. This arrangement is, of course, only ideal in a second-best sense; if moral hazard could somehow be prevented or reduced, consumers could unequivocally be made better off.

Each of the provisos in the initial statement of the proposition above is important, and it may be useful to examine in more detail exactly what would happen if each did not hold.

First, it would be necessary that every insurer know the total amount of insurance the individual has purchased. If the total amount of insurance were not known, there would be no way to accurately make the premium vary with the total amount of insurance coverage.

The insurer could still try to make the premium vary with the total amount of insurance purchased *from that firm*, but then the individual's strategy would be to buy small amounts of coverage from many different firms.

Insurance companies do generally try to obtain information on multiple policies held by policyholders, under what are called "coordination of benefit" (COB) arrangements. The direct goal of COB arrangements is to prevent double coverage, or payment twice for the same thing. But, COB is not fully effective; the "Sunday supplement" health insurance policies, in fact, advertise that their indemnity payments (usually per day of hospitalization), are paid regardless of whatever other insurance might pay. Indeed, the profit-maximizing supplemental insurer should conspire with the purchaser to keep the additional purchase a secret, because doing so reduces the net price of additional insurance to the buyer.

Even with COB, however, an *individual's* premiums are not always adjusted upward if he buys supplemental coverage from another firm. Moreover, although COB appears to work fairly well among major firms writing policies with service or assigned benefits, no analogous adjustment procedure exists for persons who supplement public insurance. We shall discuss this in more detail below; the point to be made here is that the premium for supplemental coverage of any tax-financed insurance reflects only the claims on the supplemental coverage. It does not reflect additional claims on the "basic" coverage, and so tends to underprice supplemental or shallow coverage.

A second possible source of inefficiency arises if there are economies of scale in the monitoring of actions that lead to moral hazard. Suppose, for example, that cigarette smokers have higher claims than nonsmokers. An obvious policy would be to tie premium rates to smoking. Not only would this discourage excessive smoking, it would ensure that the health costs associated with smoking are borne by smokers, rather than the entire population. In effect, the rise in premium cost would constitute a kind of tax on smoking.

But it would obviously be very difficult for individual insurance firms to monitor the cigarette consumption of their insureds. An alternative arrangement would be for the government to tax tobacco products, or other goods whose purchase is associated with higher medical expenses. The government would not need to distinguish between the customers of alternative insurance firms. Such an arrangement would not be as desirable as the infeasible direct monitoring of smoking, because it would not tie premiums to any residual higher health risk of smokers, but it might be superior to feasible alternatives.

The final question deals with possible "spillovers" between insured and uninsured patients. We emphasized above that one of the major ways in which moral hazard is manifested is through changes in the quality or style of care. A similar point has been made by Martin Feldstein,[6] who has gone on to assert that, as a matter of empirical fact, the level of health insurance in the United States is now excessive.[7] By this he means that a reduction in the average extent of coverage would produce an aggregate welfare gain, because a reduction in insurance would reduce welfare cost by more than it reduced the value of risk spreading. In other work,[8] Feldstein and Friedman indicted the tax treatment of insurance premiums as a major cause of overinsurance. This topic will be discussed by other conference papers. But the question of whether there would still be overinsurance in a neutral tax system is of some interest, especially since Harris[9] has recently reconsidered this question (and the question of overinsurance generally).

Feldstein appears to claim that there are certain kinds of spillovers inherent in the way hospitals and patients behave that have exacerbated inflation and the resultant welfare loss. He gives the following story: The price and type of health services that are available to any individual reflect the extent of health insurance among other members of the community. Even the uninsured individual will find that his expenditure on health services is affected by the insurance of others. Moreover, the higher price of physician and hospital services encourages more extensive use of insurance. For the community as a whole, therefore, the spread of insurance causes higher prices and more sophisticated services that in turn cause a further increase in insurance. People spend more on health because they are insured and buy more insurance because of the high cost of health care.

The proposition that insurance increases the demand for medical care has already been argued above. The proposition that a rise in unit price of medical care increases the demand for insurance is not necessarily true in theory, but seems to be confirmed by Feldstein's empirical work.

What do these effects of insurance on price represent, and how are they related to the presence or absence of overinsurance? There are

---

[6] Martin S. Feldstein, "Quality Change and the Demand for Hospital Care," *Econometrica*, vol. 45 (June 1977), pp. 1601–701.

[7] Martin S. Feldstein, "The Welfare Loss of Excess Health Insurance," *Journal of Political Economy*, vol. 81 (March 1973), pp. 251–80.

[8] Martin S. Feldstein and Bernard Friedman, "Tax Subsidies, the Rational Demand for Insurance, and the Health Care Crisis," *Journal of Public Economics*, vol. 7 (April 1977), pp. 155–78.

[9] Jeffrey Harris, "The Aggregate Coinsurance Rate and the Supply of Innovations in the Hospital Sector," unpublished paper, Massachusetts Institute of Technology, Department of Economics, July 1979.

three possible ways of looking at the determination of prices, quantity, and quality in the medical care sector. In fact, most analyses focus specifically on hospital care, on the logical ground that it accounts for 40 percent of health care spending, and is the largest single component of the health care dollar. This still leaves out the remaining 60 percent, and we should be careful that we do not generalize excessively from models of the hospital.

The first hypothesis, which we call (as does Harris) hypothesis A, is that health care providers take gross price and the quality of care as given, and attempt to maximize profits. Because quality is exogenously given, and because all surpluses are used up as profits, hypothesis A implies that changes in the demand for medical care, such as those induced by insurance, will not themselves change quality. If the market is competitive, choosing insurance in a "neutral" world in which the price of insurance is not subsidized or taxed, but fully reflects the actuarial value of claims at various levels of coverage, will be optimal. Of course, if there were monopoly in the medical care market, then subsidization of insurance might actually help get user prices closer to marginal cost, and so improve welfare. Unfortunately, all welfare gains in moving to such an "efficient" outcome would go to providers.

The second hypothesis (hypothesis B) was advanced initially by Feldstein in the work described above, and was extended by Harris. It supposes that providers convert earned surplus into increases in quality, taking the market levels of price and quality as given. Thus, contrary to what firms believe, an increase in insurance will (at least temporarily) lead to an increase in quality, and the increase will be spread over all consumers of care, not just those with increased insurance coverage. (Implicitly, in either hypothesis A or B, the behavior of the industry is thought to be appropriately described by analyzing that of a single firm.) The character of long-run equilibrium for this second hypothesis is a bit less certain and will be discussed below.

The final model (hypothesis C) assumes that *both* quantity and quality are in effect sold in the market, and that in most instances there is more than one provider available to consumers, so consumers do not all have to consume the same level of quality. The "market for quality" would be provided either by a given seller's willingness to supply the level of quality patients demand or by permitting patients to choose among sellers providing different levels of quality.

Russell[10] and Feldstein and Taylor also have implicitly supported hypothesis C in concluding that the high rate of technical or "quality"

---

[10] Louise Russell, *Technology in Hospitals* (Washington, D.C.: The Brookings Institution, 1979).

change in hospitals, which is the main source of real price inflation, has been caused by the spread of insurance coverage. Feldstein and Taylor argue: "This increased demand for expensive care is primarily the result of the growing share of hospital costs that is paid by public and private insurance. With insurance now paying approximately 90 percent of all hospital costs, there is a strong incentive for patients and their physicians to seek the 'best possible care' almost without concern about its cost."[11]

The basic idea behind this model is simple: When insurance lowers the user price to the consumer of an increment in "quality," the consumer will be more willing to pay for additional quality, and some provider will be willing to provide it.

The motivation for satisfying possible patient desires for higher quality could be described by orthodox consumer choice theory: Patients want higher quality care and patronize those physicians and hospitals willing to supply it. This occurs to such an extent that most hospitals, concerned either with growth (in output or physician staff) or survival, are motivated to provide the quality patients want. An obvious objection to this view is the fact that many patients do not make the choice of type of hospital: The hospital is chosen by their physician. A second view, therefore, would suggest that if the physician as agent is willing to prescribe and to influence (by hospital selection or by hospital direction) all increases in quality that benefit his patient medically and that the patient is willing to pay for, then long-run equilibrium will go at least as far as described above, and possibly farther.

If hypothesis C is valid, then "neutral" incentives in purchasing insurance will be all that is needed to achieve optimality. It follows that quantities of insurance in excess of what would be selected as if consumers made fully informed choices under neutral incentives would be nonoptimal. Insurance would be optimal in the sense that it leads to optimal levels of risk-spreading quantity and of quality. In terms of the units of quantity and quality, in Figure 1 a point such as P_1 might represent the optimal combination of medical care quantity, medical care quality, and other goods, to be accompanied, of course, by optimal insurance. We shall call this level of insurance (and copayment) r^*.

Under hypothesis B, neither the characterization of final equilibrium nor the determination of the optimality of neutral-incentive insurance coverage is quite so straightforward. In this model, recall that in the short run the hospital provides a level of quality that equates supply

---

[11] Feldstein and Taylor, *The Rapid Rise of Hospital Costs.*

FIGURE 1
WELFARE EFFECTS OF ALTERNATIVE COMBINATIONS
OF QUANTITY AND QUALITY

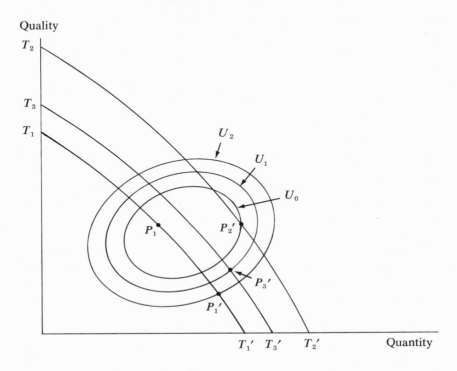

and demand and permits the hospital to break even (because all profits are "used up" in higher quality). Suppose, for example, that quantity supplied (such as admissions given length of stay, or bed-days) is perfectly fixed by the existing bed stock. Then there exists some level of quality that is consistent with demand equal to this fixed supply and a break-even pricing policy (price equals average cost) for the hospital.

With a different level of supply, there is a different equilibrium level of quality. The equilibrium combinations of quality and quantity would, therefore, be represented by a curve such as $T_1 T_1'$ in Figure 1. Note that this curve is an opportunity locus for the hospital, but not a product transformation curve for the economy; the quantity of resources devoted to hospital care is quite likely to vary along this curve. The utility contour lines, such as U_o, represent combinations of price, quality, other goods, and (not shown) insurance coverage that the consumer can purchase with his income and that yield equal utility. They are constructed so that the combinations of insurance, other goods, quantity, and quality at any quantity-quality point both yield the indicated utility *and* provide a market equilibrium.

If hypothesis C held, instead of B, the optimal level of insurance coverage would be one that yielded the curve T_1T_1', and if the industry were "competitive" in the long run, point P_1 would be chosen. Hypothesis B, however, implies that *hospitals select* the mix of quantity and quality along any line such as T_1T_1', and do not necessarily choose P_1.

Suppose, for example, that hospitals chose not P_1 but rather P_1' with insurance at the same level r^*. The contour through P_1' indicates the level of utility achieved. Feldstein and Harris present slightly different stories on how P_1' is chosen. Feldstein[12] assumes that the hospital selects the combination that maximizes some unspecified "hospital" utility function in quantity and quality. Harris assumes instead that the hospital selects the point that would have maximized net revenue of the hospital had it decided to earn profits rather than turn surpluses into quality improvements.[13] Now it is easy to see that it is *possible* that an increase in insurance in excess of the "optimal" initial level r^* may actually improve welfare. Consider an increase in coverage that shifts the opportunity locus out to T_2T_2'. If the hospital selected point P_2', the representative consumer would in fact be better off than at P_1'.

It is, however, not likely that r^* would be chosen in a B-hypothesis world. Indeed, it is quite likely that the level of coverage that would be chosen in a "neutral" (unsubsidized or taxed) insurance price environment in a B-hypothesis world would exceed r^*. The reason is that, when they chose r^* under hypothesis C, consumers were able to trade off both quantitative and qualitative moral hazard against risk reduction, whereas under hypothesis B consumers do not take qualitative moral hazard into account. No single consumer thinks that his increased purchase of insurance raises quality, and yet the net effect of an insurance-induced increase in demand is an increase in quality.

Suppose, therefore, that T_3T_3' represents the transformation curve associated with the equilibrium level of coinsurance under neutral incentives and hypothesis B. Suppose that P_3' is the quantity-quality combination the hospital selects. In this case, as in the earlier hypothetical example, an increase in coverage beyond that chosen under neutral incentives (as represented, say, by the movement from P_3' to P_2') can increase the representative consumer's utility.

---

[12] Feldstein, "Quality Change," pp. 1601–701.

[13] It does not appear that Harris's hospital equilibrium is well defined, since the conversion of profits into quality will probably shift the demand curve for quantity.

Afficionados will recognize this exercise as one in the theory of second best. We have found again that if one optimality condition is not satisfied (firms supply highest valued products), satisfaction of another condition (insurance prices reflect true cost) may not lead to optimality.

The issue of whether we can be sure we have overinsurance or not can then be reduced to the answer to one of two questions: (1) Do we live in a B-hypothesis world rather than an A-hypothesis world or a C-hypothesis world? (2) If the answer is yes, then is the marginal benefit or value of quality to the consumer greater than its cost?

It would be possible to reject hypothesis A on its face, at least for hospitals that are largely nonprofit and earn little or no net surpluses. One should be somewhat cautious, however, because the 60 percent of the health care dollar that does not go to hospitals is largely spent in markets where profits can be earned. Even in the nonprofit hospital industry, there is something other than a rise in hospital prices and costs which can equilibrate supply and demand by converting excess demand into net surplus: The fees for complementary physicians' services can rise. For instance, an excess demand for a bed for a hospital episode can be eliminated by (and can even be the cause of) higher surgeon fees under less than complete coverage.

The more plausible argument, however, is that hypothesis C is a reasonable description of long-run equilibrium for the bulk of consumers, who live in metropolitan areas in which there are choices.

Even where hypothesis B might be a better description of reality, as in a small city where consumers have few quality options, it is difficult to argue strongly for the view that quality is too low, which is necessary if increased insurance is to improve welfare. Although Harris is correct that it is invalid to conclude that physicians and hospitals "naturally burn up insurance-generated economic rents on gadgets that patients really don't need," surely the consensus of both fact and anecdote is that technology is usually carried too far. It would be hard to find any real evidence of a technology that would benefit patients but would also increase costs and that doctors and hospitals do not want to use. Moreover, the usual argument is not that doctors and hospitals provide gadgets patients don't need *at all*; rather, it is that, in their attempt to do all they can for the patient, they provide gadgets the patient does need, but only a little—that is, gadgets the patient would not choose if he had to pay the full cost. But with insurance the patient has less reason to object. It would be hard not to conclude that patients get all the quality they are willing to pay for, and possibly even a little more.

The only way to really settle the matter is to provide some direct estimates of costs and benefits of new technology—both that which has been used, and that which, because of patient unwillingness to pay the cost, has not been applied. Such research would be worthwhile, but in its absence it does seem that the overinsurance option is by far the better bet.

In all of this discussion, we have assumed that there is only one kind of consumer. If consumers have different demands for quality (or, for that matter, different demands for insurance that will lead to different demands for quality), it is likely that the market will provide a spectrum of quality levels. But if, because of some initial fixed costs, the number of product qualities falls short of the number of different ones consumers desire, we are in the world of monopolistic competition. As Spence[14] has suggested, even without distortion of the price of medical care, the competitive market does not necessarily provide the optimal number of product qualities. We are again in a second-best world; the spread of insurance *could* move us closer to the optimal number; there might be no welfare cost at all. The larger the variety of products, and the less diverse the consumer preferences, the smaller the practical problem this is. Compared to the massive distortions in the market for quality overall, it would appear that issues concerned with the mix of qualities is of less concern.

With a caution about the difficulty of making welfare judgments when there is monopolistic competition, it does appear that a neutral market for insurance should lead to optimality in an A world or a C world, whereas in a B world the best bet is that even with a neutral market we would have overinsurance.

Newhouse[15] has recently offered another argument (and some empirical evidence for it) that suggests overinsurance. He notes that insurance affects the patients' incentives to shop for a lower-cost provider. The resultant rise in price may lead to a further round of insurance coverage changes, but in any case the net effect of the spread of insurance is to reduce competition, especially if insurance is already at high levels.

Here we do have a genuine (if bizarre) externality. When a consumer buys more insurance, he does not take into account the fact that it induces him to become a less aggressive shopper. This change in search behavior in turn leads to an increase in monopoly power, *which harms all consumers*. So, at least over some range, there can be an externality leading to overinsurance even with neutral incentives.

---

[14] Michael Spence, "Product Differentiation and Welfare," *American Economic Review*, vol. 66 (May 1976), pp. 407–14.

[15] Joseph Newhouse, *The Erosion of the Medical Marketplace*, Report R-2141-1-HEW (Santa Monica, California: The Rand Corporation, 1978).

If there is overinsurance under neutral incentives, one solution is to levy a tax on the purchase of insurance. The tax is intended to reflect the costs that the insurance purchase imposes on persons other than the direct purchaser. If publicly financed partial insurance already exists in the market (such as public catastrophic insurance), then there is an additional reason to tax private supplemental insurance. The person who buys private insurance will make higher claims on the public insurance. If those claims are not to be reflected in taxes he pays for the public insurance, they should be reflected in a tax laid on the supplemental insurance itself. In principle, the tax should reflect the magnitude of additional use of catastrophic insurance for each possible level of supplementary insurance.

Controlling Moral Hazard

Up to now we have discussed the optimal extent of insurance under the assumption that moral hazard exists and must be dealt with. It should be obvious that overinsurance could be turned into optimal insurance if some way could be found to reduce moral hazard behavior. In this section I will briefly consider some such alterations.

They fall into two broad categories. One set tries to correct the distortion in user price while at the same time preserving coverage of the bulk of the financial risk by *explicit* statement of what payments will be made in what circumstances. The other approach retains the low user price on medical care, but uses consumer choice among policies that offer different *implicit* stipulations of the benefits to be provided. The first approach amounts to the use of various kinds of indemnities; the second relies on vertically integrated combinations of insurance and provision of care, as in a health maintenance organization (HMO).

As noted above, moral hazard arises because it is impossible for the insurance contract to specify precisely the different states of illness in which different payments will be made. The argument that the state of illness cannot always be measured perfectly is, of course, correct. But it does not follow that it cannot be measured at all. There are surely some types of illness for which the variation in possible conditions is sufficiently small to provide a reasonably accurate estimate of the level of expenditure that would have been chosen if the full resource cost was confronted. The insurance policy could be written to pay an indemnity of that amount, conditional upon the occurrence of the illness or condition. The consumer could then be left free to choose whatever type of care he wished. For example, in its maternity coverage the policy could pay X dollars for a normal delivery, with X dollars being set at a "reasonable" value.

Such indemnities used to be common in health insurance policies, especially those offered by commercial insurers, although inflation in medical care costs often made the benefit level too small. An easy solution to continuing inflation would be to index the indemnity benefit level to medical care prices. It would also be possible to set limits to the out-of-pocket loss (or gain), in order to avoid exposure to risk.

A less daring strategy is indemnities per unit, such as per physician visit or hospital day. Such policies do not control moral hazard with respect to quantity but they do control it with respect to quality. Although in principle the level of the indemnity could be set at any amount, there are some advantages in tying it to the cost of particular providers, as is done in the Newhouse-Taylor Variable Cost Insurance[16] or the Elwood-McClure Health Alliance. The advantage of such an approach is that the insurer performs the search process for the patient, while at the same time providing a tangible reward in the form of a larger stream of customers for a provider who keeps his charge low.

The alternative to explicit limitations on quantity or price is the implicit limitation on quantity. This usually takes the form of an HMO, which agrees to provide all the care the patient "needs" in return for a lump-sum premium. The quantity and quality of care needed is, however, to be determined by the provider. Compared to explicit limits, this approach is obviously much more flexible, since it does not require thousands of contingencies to be spelled out in advance. This advantage is, however, achieved at the cost of (a) greater difficulty in supplementation, and (b) a necessary limit to the set of providers.

Viewed from this perspective, it is likely that various combinations of benefit levels and explicit and implicit rules will appeal to different groups of people. Those who expect the nature of most illnesses involving large losses to be well defined but who like a wide range of providers to choose from should prefer explicit indemnities. Those confronting a variety of ill-defined conditions but with a reasonably well-chosen provider should prefer the HMO option. Competition is a check equally on the excesses of both groups.

Critical to efficient pluralistic choice here is a set of prices (premiums) that accurately reflect costs. Subsidies, or insulation of the choice from relative premium costs, can lead to distortions and consequent "overinsurance." Choices between options may not be made rationally, and the options that load more costs on the patient will not be preferred.

---

[16] Joseph Newhouse and Vincent Taylor, "How Shall We Pay for Hospital Care?" *The Public Interest*, no. 23 (Spring 1971), pp. 78–92.

Overinsurance and NHI

What messages do these considerations offer for the design of ideal national health insurance? First, the rationale for publicly financed or mandated insurance coverage goes beyond what has been discussed in this paper; it is usually based on some concept of consumption externality (we all feel better if everyone consumes at least adequate care) or consumer ignorance (consumers underestimate the probability of catastrophic events). It is these compulsory or tax-financed insurances designed to deal with these problems that would generally be thought to constitute a national health insurance plan.

The rationales just discussed provide the basis for the kind of income-conditioned NHI, with large deductibles and copayments for the nonpoor, that Martin Feldstein[17] and I[18] have suggested. Such arrangements are intended to deal primarily with underinsurance. But how can overinsurance be corrected under NHI? It is sometimes erroneously (at least as far as my own analysis is concerned) supposed that the tax-financed or compulsory amounts of insurance are *all* that any family is supposed to have. Getting coverage down from current high "first-dollar" levels to these much lower levels is then all that is necessary to deal with overinsurance.

A proper interpretation would, however, be that these compulsory amounts represent *basic minimums*. Coverage in excess of these amounts provides no "social benefits," but if it provides private benefits to the purchaser, there is no reason why he should be prevented from buying the insurance *as long as he pays the full cost*. Indeed, the variation in the amounts and types of insurance people buy is at present very large, a finding consistent with a wide variation in tastes for insurance.[19] There appears to be no reason not to let persons indulge their different preferences for insurance coverage.

The ideal NHI system, therefore, would provide the appropriate basic minimum coverage *and* the right "signals" for supplementary coverage. Whether the right signals are those that emerge from a neutral tax structure depends, as argued above, on whether the world is consistent with hypothesis B or hypothesis C. At a minimum, it would appear that supplementary coverage should be taxed to reflect the additional use of the basic public insurance benefit. Beyond this, there can be a case for some additional (probably moderate) taxation of

---

[17] Martin S. Feldstein, "A New Approach to National Health Insurance," *The Public Interest*, no. 23 (Spring 1971), pp. 251–80.

[18] Mark Pauly, *The Role of the Private Sector in National Health Insurance* (Washington, D.C.: Health Insurance Institute, 1979).

[19] It is also consistent with a wide variation in the net price of insurance.

supplemental insurance to take account of spillovers into quality levels or market functioning.

Removing tax subsidies and imposing a slight positive tax will obviously discourage supplementary coverage. Will it discourage coverage enough to make a difference? Arguments have been made that Americans want comprehensive coverage, and will buy it virtually no matter what. Keeler, Newhouse, and Small[20] have shown that, to the contrary, low-deductible insurance or supplementation will not, under plausible assumptions, be a rational purchase under neutral incentives. The provision of a medical loan scheme would further weaken the attraction of supplementation. There may be some people who are so risk averse, or so incapable of budgeting their expenses, that they will still adopt full coverage. But generalizing from current desire for comprehensive coverage—a desire that is quite rational for many people given current tax incentives—to an invariant taste for full insurance is probably wrong. America's love affair with comprehensive coverage is likely to go the way of America's love affair with the gas-guzzling automobile when the real costs of indulging one's preferences rise.

Conclusion

Overinsurance can occur. It usually arises from distortion in relative prices facing nonpoor purchasers of insurance. For the poor, and for catastrophic expenses, some method of encouraging coverage seems worthwhile. But for the rest of the population, an elimination of distortions, usually caused themselves by government tax policy, might also be all that is needed; a moderate tax on supplementary insurance might be called for. For those persons who presently have rational (that is, catastrophic) coverage, there surely seems to be nothing to be gained from compelling an increase in coverage under NHI, and there is much to lose in the way of waste of administrative costs and further inflationary pressure. To be sure, cost controls might moderate inflation, but they would have a greater chance of success without the demand pressure.

Up to the present, the federal government's record in redesigning the health care system has been none too successful. Perhaps a return to a more neutral position, in which individuals themselves make choices, is the best course.

---

[20] Joseph Newhouse, Emmett Keeler, and Kenneth Small, "The Demand for Supplementary Insurance or Do Deductibles Matter?" *Journal of Political Economy*, vol. 85 (October 1977), pp. 789–802.

The Tax Treatment of Health Insurance Premiums as a Cause of Overinsurance

Ronald J. Vogel

The most prevalent manner of financing government is through a tax system.[1] But any tax except a head tax[2] creates distortions in economic behavior that may have undesirable and unforeseen side effects. Likewise, health insurance affects behavior because, unlike life insurance, it is subject to moral hazard.[3] And, although health insurance reduces risk, it distorts the demand for medical care. If some economic goods are left untaxed or receive favorable tax treatment, we would expect them to be preferred to goods that receive full taxation, all other things being equal, because their effective relative prices are thereby lowered.

Health insurance is one of the economic goods that receives favorable treatment under present U.S. tax laws. Therefore, we would expect more health insurance to be purchased than if it were treated like, say, employer-paid vacations. Because the tax laws give an incentive to purchase more health insurance, and because health insurance encourages consumers to purchase more medical care than they would in the absence of health insurance, we can establish a direct link between the tax treatment of health insurance and the demand for medical care. Furthermore, the insurance-induced distorted demand for medical

NOTE: This paper was written by the author in his private capacity. No official support or endorsement by the Health Care Financing Administration or by the U.S. Department of Health, Education, and Welfare is intended or should be inferred. The author would like to thank Jeannette Austin, Roger Blair, Benjamin Bridges, Jr., Bernadette Chachere, Henry Grabowski, Mark Pauly, Harvey Sapolsky, and Robert Seidman for their thoughtful comments on two previous drafts.

[1] However, many socialist governments derive large amounts of revenue from the profits of state-owned enterprises.

[2] Yet, even a head tax could exert a negative influence on the birth rate, all other things being equal.

[3] Moral hazard is defined as a state where the insuree has control over the insured event. Even with insurance, such as life insurance, there is some moral hazard involved, but most people do not kill themselves to collect on their life insurance, and most life insurance companies will not pay for suicides. On the other hand, most persons with health insurance can obtain some form of medical care just about whenever they choose, even if it be in a hospital emergency room. See Mark V. Pauly, "The Economics of Moral Hazard," *American Economic Review*, vol. 58 (June 1968), pp. 231–37.

care is directly related to the rising cost of medical care and to what is widely perceived to be the health care "crisis."

We will first examine the history and then do an analysis of tax incentives for health insurance. Next we will review the simple analytics of the demand for medical care and the demand for health insurance, and the effects of tax subsidies. The findings of relevant empirical research in this area will then be reviewed, and estimates of total "tax expenditures" and welfare losses will be presented. Finally, we will examine the policy implications of existing tax treatment of health insurance and propose alternatives to the present situation.

History and Analysis of Tax Incentives for Health Insurance

As Table 1 indicates, private expenditures for health insurance have grown from $1.3 billion in 1950 to $39.4 billion in 1976. In the ten years between 1967 and 1976, these same expenditures grew at an average annual rate of 25.5 percent. While expenditures on health care as a percentage of GNP increased by 93 percent over the twenty-six-year period, private health insurance expenditures as a percentage of GNP increased 380 percent. And, in 1950, private health insurance expenditures were 10.7 percent of health care expenditures; by 1976, that figure had reached 28.0 percent.

Using any comparison, one sees that the private health insurance industry in the United States has been rapidly growing. One of the major reasons why private health insurance may have grown so rapidly, is that, unlike most other consumer purchases, except housing, it is heavily subsidized by the tax system.

At present, health insurance is directly subsidized by the federal income tax system in two ways. First, employer-paid health insurance premiums are fully tax deductible by the employer as business expenses, and are not considered to be taxable income of the employee. Second, up to $150 of health insurance premiums paid by the individual may be directly deducted under the individual income tax, and the rest of his health insurance premiums may be included with other medical expenses, subject to the 3 percent of adjusted gross income test, under the individual income tax. Furthermore, employer-paid health insurance premiums do not enter the Social Security tax base. And, of the forty-one states and the District of Columbia that have income taxes, all but five allow medical deductions for individuals. All allow the deduction of employer-paid premiums as business expenses. In New York City and in Maryland, medical expenses may be deducted under the local income tax.[4]

---

[4] *State Tax Reporter* (Chicago: Commerce Clearing House, 1978).

221

TABLE 1

HEALTH CARE AND PRIVATE HEALTH INSURANCE EXPENDITURES,
1950–1978

Year	(1) Gross National Product (billions of dollars)	(2) Health Care Expenditures (billions of dollars)	(3) Health Insurance Expenditures (billions of dollars)	(4) (2 ÷ 1)	(5) (3 ÷ 1)	(6) (3 ÷ 2)
1950	264.8	12,027	1,292	4.5	0.5	10.7
1955	381.0	17,330	3,150	4.5	0.8	18.2
1960	498.3	25,856	5,841	5.2	1.2	22.6
1965	658.0	38,892	10,001	5.9	1.5	25.7
1966	722.4	42,109	10,564	5.8	1.5	25.1
1967	773.5	47,897	11,105	6.2	1.4	23.2
1968	830.2	53,765	12,899	6.5	1.6	24.0
1969	904.2	60,617	14,658	6.7	1.6	24.2
1970	960.2	69,201	17,185	7.2	1.8	24.8
1971	1,019.8	77,162	19,659	7.6	1.9	25.5
1972	1,111.8	86,687	22,685	7.8	2.0	26.2
1973	1,238.6	95,383	25,196	7.7	2.0	26.4
1974	1,361.2	106,321	28,282	7.8	2.1	26.6
1975	1,454.5	123,716	33,599	8.5	2.3	27.2
1976	1,625.4	141,013	39,422	8.7	2.4	28.0
1977	1,887.2	170,000	—	9.0	—	—
1978	2,107.6	192,400	—	9.1	—	—

NOTE: Dashes indicate data are not available.
SOURCE: Robert M. Gibson and Charles R. Fisher, "National Health Expenditures, Fiscal Year 1977, *Social Security Bulletin*, vol. 41 (July 1978), pp. 3–20; Robert M. Gibson, "National Health Expenditures, 1978," *Health Care Financing Review*, vol. 1 (Summer 1979), pp. 1–36; and Marjorie Smith Carroll, "Private Health Insurance Plans in 1976: An Evaluation," *Social Security Bulletin*, vol. 41 (September 1978), pp. 3–16.

Table 2 presents Congressional Budget Office estimates of federal government direct expenditures for health care and "tax expenditures"[5] on private health insurance for fiscal 1980. It is estimated that the two types of tax expenditures mentioned above will cost the federal government $10.6 billion in fiscal year 1980. One interesting comparison here,

[5] Economists use the term "tax expenditure" for tax revenue forgone by the government due to special provisions in the tax law. In this case, the forgone tax revenue is spent by the consumer-taxpayer on the purchase of health insurance rather than by the government on, say, education or highways.

TABLE 2

TAX EXPENDITURES FOR PRIVATE HEALTH INSURANCE COMPARED
WITH DIRECT EXPENDITURE PROGRAMS FOR HEALTH CARE,
FISCAL 1980

Program	Estimated Outlays or Expenditures (billions of dollars)
Medicare	32.1
Medicaid	12.8
Tax expenditures for private health insurance	10.6
Veterans health programs	5.9
All other health services programs	5.0

SOURCE: Alice M. Rivlin, "The Effect of the Tax Laws on Health Insurance and Medical Costs," Statement by the Director of the Congressional Budget Office before the Subcommittee on Oversight, Committee on Ways and Means, and the Task Force on Tax Expenditures, Committee on the Budget, U.S. House of Representatives, July 9, 1979, p. 4.

in view of the empirical findings related to equity considerations that we shall discuss later in this paper, is that the federal government will "spend" almost as much for private health insurance as it does for the poor under the Medicaid program. The Treasury estimates that tax expenditures under the employer exclusion grew at a rate of about 19 percent a year between 1968 and 1979 and that tax expenditures under the individual income tax deduction grew 7 percent a year during the same period.[6]

The federal exclusion of the employer's contribution to health insurance premiums appears to have been allowed since the beginning of the tax law. However, a 1943 special ruling by the Internal Revenue Service supported the exclusion by declaring payments made by an employer to an employee group medical plan to be nontaxable to the employee and deductible as a business expense.[7] Formal recognition of the employer exclusion was given with the revision of the tax code in 1954.[8] The only major provision in the 1954 code was that the

[6] Eugene Steuerle and Ronald Hoffman, "Tax Expenditures for Health Care," U.S. Department of the Treasury, Office of Tax Analysis, OTA Paper No. 38, April 1979, pp. 10–11.

[7] Special Ruling, October 26, 1943, 433CCH, Federal Tax Service, paragraph 6587, as cited in Steuerle and Hoffman, "Tax Expenditures," p. 3.

[8] U.S. Department of the Treasury, Internal Revenue Service, *Internal Revenue Code of 1954* (Washington, D.C., 1954).

employee health and accident plan be employee-originated and that the insurance benefits be consumed during the period of employment. The code has remained the same since then.

On the other hand, the medical deduction under the individual income tax was not allowed until 1942, and has undergone six changes to the present, the latest in 1967. Table 3 contains a brief synopsis of the history of the medical and insurance deduction.

The limitation on what could be deducted consisted of the amount over 5 percent of "net income" between 1942 and 1948, and that amount over 5 percent of "adjusted gross income" between 1948 and 1951. From 1942 to 1951, the maximums were increased slightly and medical insurance was treated exactly as other medical expenditures. In 1951 those over sixty-five were given more generous treatment and were no longer subject to the 5 percent limitation.

The law of 1954 introduced further refinements. The 5 percent limitation was reduced to 3 percent; however, "medicine and drugs" could only be included under the 3 percent limitation to the extent that they exceeded 1 percent of adjusted gross income. Insurance premiums continued to be treated as other medical expenditures and the maximums were doubled. For the next thirteen years, the medical deduction remained basically unchanged, except that the maximums were again raised in 1961.

Medicare went into effect in July 1966 and brought sweeping changes in the medical insurance available to those aged sixty-five and over. At the same time, the medical deduction was changed in two important ways: All maximums were abolished and the treatment of health insurance was made more generous. Henceforth, half of health insurance up to $150 would be fully deductible; the other half, plus any amount over the $150, would be subject to the 3 percent limitation.[9] Beginning in 1967, those aged sixty-five and over no longer received different treatment from the rest of the population.

Before 1960, however, the tax treatment of health insurance did not consitute a "problem," because health insurance was relatively not important in the insurance industry or in the economy, and because only

---

[9] In 1978, the Carter administration tried to amend the continuous twelve-year 1967 individual income tax treatment of health insurance. The Carter proposal would have combined medical and casualty losses and would have made them deductible only to the extent that they exceeded 10 percent of adjusted gross income. All health insurance premiums would have been subject to the same floor. This proposal would not have changed the employer exclusion. The House accepted the simplification aspects of the proposal, but rejected the 10 percent floor in favor of the present 3 percent floor. However, no change was included in the Revenue Act of 1978, because the Senate rejected the House version.

TABLE 3

HISTORY OF MEDICAL DEDUCTION

Year of Enactment	Limitations	Maximum	Treatment of Insurance
1942	Medical expenses over and above 5 percent of "net income."	$2,500 for family or head of household; $1,250 for all others.	All insurance deductible over 5 percent of "net income," subject to maximums.
1948	Same treatment as in 1942, except "adjusted gross income" is substituted for "net income."	Deduction could not exceed $1,250 multiplied by the number of exemptions (excluding those for age and blindness) with a maximum deduction of $2,500. $5,000 maximum for joint return of husband and wife with dependents.	Same treatment as in 1942.
1951	Same as 1948 for those under 65 years. For those over 65, no 5 percent limitation and they can deduct dependent medical deductions which exceed 5 percent of AGI.	Same as 1948.	Same as 1948.
1954	For the first time a distinction is made between "medicine and drugs" and "medical expenses." For those under 65, medicine and drugs could be included only to the extent that they	Allowed in any case: $2,500 multiplied by number of exemptions (excluding those for age and blindness) with maximum of $10,000 for husband and wife filing jointly,	Premiums deductible to the extent that they exceed 3 percent of AGI for those under age 65. For those 65 and over, no limitation on health insurance deductibility.

225

TABLE 3—Continued

Year of Enactment	Limitations	Maximum	Treatment of Insurance
	exceed 1 percent of AGI. Medical expenses deductible if they exceed 3 percent of AGI. For those over 65, no limitation; full amount of medical expenses deductible, but "medicine and drugs" limited to amount over 1 percent of AGI. For dependents of those over 65, the 3 percent of AGI rule holds.	head of household, or surviving spouse. Could not exceed $5,000 for a single person or for a married person filing a separate return.	
1961	Same as 1954.	Maximum raised to $5,000 times the number of exemptions (excluding those for age and blindness) with a maximum of $20,000 for a joint return, head of household, or surviving spouse and $10,000 for single persons. Taxpayers 65 and older and both disabled, maximum was $40,000 if they filed jointly with a $20,000 limit for each.	Same as 1954.
1964	Same as 1954 except that for those 65 and over all expenses again fully deductible, as in 1951.	Same as 1961.	Same as 1954.
1967	1 percent on medicine and drugs and	All maximum limitations on medi-	Half the cost of medical insurance

226

3 percent on medical expenses apply to *all* taxpayers regardless of age.

cal expenses previously in effect were eliminated.

up to $150 fully deductible as a medical expense without regard to the 3 percent limitation. The remaining cost plus excess over $150 deductible as a regular medical expense. For those 65 and over payments for supplementary medical insurance under Medicare are deductible.

SOURCE: Bridger M. Mitchell and Ronald J. Vogel, *Health and Taxes: An Assessment of the Medical Deduction*, R-1222-OEO (Santa Monica, California: The Rand Corporation, 1973), p. 2.

a relatively small percentage of taxpaying families were able to itemize deductions.[10]

By examining a simple model, we can see why employers would be indifferent about paying health insurance premiums in lieu of wages and why employees would prefer to receive income in the form of health insurance premiums rather than as wages. Assume a world where the following conditions exist:

- Income may be received in money or in kind, such as employer-paid health insurance premiums.
- Labor is perfectly mobile and can move from firm to firm, depending upon opportunities for money income and income in kind.
- Labor has full knowledge of the available proportions of money income and income in kind.
- There are a large number of firms in which the individual may find employment.
- Competition and a given state of technology dictate the size of firms and the number of employees which they can hire.
- Money income is flexible both upward and downward.

Also, assume a perfectly competitive firm with the production function:

$$Q = f(K,L) \qquad (1)$$

where Q is output, K is capital, and L is labor. To maximize profits, the firm will hire the inputs K and L to the point where the value of their marginal products is just equal to the market price of K and L. The state of perfect competition makes it necessary for every firm to pay each factor input the exact value of its marginal product.

If one introduces a "fringe benefit," such as employer-provided health insurance,[11] for L, one may write:

$$W = W_M + W_I \qquad (2)$$

where W is total wages, W_M is nominal money wages and W_I is wages in kind, in the form of employer-paid health insurance premiums. Because of the assumption of perfect competition in both product and labor markets, W must be equal to the value of the marginal product of L.

---

[10] John Krizay and Andrew Wilson, *The Patient as Consumer: Health Care Financing in the United States* (Lexington, Mass.: D.C. Heath and Company, 1974), p. 3; and U.S. Bureau of the Census, *Statistical Abstract of the United States, 1978*, 99th edition, Washington, D.C., 1978, p. 269.

[11] For the moment, we leave aside the question of why something like a "fringe benefit" would arise in a perfectly competitive market. (See note 14.)

In a world where there is, for simplicity's sake, a proportional tax on money income, but not on nonmoney income or income in kind,

$$W_{NET} = W_M(1 - t) + W_I \qquad (3)$$

where W_{NET} is after-tax income and t is the tax rate on money income in the form of wages. Clearly, in this case, the employee has an incentive to channel income from W_M to W_I.[12]

Firms attempt to maximize the following objective function:

$$Y = pQ - cK - (W_M L + W_I L) \qquad (4)$$

where Y is profits, p is output price, and c is the cost of capital.

If we introduce a proportional normal profits tax with all production costs deductible, then:

$$Y_{NET} = (pQ - cK - W_M L - W_I L) \cdot (1 - t) \qquad (5)$$

where Y_{NET} is after-tax profits. Therefore, it makes no difference to the firm whether it pays employees W in the form *of* W_M or W_I because *all* production costs are deductible for tax purposes.[13]

In this simple model, which approximates the real world, we find that the employee has a positive incentive to receive income in kind, in the form of employer-paid health insurance premiums with or without a tax on those premiums.[14] The higher the tax rate on money income, the stronger that incentive; with a high income, high rates of inflation, or rising incomes, and with a progressive tax on money income, the incentive becomes even stronger.[15]

---

[12] The extent to which he will want to do this will depend upon his indifference mapping between W_M and W_I. See Peter E. Kennedy and Ronald J. Vogel, "A Theory of the Determinants of Fringe Benefits," Working Paper, Health Care Financing Administration, Washington, D.C., July 1979, pp. 7–10.

[13] The employer may see positive advantages in paying W_I if such payments enabled him to reduce labor turnover costs and, consequently, labor training costs. See Kennedy and Vogel, "A Theory of the Determinants," pp. 4–6. Even if W_I were taxed at the same rate as W_M, employees might not be indifferent to receiving income either in the form of W_M or W_I, even when there is a load factor on W_I. If there are economies of scale in the functions of providing health insurance, then the employee might receive a greater amount of health insurance protection for a given W_I, if it were bought through the group formed by the employer rather than if he had bought the insurance himself. To the extent that the load factor on "employer-provided" insurance is lower than the load factor on individual insurance, the employee has an incentive to receive some of W in the form of W_I even in the absence of tax advantages.

[14] This model thus shows why "fringe benefits" could arise in a perfectly competitive market.

[15] There is ample empirical evidence that, in the long run, "employer-paid" benefits, such as half the social security tax and health insurance premiums, are shifted backward onto the employee (as in the above model) in the form of lower W_M than would be the case without W_I. See Joseph A. Pechman, Henry J. Aaron, and

Because, in the model, the employer remains indifferent about W_I,[16] we presume that he bends to the incentives presented to his employees by government and pays what they ask in the form of W_I.

The Simple Analytics of the Demand for Medical Care and Health Insurance, and the Effects of Tax Subsidies

Following Feldstein and Friedman,[17] we posit an individual's demand for the quantity of health services, *at the time of illness*, to be a function of price. The situation is depicted in Figure 1. In the absence of health insurance, the individual would pay price P_1, and consume quantity Q_1 of health services.

People buy health insurance to protect their own wealth position at the time of illness. That is, they pay a set and known amount against an unknown future random event that, if uninsured and large enough, could wipe them out completely or leave them in serious financial difficulty. Depending upon their degree of risk aversion, they will be willing to share in the cost of that future random event in order to hold their initial health insurance premium at a lower level than it would be had they not shared. Thus, individuals are willing to pay coinsurance.[18]

Referring back to Figure 1, *at the time of illness*, this particular consumer would consume Q_2 of medical services with a coinsurance rate of C_2, or even Q_3 at the lower coinsurance rate of $C_2 \cdot P_1 (1 - t)$ (to which we will return shortly). He would consume quantities of medical care greater than Q_1, because, at the time of purchase of the medical

---

Michael K. Taussig, *Social Security: Perspectives for Reform* (Washington, D.C.: The Brookings Institution, 1968), pp. 175–78; John A. Brittain, "The Incidence of Social Security Payroll Taxes," *American Economic Review*, vol. 61 (March 1977), pp. 110–25; and Bridger M. Mitchell and Charles E. Phelps, "National Health Insurance: Some Costs and Effects of Mandated Employee Coverage," *Journal of Political Economy*, vol. 84 (May/June 1976), pp. 553–71. Even when shifted, as in the above model, tax incentives to receive W_I from the employer remain strong. If the employees do not perceive the shifting of the employer-paid premiums and count them as "extra income," the strength of the incentives for this "fringe benefit," apart from the tax subsidies, also becomes even more pronounced.

[16] It is also assumed that the employer passes any administrative costs that he may have with W_I onto his employees, just as he shifts W_I onto them.

[17] Martin S. Feldstein and Bernard S. Friedman, "Tax Subsidies, The Rational Demand for Insurance and the Health Care Crisis," *Journal of Public Economics*, vol. 7 (April 1977), pp. 155–78.

[18] Coinsurance refers to that percentage of the health services bill paid by the consumer himself. For example, with a coinsurance rate of 25 percent and no deductible, a consumer of $500 worth of health services would have to pay $125 out of his own pocket; the insurer would pay the remainder.

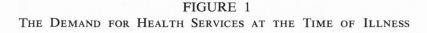

FIGURE 1

THE DEMAND FOR HEALTH SERVICES AT THE TIME OF ILLNESS

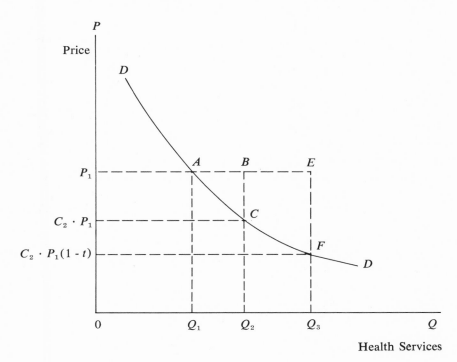

Health Services

services and due to his insurance protection, the *net* price for medical services that he faces is lower than if he had no health insurance.[19]

The area Q_1Q_2CA under the demand curve represents the value to the consumer of this additional consumption of medical services, which he would not have bought without health insurance; in this sense, we can say that he has "overpurchased" medical services. The area ABC

---

[19] Of course, this would not be true if the demand curve for medical services were perfectly inelastic—in other words, if the demand curve were perfectly vertical. Empirical studies have shown that the demand curve for medical care is not perfectly inelastic. See Martin S. Feldstein, "The Rising Price of Physicians' Services," *Review of Economics and Statistics*, vol. 52 (May 1970), pp. 121–33; Martin S. Feldstein, *The Rising Cost of Hospital Care* (Washington, D.C.: Information Resources Press, 1971); Charles E. Phelps and Joseph P. Newhouse, "The Effects of Coinsurance: A Multivariate Analysis," *Social Security Bulletin*, vol. 35 (June 1972), pp. 20–28; Joseph P. Newhouse and Charles E. Phelps, "New Estimates of Price and Income Elasticities," in Richard Rosett, ed., *The Role of Health Insurance in the Health Services Sector* (New York: National Bureau of Economic Research, 1976).

over the demand curve represents the "welfare loss" to society of this additional consumption.[20]

If a tax subsidy for the purchase of health insurance is introduced, and the demand function for health insurance is downward sloping, we would expect more health insurance to be purchased. This is because, at the margin, the tax subsidy has made the price lower per unit of health insurance purchased. Table 4 shows a hypothetical example of the arithmetic involved. If there were no insurance deduction and the employer-paid insurance premiums of $250 were treated as taxable income to the employee, this person's taxable income, after he deducted medical expenses, would be $24,612.50. He would owe a tax of $4,179. With no health insurance deduction for the premiums which he himself pays, his tax bill would be $70 less. Given the present treatment of health insurance under the income tax, his tax is only $4,011, so he receives a tax discount of $168 for the purchase of health insurance. Referring back to Figure 1, his tax discount can be translated into price $C_2 \cdot P_1 (1 - t)$.[21]

Before the tax subsidy, health insurance enabled the consumer to purchase Q_2 of medical services, *at the time of illness*. With the tax subsidy to his purchase of health insurance, he can now purchase Q_3 of medical services, at the time of illness. Therefore, in Figure 1, we can identify a further welfare loss of the amount *BEFC*. The consumer is now "overinsured" in the sense that he does not *fully* value the additional amount of insurance that he possesses due to the tax subsidy. His own full valuation is measured by the area under his demand curve. In a world where there were only head taxes and all income transfers were in cash (in other words, welfare recipients were given cash rather than food stamps or subsidized housing), there would be no welfare losses, because economic behavior would not be distorted. Here, in the

---

[20] Because the representative individual does pay the full actuarial cost of Q_2, "welfare loss" here refers to the excess over the value received of quantity times the price of the subsidized units of purchase, which this consumer would not buy if he had to pay all of it out of his own pocket, at the time of purchase—that is, the area *ABC* over his demand curve. See Mark V. Pauly, "A Measure of the Welfare Cost of Health Insurance," *Health Services Research*, vol. 4 (Winter 1969), pp. 281–91; Martin S. Feldstein, "The Welfare Loss of Excess Health Insurance," *Journal of Political Economy*, vol. 81 (March/April 1973), pp. 251–280; and Charles E. Phelps and Joseph P. Newhouse, *Coinsurance and the Demand for Medical Services*, R-964-1-OEO (Santa Monica, California: The Rand Corporation, 1974).

[21] Most insurance policies contain both a deductible and a coinsurance rate. Here, for analytical simplicity, we view the C as average coinsurance rates. Also, the present United States income tax is progressive, but for simplicity of exposition it is more convenient to think of it as being proportional. These simplifying assumptions do not invalidate the theoretical argument when the theoretical argument is applied to the world as it actually exists.

chain of progression from tax subsidy to overinsurance and from over-insurance to the overpurchase of medical services, we have identified two economic distortions through subsidies, and, consequently, two welfare losses to society as a whole.[22]

Do these analytic findings imply that tax subsidies for the purchase of health insurance should be abolished, and even, indeed, that the sale of health insurance in its present form should not be allowed? The answer to those two questions depends upon how much economic inefficiency society is willing to bear in order to achieve other goals that it may have. For example, if equity is seen as an important goal, and the tax subsidy achieves the goal better than any other instrument, then society may be willing to bear the welfare losses that the tax subsidy produces in the achievement of a more equitable society.

The economist, *qua* economist, cannot answer those questions. All the economist can do is point out the economic consequences of certain policies and then point to less costly policies for achieving designated objectives. In the next section, we attempt to quantify the consequences of the present tax–health insurance–medical purchase chain of events.

Empirical Findings

The present tax deduction under the individual income tax can be expressed formally as:

$$D = \tfrac{1}{2}I + \max\left\{(M_M - 0. \cdot 01 Y_G), 0\right\} + \max\left\{(M_H - 0. \cdot 03 Y_G), 01\right\} \tag{6}$$

where M_M is expenditures on medicine and drugs, and M_H is health care expenditures not covered by insurance plus insurance expenditures not included in the $\tfrac{1}{2}I \leq \$150$, which is health insurance expenditures. Y_G is adjusted gross income. The constraints on D, the medical deduction, is that $0 \leq D \leq Y_G$. At the margin, the individual's tax liability is defined as:

$$Y_N = Y_G - D_M \tag{7a}$$
$$T = t x Y_N \tag{7b}$$

where T is the person's tax liability after D_M, the medical deduction, has been taken; t is his marginal tax rate; and Y_G and Y_N are, respectively, adjusted gross and net income. As the question is formulated in

---

[22] Because there are benefits from risk reduction, the total welfare loss is less than the geometric area $ABC + BEFC$ in Figure 1. At the margin, at $C_2 \cdot P_1$, the reduction in risk is just equal in value to BC. Even in the area $BEFC$, there remain some benefits from risk reduction.

TABLE 4

HYPOTHETICAL INDIVIDUAL TAX RETURN

	Total Amount	Amount Spent Out of Pocket
Adjusted gross income (AGI)	$25,000	$4,000 (deductible)
Medical expenses	4,000	− 250
Medicine and drugs	450	$3,750
Self-paid insurance premiums	350	× 0.25 (coinsurance rate)
Employer-paid insurance premiums	250	$937.50
Deductible on insurance policy	250	+ 250.00 (deductible)
Coinsurance rate	25%	$1,187.50

Medical Deduction on Form 1040

Medical and dental expenses (not paid by insurance or otherwise):

		Amount
1.	One-half (but not more than $150) of insurance premiums you paid for medical care	$ 150.00
2.	Medicine and drugs	450.00
3.	Enter 1 percent of Form 1040, line 31 (AGI)	250.00
4.	Subtract line 3 from line 2	200.00
5.	Balance on insurance premiums for medical care not entered on line 1	200.00
6.	Other medical and dental expenses	1,187.50
7.	Total (add lines 4 through 6)	1,587.50
8.	Enter 3 percent of Form 1040, line 31 (AGI)	750.00
9.	Subtract line 8 from line 7	837.50

10. Total medical and dental expenses (add lines 1 and 9) 987.50

Tax Discount	Above Example	No Insurance Deduction	No Insurance Deduction and Employer Contribution Treated as Taxable Income
Taxable income	$24,012.50	$24,362.50	$24,612.50
Tax[a]	4,011.00	4,109.00	4,179.00
Tax discount on insurance	168.00	70.00	0.00

[a] Married couple, filing a joint return. The source of the tax computation is: U.S. Department of the Treasury, Internal Revenue Service, *Your Federal Income Tax: 1979 Edition*, Publication 17, Washington, D.C., 1978, tax table B, p. 175.
SOURCE: Author's calculations.

equations (6), (7a), and (7b), it is clear that the insurance portion of the medical deduction has the same effect as an insurance policy with a coinsurance rate of $(1 - t)$. Then comes a deductible proportional to income, after which there is a second coinsurance rate equal to $(1 - t)$. Unlike with ordinary health insurance policies, the deductible is proportional to income, while both coinsurance rates are regressive to income, because under a progressive income tax system $\delta t/\delta Y_G > 0$.

Tax experts usually judge taxes on the basis of three effects: efficiency, equity, and stabilization.[23] We may judge the tax treatment of health insurance using the same criteria. In the previous section, we analyzed the distortions brought about by the subsidy of a subsidy in health insurance-medical services, and the consequent efficiency loss. The previous paragraph showed that, because the health insurance subsidy is a function of the marginal tax rate under a progressive income tax system, it can be regressive.[24] As yet, we have not discussed its stabilization effects.[25] We will do so following the discussion concerning the empirical findings on efficiency and equity effects.

For the purpose of this paper, there have been three important contributions to the literature on the topic of taxation, health insurance, and medical services. Feldstein and Allison, Mitchell and Vogel, and Feldstein and Friedman have all explicitly addressed the tax issue empirically.[26]

Using 1969 data, Feldstein and Allison found that the exclusion of employers' premium payments for health insurance resulted in a tax expenditure of $1.63 billion. The distribution of the employer contribu-

---

[23] Richard A. Musgrave and Peggy B. Musgrave, *Public Finance in Theory and Practice* (New York: McGraw-Hill, 1976), chapter 1.

[24] Its ultimate regressivity is a function of the interplay between the deductible and the tax-produced coinsurance rate. At a very low deductible with steep progressivity of the tax schedule, it would be more regressive than at a high deductible that few people could meet, or with any deductible and no progressivity in the tax system. Also, its value as a subsidy may be more now than in 1967, because of rising prices and incomes. If the price level of insurance rises faster than the income upon which the deductible is based, the subsidy is worth more in real terms for those in higher marginal tax brackets.

[25] By "stabilization" we mean here its effects upon the dynamics of the price system. The relative price of the medical care system has an effect upon the absolute price system, of which it now constitutes almost 10 percent. See Robert M. Gibson, "National Health Expenditures, 1978," *Health Care Financing Review*, vol. 1 (Summer 1979), pp. 1–36.

[26] Martin S. Feldstein and Elizabeth Allison, "Tax Subsidies of Private Health Insurance: Distribution, Revenue Loss and Effects," in U.S. Congress, Joint Economic Committee, *The Economics of Federal Subsidy Programs*, Part 8—Selected Subsidies (Washington, D.C., 1974); Bridger M. Mitchell and Ronald J. Vogel, "Health and Taxes: An Assessment of the Medical Deduction," *Southern Economic Journal*, vol. 41 (April 1975), pp. 660–72. Feldstein and Friedman, "Tax Subsidies, The Rational Demand for Insurance," pp. 155–78.

tion by family income rose from $96 for those earning less than $1,000 to about $170 for those earning $10,000 or more. Tax savings per family as a result of the exclusion ranged from $12.10 at the lowest level of income to $58.81 for those earning more than $25,000. Feldstein and Allison also found that 29 percent of these families had incomes below $6,000, but these same families had only 19.2 percent of the cumulative percentage of the tax reduction. On the other end of the distribution, the top 16 percent of families received 23 percent of the tax reductions.

Feldstein and Allison next analyzed the $\frac{1}{2}I$ portion of the health insurance deduction under the individual income tax. Tax reductions here were estimated to be $389 million using a statutory tax rate method, and $339 million using an effective tax rate method.[27] Feldstein and Allison refer to the regressivity of this part of the tax deduction as "striking." For example, they found that a third of the tax reduction goes to the 10 percent of taxpaying families with incomes above $15,000, and that taxpaying families with incomes less than $6,000 account for 50 percent of the returns but only receive 10 percent of the tax reduction.

After a discussion of the effects of these two subsidies on the demand for insurance and health services, they come to the conclusion that the subsidy causes "a substantial revenue loss, distributes these tax reductions very regressively, encourages an excessive purchase of insurance, distorts the demand for health services, and thus inflates the prices of these services."[28]

The one flaw in their analysis is that they underestimate the size of the tax subsidy for the purchase of health insurance because, in analyzing the health insurance deduction under the individual income tax, they did not account for that portion of the health insurance premium which may be included under the max $\{(M_H - 0.03Y_G), 0\}$ rubric.

Using Internal Revenue Service data for 1970, Mitchell and Vogel corrected that oversight. They estimated total tax subsidies for the purchase of health insurance to be $2.5 billion for the employer exclusion and $600 million from personal income tax deductions. Consistent with the Feldstein and Allison results, Mitchell and Vogel found a mean subsidy per taxpayer ranging from $1.06 for a person with an adjusted gross income (AGI) below $3,000 to $40.03 for a person with a AGI greater than $50,000. The mean subsidy per

---

[27] See Feldstein and Allison, "Tax Subsidies of Private Health Insurance," pp. 977 and 979, for the conceptual difference in the two methods.

[28] Feldstein and Allison, "Tax Subsidies of Private Health Insurance," p. 984.

itemizing taxpayer ranged from $9.51 to $40.72 for the same AGI groups respectively.

If one restricts the tabulations to only those taxpayers having personal insurance premiums, the tax subsidy becomes even more regressive. The subsidy per insurance policy rose from $15 for adjusted gross income below $3,000 to $62 for income above $50,000. Moreover, the subsidy as a percentage of the health insurance premium rose from 8.4 percent to 25.6 percent for the same AGI classes.

The importance of this finding stems from the fact that for employees who work in a group of 100 or more, a 10 percent subsidy is sufficient to cover the entire loading cost (administrative costs and profits of the insurer) of the policy.[29] Personal income tax subsidies reach 10 percent of the premium at an AGI of $6,000, so that anyone with an income of $6,000 or more has a positive incentive to purchase group health insurance at no loading cost to himself. Furthermore, because the percentage subsidy increases with income, current tax policy toward health insurance allows middle- and upper-income taxpayers to make money by buying group health insurance rather than paying their medical expenses directly. Mitchell and Vogel conclude that, because of present tax treatment, "employees have a financial incentive to buy the most comprehensive insurance they can obtain through their employer's group policy (even when their employer makes no contribution to the premium charged)."[30] If the employer contributes to the plan, and even if 100 percent of the employer-paid premium is shifted back to the employee, the employee gains an even larger tax subsidy because there is no tax whatever on the employer contribution.

Feldstein and Friedman present a comprehensive analysis of the total "problem." As they point out, the consumer's optimal purchase of health insurance is a balance of his gain from eliminating risk against his loss from distortions of his behavior. Their theoretical analysis proceeds along the lines of the previous section of this paper. Then they estimate what optimal coinsurance rates would be with the tax subsidy at different marginal tax rates, and what they would be without the tax subsidy,[31] assuming combinations of three different price elasticities and three different degrees of risk aversion.

They find, for example, that with moderate risk aversion and with a moderate price elasticity of demand for health insurance, a family

---

[29] Charles E. Phelps, *The Demand for Health Insurance: A Theoretical and Empirical Investigation*, R-964-1-OEO (Santa Monica, California: The Rand Corporation, 1974).

[30] Mitchell and Vogel, "Health and Taxes," p. 669.

[31] Examining different coinsurance rates is one measure of the differences in *quantities* of health insurance purchased.

with a combined marginal tax rate of 21 percent would want a coinsurance rate of 80 percent with no tax subsidy; with the tax subsidy, this family would want a coinsurance rate of 58 percent. For such a family, the tax subsidy more than doubles the amount of the insured proportion. On an aggregate basis, their calculations show that average effective coinsurance rates would rise from about 40 percent with the tax subsidy to between 55 and 60 percent without the tax subsidy. This represents about a 50 percent increase in the share paid by health insurance, because of the tax subsidy.

Finally, Feldstein and Friedman analyze the dynamics of the growth of health insurance and the price of care. They conclude their paper with a short discussion of the loss in welfare due to the tax and insurance subsidies. They conclude that in 1970 alone, the welfare loss was approximately $8 billion—a substantial amount, because the total subsidy was $4 billion.

The findings in these three empirical studies indicate that the present tax treatment of health insurance premiums leaves much to be desired under any of the three tax criteria mentioned earlier in this section. On efficiency grounds the tax treatment generates extremely large welfare losses in relation to the size of the subsidy; it must, therefore, be judged to be an inefficient subsidy. Because part of the subsidy is an increasing function of the marginal tax rate, which increases with income, and because the other part of the subsidy leaves completely untaxed nonmoney income which increases as income increases,[32] the tax subsidy violates the canons of both horizontal and vertical equity within the income tax system.[33]

Finally, this subsidy has been responsible for substantial price increases within the health care system, because physicians and hospitals have been induced by it to produce a different and more expensive product.[34] The nature and "quality" of medical care has changed as patients demand more of it because of its relatively lower net price at the time of illness, due to insurance, even though these changes may not affect the efficacy of medical care. One example of this phenomenon would be patients who, because of a lower net price due to health insurance, choose a private room rather than a semiprivate room. Another example is a physician ordering a myriad of tests on the

---

[32] See Kennedy and Vogel, "A Theory of the Determinants," p. 13.

[33] Horizontal equity states that individuals in similar situations should be treated similarly. Vertical equity states that individuals in dissimilar situations should be treated dissimilarly.

[34] Martin S. Feldstein, "Hospital Cost Inflation: A Study in Non-Profit Dynamics," *American Economic Review*, vol. 61 (December 1971), pp. 853–72; and Feldstein, *The Rising Cost of Hospital Care*.

patient rather than only two or three commonly known effective tests, "because insurance will pay for it." Such choices create inflation in the medical market by driving up the gross price of a day in the hospital. Their effect on health per se is oftentimes debatable. To the extent that the health sector constitutes almost 10 percent of gross national product,[35] inflationary pressures are exerted on the rest of the economy.

Alternatives to the Present Tax Treatment of Health Insurance Premiums

Both the tax credit and the deduction are instruments for decreasing tax liability, and, because they produce income and substitution effects, they influence taxpayer behavior. A flat credit of $100 will always have a greater effect than a deduction of $100,[36] because the deduction is a function of the marginal tax rate, whereas the credit is not. With a credit, there is only a positive income effect; with a deduction, there is a positive income effect and a negative substitution effect. As one authority on deductions sees it, the criterion for the choice of a credit or a deduction turns on whether the Congress or the policy maker wishes to subsidize a certain form of expenditure (a credit), or wishes to further refine taxable income (a deduction).[37]

In the public finance literature, discussion of the credit versus the deduction has centered upon the incentive power of the credit and the consequent loss of tax revenue. The largest single problem with the deduction is that the percentage of an individual's deductible expenses paid by government depends directly upon his marginal tax rate. As a result, the rich benefit more than the poor.

The medical deduction has been in existence since 1942, and although a medical credit has never been allowed, the specification of the medical deduction has gradually moved toward a policy of subsidizing more health insurance and more medical care, thus moving closer to the intent of a credit.[38] However, given the historical evolution of the health insurance subsidy under the insurance portion of the medical deduction, and especially under the employer exclusion, the effects have become quite unlike any other provision within the entire individual income tax system. If efficiency and equity in this sector are to be restored, revision of this provision in the tax law is needed.

---

[35] Robert M. Gibson, "National Health Expenditures, 1978," pp. 1–36.

[36] Assuming that the marginal tax rate never reaches 100 percent or more.

[37] C. Harry Kahn, *Personal Deductions in the Federal Income Tax* (Princeton, N.J.: Princeton University Press, 1960), p. 174.

[38] One could continue to make a case for the use of the medical deduction for refining income for tax purposes. It seems difficult to make a similar case for health insurance as it is now treated under the tax laws.

Recently, the Congressional Budget Office (CBO)[39] and staff of the Treasury's Office of Tax Analysis[40] have put forward possible alternatives to the present federal tax treatment of health insurance premiums.

In her congressional testimony, CBO Director Alice Rivlin posed the following alternatives, which she said were not mutually exclusive: (1) repealing the separate deduction for health insurance premiums; (2) limiting the employer exclusion to a fixed dollar amount; (3) requiring firms to offer a choice of health plans and to make equal contributions to each; and (4) requiring that all tax-subsidized health plans contain deductibles or coinsurance requirements or both.

Steuerle and Hoffman discuss three other possibilities: (1) including employer contributions as income to his employees; (2) increasing the deduction floor, now 3 percent of adjusted gross income; and (3) converting the personal deduction to a personal credit.

Each of these proposals has its pros and its cons, but their ultimate acceptance can only be judged from the point of view of the policy goals they hope to achieve. For example, Rivlin's first alternative would, at the margin, reduce the tax subsidy to purchase health insurance, but by only a minimal amount. Steuerle and Hoffman's first alternative would still allow an insurance deduction for those taxpayers who itemize their deductions. The point is that there are a multiplicity of permutations and combinations of policy alternatives such as the seven presented above, each carrying its own efficiency, equity, and price stabilization effects.

This paper points to the present tax treatment of health insurance as a cause of "overinsurance." Technically, we have defined "overinsurance" as the quantity of health insurance over and above that amount of health insurance that the consumer would buy in the absence of tax subsidies. Therefore, the solution to "technical overinsurance" is a simple one: the legislative elimination of all tax subsidies. Furthermore, restoration of equity requires that the treatment of health insurance cease to be a function of the marginal tax rate.

Theoretically, then, health insurance would most likely evolve into a form much like other types of insurance such as life or casualty. In other words, people would only insure against those medical events which have a small probability of happening, but which, when they do

---

[39] Alice M. Rivlin, "The Effects of the Tax Laws on Health Insurance and Medical Costs," Statement by the Director of the Congressional Budget Office before the Subcommittee on Oversight, Committee on Ways and Means, and the Task Force on Tax Expenditures, Committee on the Budget, U.S. House of Representatives, July 9, 1979, pp. 7–13.

[40] Steuerle and Hoffman, "Tax Expenditures for Health Care," pp. 24–31.

241

happen, have financially catastrophic consequences. This would imply the evolution of relatively higher deductibles and higher coinsurance payments, as with casualty insurance. If it were deemed financially difficult for some members of society, such as those in low-paying marginal jobs, to purchase this new form of health insurance, there is no reason why government payments in cash could not be made to them so that they might still purchase health insurance. Thus, efficiency and equity would be preserved, as would a greater chance for price stability.

Because of the existence of moral hazard, the subsidy inherent in health insurance itself can never be eliminated. However, the existence of high deductibles and high coinsurance rates considerably mitigates moral hazard. In the end, it appears that the "optimal" amount of health insurance purchased depends on the balancing of the consumers' gain through avoiding risk against the welfare losses due to the distortions in their behavior caused by health insurance.

Thus far, we have ignored the institutional environment in which health insurance has grown so rapidly in recent years. Enthoven emphasizes the importance of federal tax subsidies in conjunction with unionization and collective bargaining, plus other government policies that encourage *job-related* health insurance.[41] Although, in a time-series regression, Kennedy and Vogel could find no statistical significance on a dummy variable for years when wage-price controls were in effect,[42] it has often been alleged by anecdote that unions sought increases in pay for their members via fringe benefits such as health insurance, which were exempt from wage-price controls.

Be that as it may, union leaders now do bargain aggressively for health insurance benefits because both unions and employers recognize the importance of tax-sheltered income for employees. Union leaders may use increases in fringe benefits to bind members to the union.[43] They may also recognize that fringe benefits like health insurance are more visible to the membership if they are spread broadly among the membership in the form of shallow coverage for the many small events of illness rather than centered on the relatively few events of serious illness. Thus, the tax incentives together with the union leadership's incentives create an atmosphere where broader, and consequently more costly, health insurance is purchased.

It is an open question whether the removal of all tax subsidies for the purchase of health insurance would eliminate the job-centered purchase of health insurance. At the margin, health insurance would

---

[41] Alain C. Enthoven, "Consumer-Centered vs. Job-Centered Health Insurance," *Harvard Business Review*, vol. 57 (January/February 1979), pp. 141–52.

[42] Kennedy and Vogel, "A Theory of the Determinants," p. 12.

[43] Ibid., pp. 4–6.

become more costly for the tax-itemizing employee and we would expect him to consume less of it. If employers were no longer able to deduct their "contributions" to employee plans as business expenses, their after-tax profits would be lowered, and we would expect employers and their stockholders to offer much more resistance to union demands.

Eliminating the deduction would also tend to lower the demand for health insurance. If employer "contributions" were attributed to employee income as taxable income, then employees might then want to take more income in the form of cash, rather than in the form of shallow health insurance. Such a course of action might also change employee perception about who actually does pay for all of the health insurance protection provided. This in turn might convince employees to shop around for less costly forms of health insurance, make them less reliant on the union, and make the purchase of health insurance less job-oriented and more like the purchase of other consumer goods.

One could argue that the purchase of health insurance would then move toward the more expensive *individual* health insurance policies. But this need not be the case at all. The union could still be the group bargaining agent for *group* health insurance from commercial insurers. At this juncture, however, employees would bear all or most of the cost of the health insurance, would perceive that fact, and would make their decisions about the quantity of health insurance to be purchased accordingly.

It seems likely that the United States will eventually have some form of national health insurance. Many of the bills introduced in Congress have the same structural defects as those forms of health insurance discussed in this volume. With the exception of three bills, all of the bills also assume the continued present tax treatment of health insurance premiums.[44] Because the employer exclusion is a much larger tax subsidy for the purchase of health insurance than is the personal deduction, those bills that rely primarily on "employer contributions" would encourage a further overpurchase of health insurance under present tax treatment. Less distortion would be created by placing more reliance on employee contributions, but this course of action might not be possible politically, because many of the present bills aim at broader insurance coverage for the entire population, with either the employer or government footing most of the cost.

To solve the problem of overinsurance as analyzed in this paper,

---

[44] Saul Waldman, *National Health Insurance Proposals*, HEW Publication No. (SSA) 76-11920, Washington, D.C., 1976; Gordon R. Trapnell, *A Comparison of the Cost of Major National Health Insurance Proposals*, Report No. PB-259-153 (Springfield, Va.: National Technical Information Service, 1976); Congressional Budget Office, *Controlling Rising Hospital Costs*, Washington, D.C., 1979, p. 67.

Feldstein and Friedman have proposed their own national health insurance program.[45] They would completely eliminate all tax subsidies for the purchase of health insurance. National health insurance would have high deductibles and high coinsurance rates. Furthermore, it would not be possible to buy health insurance supplemental to national health insurance because the deductibles and coinsurance payments would have to be paid in cash and would *not* be reimbursable under any other privately supplied supplementary health insurance system. From an economic point of view, this would be an interesting health insurance system. Whether it could emerge under present institutional arrangements, and given the politics of the debate on national health insurance, is another matter.

Concluding Remarks

In public discussions,[46] it is not generally recognized that the United States has had a rapidly progressing form of national health insurance since 1942. However, initially, this form of health insurance could barely be described as "national." Only 12 percent of taxpayers itemized deductions.[47] Health insurance constituted only a small percentage of GNP,[48] so the employer exclusion was relatively unimportant. There were few state income taxes, the social security tax rate was low, and the tax had a small base.

The Congressional Budget Office projects that by 1984, if current tax treatment is continued, federal tax expenditures for health will be $25 billion, the bulk of which are subsidies for the purchase of health insurance.[49] Today more than 20 million households, or 24 percent of all taxpayers, have a health insurance subsidy under the individual income tax,[50] and about 80 percent of the work force benefits from the employer exclusion.[51] Furthermore, state income taxes, which contain

---

[45] Feldstein and Friedman, "Tax Subsidies, The Rational Demand for Health Insurance," p. 177.

[46] American Enterprise Institute, *Rising Health Costs: Public and Private Responses*, Round Table Discussion, April 26, 1979, (Washington, D.C.: American Enterprise Institute, 1979).

[47] U.S. Department of the Treasury, Internal Revenue Service, *Statistics of Income for 1943*, Washington, D.C., 1943, pp. 21 and 101.

[48] Krizay and Wilson, *The Patient as Consumer*, p. 198.

[49] Congressional Budget Office, *Five-Year Budget Projections and Alternative Budgetary Strategies for Fiscal Years 1980–1984, Supplemental Report on Tax Expenditures*, Washington, D.C., 1979, table 1, p. 18.

[50] U.S. Department of the Treasury, *Statistics of Income: Individual Income Tax Returns*, Washington, D.C., 1976, pp. 3 and 58.

[51] Walter Kolodrubetz, "Group Health Insurance Coverage of Full-Time Employees, 1972," *Social Security Bulletin*, vol. 37 (April 1974), p. 17.

the same provisions as federal tax law, prevail. The employer exclusion is even more valuable today because of inflation and rising real incomes, and because the social security tax is high and the employer exclusion escapes the social security tax too. Thus, for example, a person who is in the 25 percent federal tax bracket, is in the 10 percent state tax bracket, and is subject to an 11 percent social security tax[52] has an effective subsidy (or discount) for the purchase of health insurance through his employer of about 46 percent, at the margin. It is not surprising, then, that employer-provided health insurance has been the most rapidly growing fringe benefit in recent years.[53]

Musgrave first coined the term "merit good"[54] for wants that, in theory, the private sector could supply and demand but that the body politic deemed to be supplied or demanded not at all or in too small quantities. Examples would be free school lunches and subsidized housing. The present tax treatment of health insurance implies that health insurance is a merit good, because much more of it is sold and bought than the private sector would either supply or demand in the absence of the large tax subsidy.

However, if Congress chooses to continue the present tax treatment for this "merit good," then it should realize that it is doing so at an extremely large cost. Feldstein calculated that the welfare loss of $4 billion health insurance tax subsidy was $8 billion in 1970.[55] If we use simple proportions, then the welfare loss of the $10.6 billion tax subsidy will be $21.2 billion in 1980 and $50 billion in 1984.[56] By way of contrast, the value of all imported petroleum products into the United States was $25 billion in 1975 and $42 billion in 1977.[57]

This paper has detailed the substantial inefficiencies involved in the present approach. Moreover, the present tax treatment of health

---

[52] We assume here, as in our history and analysis section, and bolstered by the empirical evidence cited there, that the employer's half of the social security tax is shifted back onto the employee.

[53] Kennedy and Vogel, "A Theory of the Determinants," table 3.

[54] Richard A. Musgrave, *The Theory of Public Finance* (New York: McGraw-Hill, 1959), pp. 13–14.

[55] Feldstein, "The Welfare Loss of Excess Health Insurance," pp. 251–80.

[56] A simple geometric demonstration will show that to assume proportionality, with a linear demand curve, will *understate* the true welfare loss. If the demand curve is convex to the origin, it will understate the welfare loss even more. See Pauly, "A Measure of the Welfare Cost," p. 287. Also, current estimates of the welfare loss from excess health insurance may be greatly understated because these estimates are based on the assumption of a competitive supply curve in the medical care sector. See Joseph P. Newhouse, *The Erosion of the Medical Market Place*, R-2141-1-HEW (Santa Monica, California: The Rand Corporation, 1978), p. 32.

[57] Bureau of the Census, *Statistical Abstract of the United States: 1978*, overleaf.

insurance is also extremely inequitable and violates the intent of a progressive income tax. Finally, it makes little sense to try to control inflation at the national level and at the same time to subsidize health insurance. The reason is that such insurance is one of the major causes of inflation in a sector of the economy that is becoming increasingly more important as it approaches 10 percent of GNP.

These three overwhelming deficiencies in the present tax treatment of health insurance make it seem desirable to eliminate or greatly modify such tax treatment. If health insurance continues to be viewed as a merit good by society, then there are other more efficient, more equitable, and more price-stabilizing ways of providing it through the public sector than is now being done through the tax system.

Bibliography

American Enterprise Institute. *Rising Health Costs: Public and Private Responses*. Round Table Discussion. Washington, D.C.: American Enterprise Institute, 1979.

Arrow, Kenneth J. "Uncertainty and the Welfare Economics of Medical Care." *American Economic Review* 53 (December 1963): 941–974.

Brittain, John A. "The Incidence of Social Security Payroll Taxes." *American Economic Review* 61 (March 1971): 110–125.

Brittain, John A. *The Payroll Tax for Social Security*. Washington, D.C.: The Brookings Institution, 1972.

Carroll, Marjorie Smith. "Private Health Insurance Plans in 1976: An Evaluation." *Social Security Bulletin* 41 (September 1978): 3–16.

Commerce Clearing House. *State Tax Reporter*. Chicago: Commerce Clearing House, 1978.

Congressional Budget Office. *Controlling Rising Hospital Costs*. Washington, D.C.: 1979.

Congressional Budget Office. *Five-Year Budget Projections and Alternative Budgetary Strategies for Fiscal Years 1980–1984, Supplemental Report on Tax Expenditures*. Washington, D.C.: 1979.

Enthoven, Alain C. "Consumer-Centered vs. Job-Centered Health Insurance." *Harvard Business Review* 57 (January/February 1979): 141–152.

Feldstein, Martin S. "Hospital Cost Inflation: A Study in Non-Profit Dynamics." *American Economic Review* 61 (December 1971): 853–872.

Feldstein, Martin S. *The Rising Cost of Hospital Care*. Washington, D.C.: Information Resources Press, 1971.

Feldstein, Martin S. "The Rising Price of Physicians' Services." *Review of Economics and Statistics* 52 (May 1970): 121–133.

Feldstein, Martin S. "The Welfare Loss of Excess Health Insurance." *Journal of Political Economy* 81 (March/April 1973): 251–280.

Feldstein, Martin S., and Elizabeth Allison. "Tax Subsidies of Private Health Insurance: Distribution, Revenue Loss and Effects." In *The Economics of Federal Subsidy Programs*, U.S. Congress, Joint Economic Committee. Washington, D.C.: 1974.

Feldstein, Martin S., and Bernard Friedman. "Tax Subsidies, the Rational Demand for Insurance and the Health Crisis." *Journal of Public Economics* 7 (April 1977): 155–178.

Gibson, Robert M. "National Health Expenditures, 1978." *Health Care Financing Review* 1 (Summer 1979): 1–36.

Gibson, Robert M., and Charles R. Fisher. "National Health Expenditures, Fiscal Year 1977." *Social Security Bulletin* 41 (July 1978): 3–20.

Jensen, James E. "Medical Expenditures and Medical Deduction Plans." *Journal of Political Economy* 60 (December 1952): 503–524.

Jensen, James E. "Rationale of the Medical Expense Deduction." *National Tax Journal* 7 (September 1954): 274–284.

Kahn, C. Harry. *Personal Deductions in the Federal Income Tax.* Princeton: Princeton University Press, 1960.

Kennedy, Peter E., and Ronald J. Vogel. "A Theory of the Determinants of Fringe Benefits." Working paper. Washington, D.C.: Health Care Financing Administration, July 1979.

Kolodrubetz, Walter. "Group Health Insurance Coverage of Full-Time Employees, 1972." *Social Security Bulletin* 37 (April 1974): 17–35.

Krizay, John, and Andrew Wilson. *The Patient as Consumer: Health Care Financing in the United States.* Lexington, Mass.: D. C. Heath, 1974.

Meyer, Jack A. *Health Care Cost Increases.* Washington, D.C.: American Enterprise Institute, 1979.

Mitchell, Bridger M., and Charles E. Phelps. "National Health Insurance: Some Costs and Effects of Mandated Employee Coverage." *Journal of Political Economy* 84 (May/June, 1976): 553–571.

Mitchell, Bridger M., and Ronald J. Vogel. *Health and Taxes: An Assessment of the Medical Deduction.* R–1222–OEO. Santa Monica, California: The Rand Corporation, 1973.

Mitchell, Bridger M., and Ronald J. Vogel. "Health and Taxes: An Assessment of the Medical Deduction." *Southern Economic Journal* 41 (April 1975): 660–672.

Musgrave, Richard A. *The Theory of Public Finance*. New York: McGraw-Hill, 1959.

Musgrave, Richard A., and Peggy B. Musgrave. *Public Finance in Theory and Practice*. New York: McGraw-Hill, 1976.

Newhouse, Joseph P. *The Erosion of the Medical Market Place*. R–2141–1–HEW. Santa Monica, California: The Rand Corporation, 1978.

Newhouse, Joseph P., and Charles E. Phelps. "New Estimates of Price and Income Elasticities." In *The Role of Health Insurance in the Health Services Sector*, edited by Richard Rosett. New York: National Bureau of Economic Research, 1976.

Pauly, Mark V. "The Economics of Moral Hazard." *American Economic Review* 58 (June 1968): 231–237.

Pauly, Mark V. "A Measure of the Welfare Cost of Health Insurance." *Health Services Research* 4 (Winter 1969): 281–291.

Pauly, Mark V. "Overinsurance and Public Provision of Insurance." *Quarterly Journal of Economics* 88 (February 1974): 44–62.

Pechman, Joseph A.; Henry J. Aaron; and Michael K. Taussig. *Social Security: Perspectives for Reform*. Washington, D.C.: The Brookings Institution, 1968.

Phelps, Charles E. *The Demand for Health Insurance: A Theoretical and Empirical Investigation*. R–1054–OEO. Santa Monica, California: The Rand Corporation, 1973.

Phelps, Charles E., and Joseph P. Newhouse. *Coinsurance and the Demand for Medical Services*. R–964–1–OEO. Santa Monica, California: The Rand Corporation, 1974.

Phelps, Charles E., and Joseph P. Newhouse. "The Effect of Coinsurance: A Multivariate Analysis." *Social Security Bulletin* 35 (June 1972): 20–28.

Rivlin, Alice M. "The Effect of the Tax Laws on Health Insurance and Medical Costs." Statement by the Director of the Congressional Budget Office before the Subcommittee on Oversight, Committee on Ways and Means, and the Task Force on Tax Expenditures, Committee on the Budget, U.S. House of Representatives, July 9, 1979.

Rosett, Richard N., and Lien-fu-Huang. "The Effect of Health Insurance on the Demand for Medical Care." *Journal of Political Economy* 81 (March 1973): 281–305.

Steuerle, Eugene, and Ronald Hoffman. "Tax Expenditures for Health Care." U.S. Department of the Treasury, Office of Tax Analysis. OTA Paper No. 38, Washington, D.C., April 1979.

Trapnell, Gordon R. *A Comparison of the Costs of Major National Health Insurance Proposals*. Report No. PB–259–153. Springfield, Va.: National Technical Information Service, 1976.

U.S. Bureau of the Census. *Statistical Abstract of the United States: 1978*. Washington, D.C., 1976.

U.S. Department of the Treasury, Internal Revenue Service. *Internal Revenue Code of 1954*. Washington, D.C., 1954.

U.S. Department of the Treasury, Internal Revenue Service. *Statistics of Income for 1943*. Washington, D.C., 1943.

U.S. Department of the Treasury, Internal Revenue Service. *Statistics of Income: Individual Income Tax Returns, 1976*. Pub. No. 79 (4–79). Washington, D.C., 1978.

U.S. Department of the Treasury, Internal Revenue Service. *Your Federal Income Tax: 1979 Edition*. Publication 17. Washington, D.C., 1978.

Waldman, Saul. *National Health Insurance Proposals*. HEW Publication No. (SSA) 76–11920. Washington, D.C., 1976.

Blue Cross, Blue Shield, and Health Care Costs: A Review of the Economic Evidence

H. E. Frech III

Blue Cross hospital insurers and Blue Shield physician insurers occupy a special place in American medicine. They were organized and are heavily influenced by the medical providers whose care they insure. They have many special tax and regulatory advantages. And they insure a large proportion of Americans, about 45 percent of those with private health insurance. Organized as nonprofit, public service corporations, the Blues have long maintained a favorable image as powerful and beneficial institutions serving the public good.

However, recent economic research has cast doubt on the validity of this image, and the Blues are now being critically studied by researchers and attacked by antitrust authorities.[1] The basic theme of the new view is that the Blues, largely as a result of their special position in medicine, hold some market or monopoly power, and that they use this power to benefit the providers of care and those operating the Blue Cross and Blue Shield plans, at the expense of consumers in general.

The research that underlies this new belief that Blue Cross and Blue Shield market power is socially harmful is still going on. There are serious disagreements on many points. However, I find the overall picture painted by the critics of the Blues' power convincing. In this paper I will describe the industry and its regulatory and tax environment, sketch the main lines of past research in the area, and summarize the research results.

The Industry and Its Environment

The health insurance industry is largely composed of two types of firms.[2] About half of the industry is made up of the commercial insurers. This category includes profit-seeking firms and mutual insurers, nominally

---

[1] "Rx for Insurers: Washington Believes It Can Control Medical Costs by Reducing Influence of Doctors in Blue Shields," *Wall Street Journal*, March 13, 1979.

[2] More details and references to supporting documents can be found in H. E. Frech III and Paul B. Ginsburg, "Competition Among Health Insurers," in Warren Greenberg, ed., *Competition in the Health Care Sector: Past, Present, and Future*

owned by their policyholders. This part of the insurance industry is best thought of as being reasonably competitive, offering many types of insurance at competitive prices.

The commercial firms number more than 300 and entry is easy. Concentration is low. Further, about 85 percent of health insurance is purchased by groups, particularly employment groups. This indicates that most purchases are made by informed buyers, with strong incentives to search out competitive offers.

Blue Cross and Blue Shield plans make up the other half of the health insurance industry. The Blues are controlled by boards of directors with heavy representation of the hospitals and physicians. In most states, Blue Cross and Blue Shield firms are organized under special legislative enabling acts.

With few exceptions, Blue Cross and Blue Shield insurers do not compete with each other. Assisted by the national associations, the firms collude on geographic market areas. Further, Blue Shield and Blue Cross plans for the same area rarely compete. In all but a few instances, Blue Shield plans insure only physician expenses, while Blue Cross plans cover hospital expenses alone.

Since the Blues' collusion is so nearly perfect, one should treat the entire Blue Cross/Blue Shield complex as one collusion or cartel for analysis of competition and monopoly. Naturally, this includes investigations directed at possible antitrust violations.

To summarize, the health insurance industry has an interesting structure. In spite of the existence of many firms, it is not perfectly competitive. There are two distinct sectors. The commercial sector is reasonably competitive, but the Blue Cross/Blue Shield sector has a degree of monopoly power, which varies immensely across the states. There are states with virtually no Blue Cross or Blue Shield insurance and those in which the Blues hold more than 80 percent of the market. Further, the tax and regulatory advantages that form the basis of the Blues' market power also vary from state to state.

Insurance regulation is almost entirely a state function. Further, many states impose special taxes on insurance premiums in addition to the usual state income and property taxes.

Typically, the Blue Cross and Blue Shield plans pay no premium

(Germantown, Md.: Aspen Systems Corporation, 1978), pp. 168–172; H. E. Frech III, "The Regulation of Health Insurance," Ph.D. dissertation, University of California, Los Angeles (September 1974); Nancy (Greenspan) Thorndyke, "The Effects of Regulation in the Private Health Insurance Market," M.A. thesis, University of North Carolina (1976); and Ronald J. Vogel and Roger D. Blair, *Health Insurance Administrative Costs*, U.S. Department of Health, Education, and Welfare, Social Security Administration, Office of Research and Statistics, Staff Paper No. 21, Washington, D.C., 1976.

tax while the commercial insurers pay 2 percent or so. As a percentage of the insurance firms' costs, this 2 percent represents an enormous advantage for the Blues. For example, only 5 percent of Blue Cross premiums are kept to pay expenses. Thus, the typical tax advantage lowers Blue Cross costs by more than 30 percent. Blue Shield expenses are a larger percentage of premiums, but even for Blue Cross and Blue Shield combined, only about 8 percent of premium income pays expenses, so that the premium tax break alone lowers costs by more than 20 percent.[3]

Furthermore, many states exempt the Blues from other taxes that commercial insurers must pay, such as property taxes. Some states regulate the ratio of benefits to premiums for commercial insurance sold to individuals. This eliminates sales of certain types of commercial policies with high selling costs or administrative costs or both. Some states regulate the total premiums (but not premium/benefit ratios) of Blue Cross and Blue Shield plans.

Based on these important cost advantages and the evidence that diseconomies of scale are minor at best,[4] one would expect the Blues to eliminate their commercial competition entirely. In fact, their market share has hovered between 40 and 50 percent for the last fifteen years.

Theory and Evidence: How Might Blue Cross/Blue Shield Market Power Raise Health Care Costs?

It has been argued by Frech[5] and Frech and Ginsburg[6] that where the Blues have more market power, they will induce consumers to hold more complete insurance. The more complete insurance lowers the net price to consumers for purchasing more medical care and thus raises the demand for care. The higher demand for care is valued by the hospitals and physicians who provide the care in two ways. First, higher demand makes for higher income by allowing higher pricing, making it easier for providers to avoid slack times of inactivity and so on. Second, the higher demand makes it possible for providers to exercise

---

[3] Health Insurance Institute, *Source Book of Health Insurance Data, 1976–77* (New York: 1977).

[4] Roger D. Blair, Paul B. Ginsburg, and Ronald J. Vogel, "Blue Cross-Blue Shield Administration Costs: A Study of Non-Profit Health Insurers," *Economic Inquiry*, vol. 13, no. 2 (June 1975), pp. 237–251.

[5] Frech, "The Regulation of Health Insurance," and H. E. Frech III, "Market Power in Health Insurance, Effects on Insurance and Medical Markets," *Journal of Industrial Economics*, vol. 27 (September 1979).

[6] Frech and Ginsburg, "Competition Among Health Insurers," and H. E. Frech III and Paul Ginsburg, "Property Rights and Competition in Health Insurance: Multiple Objectives for Nonprofit Firms," Working Paper no. 136 (Santa Barbara: University of California, Department of Economics, July 1979).

more personal choice in the type of patients they prefer to deal with, the type of practice, location, and so on. For hospitals, higher demand makes it possible to finance high-technology medicine. All of these responses of providers lead to higher health care costs. Based on this hypothesis, one would expect higher monopoly power of the Blues to lead to higher health care prices and quantities and also to the practice of a more service-intensive and higher technology type of medical care.

The second stage of the argument—that more insurance leads to higher health-care costs—is well established by now. Of more interest is the first stage of the analysis—the argument that more monopoly power for the Blues leads to more complete insurance. First, it is well known that the Blues prefer more complete insurance. Indeed, Howard Berman, former vice president of the Blue Cross Association, has stated,

> . . . as a matter of philosophy, Blue Cross plans have from the outset been committed to the provision of service benefits and comprehensive coverage. This commitment . . . is one of the factors which distinguishes Blue Cross plans from commercial insurers. . . .[7]

There is no question that this (more complete insurance than commercial insurers) is the Blue Cross plan goal.

Another way to approach the Blues' preferences for more complete insurance is to examine the actual completeness of the Blues' insurance in comparison with the type of insurance supplied by their commercial competitors. Frech and Ginsburg[8] did this, based on the Andersen and Andersen survey.[9] Both Blue Cross hospital insurance and Blue Shield physician insurance were found to be substantially more complete than that of the commercials. For example, Blue Cross insurance paid 90 percent or more of the hospital bills for 73 percent of Blue Cross admissions. The comparable figure for the commercial hospital insurers was only 59 percent. The percentages of admissions for whom 90 percent or more of the surgical bill was paid by insurance were 53 percent for Blue Shield and 41 percent for commercial surgical insurance.

This comparison is illuminating, but it is far from conclusive. It is theoretically possible that cost and demand variations explain the greater completeness of the Blues' insurance. One needs to know if greater

---

[7] Howard Berman, "Comment: Competition Among Health Insurers," Warren Greenberg, ed., *Competition in the Health Care Sector*, pp. 189–194.

[8] Frech and Ginsburg, "Competition Among Health Insurers," pp. 167–168.

[9] Ronald Andersen and Odin W. Anderson, *A Decade of Health Services* (Chicago: University of Chicago Press, 1970).

Blue Cross/Blue Shield market power leads to more complete insurance holding constant the relevant demand and cost variables. Frech[10] and Frech and Ginsburg[11] have examined this question directly.

Using state data, Frech found that greater Blue Cross market power, as measured by the Blue Cross market share of hospital insurance in a state, led to more complete hospital insurance, as measured by the proportion of the bills paid by insurers. This held true even though demand and cost variables were held constant statistically.[12]

Specifically, a halving of the Blue Cross market share from its average of 43 percent to 22 percent would reduce the average percentage of hospital bills subsidized by insurers by 8 percent. As we know from the literature on the demand for medical care, this reduction in health insurance completeness would substantially lower hospital prices. For example, Frech[13] estimates that such a reduction would lower average hospital prices also by about 8 percent.

In a study based on data for Blue plan market areas, Frech and Ginsburg[14] took a different approach. They assumed that the Blues' insurance was more complete than commercial insurance and did not vary substantially over Blue plans. On this assumption, a market area with a larger Blue Cross or Blue Shield market share would have more complete insurance, everything else constant. The measure of market power used here was more fundamental, though less complete than that used in Frech.[15] Market power was measured by the tax advantages held by the local Blue Cross or Blue Shield plan. Again, in a statistical test where demand and cost variables were held constant, greater tax

---

[10] Frech, "Market Power in Health Insurance," pp. 62–66.

[11] Frech and Ginsburg, "Competition Among Health Insurers," pp. 174–180, and "Property Rights and Competition in Health Insurance: Multiple Objectives to Nonprofit Firms," pp. 19–23.

[12] Frech, "Market Power in Health Insurance," pp. 62–66. Using state data, Frech estimated a demand equation for hospital insurance where the quantity of insurance was defined as the proportion of hospital bills paid by insurers. The equation included the price of insurance, income, the price of hospital care, and a measure of Blue Cross market power. The monopoly power of the local Blue Cross was measured by the market share of the Blue Cross plan. The Blue Cross market power variable was taken as endogenous so that any backwards causation would be eliminated. The instruments included tax and regulatory variables which were also used in Thorndyke, "The Effects of Regulation"; Nancy T. Greenspan and Ronald J. Vogel, "An Econometric Aanalysis of the Effects of Regulation on the Private Health Insurance Market," unpublished paper, Health Care Financing Administration, U.S. Department of Health, Education, and Welfare, April 1979; and Frech and Ginsburg, "Competition Among Health Insurers," and "Property Rights and Competition in Health Insurance."

[13] Frech, "The Regulation of Health Insurance," p. 105.

[14] Frech and Ginsburg, "Competition Among Health Insurers," and "Property Rights and Competition in Health Insurance."

[15] Frech, "Market Power in Health Insurance," pp. 62–66.

and regulatory advantages for the Blues were found to cause higher Blue Cross market shares, thus more complete insurance.[16] The typical 2 percent tax difference raised Blue Cross market share by about 6.7 percent. Blue Shield market share seemed almost unaffected by the regulatory and tax advantages.

So far, some writers have argued that monopoly power for the Blues leads to excessively complete insurance. This may be the most important effect, but it does not exhaust the cost-raising effects for which this market power has been held responsible. The Blues' power has been implicated in inefficiency of management and in directly raising physician fees and suppressing insurer cost controls.

On the matter of Blue Cross/Blue Shield market power and inefficiency, there are two types of analyses. Frech[17] compares the costs of administering Medicaid claims for Blue Shield firms, mutual insurers, and profit-seeking insurers. As one would expect, the profit-seeking firms have substantially lower costs than the other two types. Mutual insurers (owned by policyholders) have processing costs about 20 percent above the profit-seeking firms, while Blue Shield firms' costs are about another 20 percent higher still.[18] Comparison of performance in processing speed and accuracy also showed the Blue Shield and mutual plans to be inferior to the profit-seeking firms. Of course, this comparison lumps together all the Blue Shield firms whether they have a great deal of market power or not. It also ignores the degree of physician domination, which more recent work shows to matter.

These results were supported by similar findings based on more complex regression analysis of similar data for 1971 by Ronald Vogel and Roger Blair.[19] However, the work of Kuo-Cheng Tseng finds Blue Cross intermediaries in Medicare part A (hospital insurance) performed better than commercial insurers for some elements of costs and worse

---

[16] Three tax regulatory variables were entered in a reduced-form equation for market share containing demand and cost variables. In particular, the variable for the difference between Blue Cross premium tax and the commercial premium tax had a strong effect on market share.

[17] H. E. Frech III, "The Property Rights Theory of the Firm," *Journal of Political Economy*, vol. 84, no. 1 (January 1976), pp. 143–152; and H. E. Frech III, "Health Insurance, Private, Mutuals, or Government," *Research in Law and Economics*, Supplement 1, pp. 61–73.

[18] These percentages are based on a comparison of means in Frech, "Health Insurance," pp. 61–73. In Frech, "The Property Rights Theory of a Firm," differences between the profit-seeking firm and a category combining Blue Shield and mutual insurers were explored in a simple regression model controlling for some dimensions of scale. Some of the performance differences were accounted for by the lower scale of the Blue Shield firms, but a large and statistically significant difference remained.

[19] Vogel and Blair, *Health Insurance Administrative Costs*, pp. 90–93, 106.

for others.[20] The author states that total costs were lower for Blue Cross plans, but statistics and statistical tests were not provided for total costs. Also, comparisons were per bill, rather than per dollar processed. If the commercials process larger bills (for which there is some evidence),[21] costs per dollar processed may be higher for the Blue Cross plans. Performance measures other than cost were not examined.

In related work, William Hsiao showed that the private insurers (largely Blue Cross/Blue Shield) were far more efficient than the Department of Health, Education, and Welfare in administering health insurance.[22] For similar tasks, the private insurers had costs 26 percent lower. Thus, nonprofit firms that compete to some extent are far more efficient than governmental processing.

A different approach is taken in the early work of Roger Blair, Paul Ginsburg, and Ronald Vogel.[23] They estimated cost functions for the Blue plans. They interpreted the finding of no scale economies and especially the finding that most Blue Shield and Blue Cross plans had failed to merge, even though the evidence showed great cost savings, as indirect evidence that the Blues were operated inefficiently.

The other line of analysis takes explicit note of the variation in the Blues' market power. Ronald Vogel[24] modified the cost analysis of Blair, Ginsburg, and Vogel by adding a variable for the premium tax advantage of the Blue Cross and Blue Shield plans as a proxy for the government-granted market power of the plan. He found that lower taxes on the Blues were correlated with higher costs of administering the Blue Cross and Blue Shield plans.

Frech and Ginsburg used similar data, more accurate measurement of the premium tax advantage of the Blues, and some other regulatory variables.[25] They found Blue Cross plans with a typical 2 percent advantage in premium taxation to have costs per enrollee about 13 percent higher than plans that pay the same taxes as commercial in-

[20] Kuo-Cheng Tseng, "Administrative Costs of Medicare Contractors: Blue Cross Plans Versus Commercial Intermediaries," *Economic Inquiry*, vol. 15, no. 4 (December 1978), pp. 371–378.

[21] Frech, "The Property Rights Theory of the Firm," pp. 143–152.

[22] William Hsiao, "Public Versus Private Administration of Health Insurance: A Study in Relative Economic Efficiency," *Economic Inquiry*, vol. 15, no. 4 (December 1978), pp. 379–387.

[23] Roger D. Blair, Paul B. Ginsburg, and Ronald J. Vogel, "Blue Cross-Blue Shield Administration Costs: A Study of Non-Profit Health Insurers," *Economic Inquiry*, vol. 13, no. 2 (June 1975), pp. 237–251.

[24] Ronald J. Vogel, "The Effects of Taxation on the Differential Efficiency of Nonprofit Health Insurers," *Economic Inquiry*, vol. 15, no. 4 (June 1977), pp. 605–609.

[25] Frech and Ginsburg, "Competition Among Health Insurers," and Frech and Ginsburg, "Property Rights and Competition," p. 178.

surers. A slightly greater effect was found for Blue Shield. Regulation of commercial group insurance was found to raise Blue Cross costs substantially as well, but had virtually no effect on Blue Shield costs.[26]

Although the effect of the premium tax difference was greater for Blue Shield than Blue Cross in this work, generally the Blue Shield regressions did not predict costs as well as the Blue Cross ones.

Eisenstadt and Kennedy[27] believe that the poorer Blue Shield regression predictions are due to ignoring variation in the extent of physician control among Blue Shield plans. They reason that even where the local Blue Shield plan has market power, if the physicians dominate they have incentives to hold down costs. Physicians can transfer wealth to themselves from the Blue Shield plan in the form of overpayment of fees. So greater physician control leads to physicians being more like the residual claimants of the typical profit-seeking, private-property firm and therefore will lead to greater efficiency.

The empirical results are consistent with this view. The authors report that for Blue Shield plans with a premium tax advantage, a higher percentage of physicians on the boards of directors significantly lowers costs. Specifically, a 10 percent increase in the proportion of physicians on the board leads to a cost decrease of about 0.7 percent. For Blue Shield plans without premium tax advantages, physician control lowered costs, but only by about half as much.[28]

The relationship between physician control and efficiency is the subject of ongoing and currently secret work by the Federal Trade Commission, the General Accounting Office, and the Blue Shield/Blue

---

[26] Cost was regressed on the same variables as in the equations for Blue Cross and Blue Shield market share reported above. On a one-tail test, the Blue Cross results for the premium tax difference were significant at the 3 percent level, while the Blue Shield coefficient was significant at about the 5 percent level. In these equations, administrative costs were deflated by the number of enrollees. In Frech and Ginsburg, "Property Rights and Competition," results for underflated costs are reported and found to be very similar. However, the deflation is found to eliminate heteroskedasticity, which is very evident in the underflated equations.

[27] David Eisenstadt and Thomas E. Kennedy, "Control and Behavior of Nonprofit Firms: The Case of a Blue Shield," unpublished paper, University of Missouri, Department of Economics, June 1979.

[28] Eisenstadt and Kennedy, in "Control and Behavior of Nonprofit Firms," estimated a pooled regression for thirty-nine plans for the years 1974–1976 using an error components model to account for correlation among the errors. The cost reductions from physician control for plans with tax advantages were statistically significant at the 1 percent level on a one-tail basis. The cost advantages of physician control were a bit less than half in magnitude where there was no premium tax advantage. These coefficients were significant at about the 15-percent level on a one-tail basis. The finding of some cost benefits, even where there is no premium tax advantage, indicates that these Blue Shield plans have some market power as a result of other regulatory and tax advantages or perhaps the support of organized medicine.

Cross Association. At the same time, these groups are analyzing the effect of physician control on the fees Blue Shield pays to physicians. Much of this work is taking place in connection with a proceeding of the Federal Trade Commission, which is considering a rule limiting physician control of Blue Shield.[29] A recent antitrust case in Ohio had a similar outcome—physician influence was reduced.[30] If physician control were found to both lower costs and raise fees, the administrative decision to limit such control would be more difficult and less clear.

Another way in which powerful Blue Shield plans might increase health-care costs is the most direct. They may simply pay higher fees to physicians who treat Blue Shield patients. Further, if there is poor enough information in the physician services market, the high Blue Shield fees may act as a convenient signal and lead to higher fees for patients who do not hold Blue Shield insurance.

The same secret work at the Federal Trade Commission, the General Accounting Office, and the Blue Cross/Blue Shield Association on the matter of physician control and efficiency is also (in fact, primarily) pursuing the issue of physician control and fees. The only public work so far is early research of Lynk.[31] Based on a small and unusual sample of plans, he finds that physician control (measured by the fraction of a plan's board occupied by physicians) generally tends to lower the Blue Shield allowable fees.[32] This result is very preliminary and is sure to be subject to revision, as Lynk and others are now working with much bigger and better data sets.

As discussed above, less complete insurance lowers health-care costs by improving the incentives facing consumers and medical providers. An alternative to less complete insurance is administrative con-

---

[29] Federal Trade Commission, Bureau of Competition, *Medical Participation in Control of Blue Shield and Certain Other Open-Panel Medical Prepayment Plans,* Staff Report to the Federal Trade Commission and Proposed Trade Regulation Rule, Washington, D.C., April 1979.

[30] "Ohio Medical Group Must Divest Itself of State Blue Shield," *Wall Street Journal,* March 26, 1979.

[31] William Lynk, "Physician Influence on Blue Shield Plans: A Reexamination of the Findings," unpublished paper, Blue Shield and Blue Cross Associations, March 1979.

[32] Some of Lynk's work involves pooling the data for several medical procedures. This procedure leads to serious econometric problems. First, the errors for the more expensive procedures are much larger than those for the more minor ones. Second, a plan with high fees for one procedure is very likely to have high fees for others, so the errors will be correlated. If such pooling is to be done, some very careful adjustments and other techniques would be necessary to preserve reasonable statistical properties for the estimates. Lynk recognizes these problems, so he also reports regressions for each of the procedures individually and finds the same basic results.

trols by the insurer. Review of medical care use and prices both before and after the fact are important examples.

Arguing on a priori grounds, Clark Havighurst stated that a competitive insurance industry would be more likely to institute effective administrative cost controls than one dominated by Blue Cross and Blue Shield.[33] This idea has been followed up by Lawrence Goldberg and Warren Greenberg, who examined the history of the Oregon Blue Shield plan.[34] They found that before the Blue Shield plan was founded, physicians were seriously restricted by claims review on the basis of appropriateness of care and prices and also by requirements for insurer approval before delivery of elective care. These policies of the commercial insurers reduced costs, but angered the physicians. Goldberg and Greenberg believe that the foundation of the Oregon Blue Shield gave the physicians a rallying point to induce the commercial insurers to reduce their cost-control efforts. The physicians and Blue Shield were apparently successful. Goldberg and Greenberg conclude:

> The experience in Oregon suggests that competition among insurers was most effective in health insurance in the absence of physician control of the carriers. The existence of a competitive insurance market was an effective force in restraining rather than adding to health costs.[35]

On the other hand, an alternative explanation of the same history of Oregon's Blue Shield plan has been proposed by William Lynk.[36] He argues that an explicit or implicit cartel of the commercial insurers had effectively reduced output below the competitive level by the device of the administrative cost controls. In a sense, insurance with numerous and effective cost controls provides less insurance than a less controlled plan. The physicians introduced the Oregon Blue Shield to break the cartel and attain the competitive equilibrium (effectively, more insurance) by reducing the cost controls of the competing commercial insurance firms, as well as by providing its own relatively uncontrolled insurance. In agreement with earlier work, Lynk states that physicians gain when consumers have more insurance. Therefore, Lynk argues, they would have an incentive to form an insurance firm to avoid a monopolistic bottleneck in the production of health insurance.

---

[33] U.S. Congress, Senate Subcommittee on Antitrust and Monopoly of the Committee on the Judiciary, *Competition in the Health Services Market*, Parts 1–3, 93rd Congress, 2nd session, 1974, p. 1076.

[34] Lawrence G. Goldberg and Warren Greenberg, "The Emergence of Physician Sponsored Health Insurance: A Historical Perspective," *Competition in the Health Care Sector*, pp. 231–254.

[35] Ibid., p. 249.

[36] William Lynk, "The Emergence of Physician-Sponsored Health Insurance," unpublished paper, Blue Cross and Blue Shield Associations, June 1978.

However, the question remains: Why would the physicians stop increasing the supply of insurance when they happened to hit the competitive level? Why not continue to increase the effective extent of insurance as far as the underlying tax and regulatory advantages of Blue Shield would allow?

There is also the historical question of the alleged cartel of commercial health insurers in Oregon. In an industry with easy entry like health insurance, how plausible is a collusion of any kind? And even if there were a collusion, would an agreement to reduce the effective supply of insurance by strict cost controls be reasonable? It would seem not, because this sort of agreement could be easily violated. It would be very difficult for one insurer to know how carefully other insurers are enforcing their administrative cost controls. An agreement to certain prices for certain coverage would appear much more likely. Lynk makes the valid point that the implications for changes in financial variables after the introduction of physician-sponsored medical insurance are identical for the competing theories of Goldberg and Greenberg versus Lynk. However, this does not mean that the two explanations are equally likely to be true. One can and should use additional evidence and considerations beyond these predictions for observable financial variables.

Blue Market Power Can Lower Costs by Administrative Controls

So far we have presented a number of theories and evidence that the Blues' monopoly power leads to higher medical care costs. However, it is possible that even though each of these theories is correct and all the evidence has been correctly interpreted, the net effect of the market power of the Blues is nevertheless to *reduce* medical care costs.

As recounted in Frech and Ginsburg, defenders of powerful Blue Cross and Blue Shield plans have argued that the size and influence of these large plans is necessary for effective administrative cost controls.[37] William Ellicott has argued: "The track record of Blue Cross Plans in cost containment activities far exceeds the performance of their commercial insurance company counterparts."[38]

There are sound theoretical reasons why administrative cost controls might be more effective for a monopolistic insurer. One of the effects is beneficial to economic efficiency; the other probably is not.

First, take the example of a small insurer considering administrative cost controls. Some of the benefit of these controls (say a limitation

---

[37] Frech and Ginsburg, "Competition Among Health Insurers," p. 180.
[38] William B. Ellicott, "Technical Appendix Comment: Competition Among Health Insurers," in *Competition in the Health Care Sector*, p. 198.

on a costly surgical procedure to only a limited number of the cases) will spill over to other insurers. This occurs if the limitation has some effect in changing the normal standard of care in the community to a more conservative one. The fact that the small insurer's cost controls benefit its competitors discourages the efforts in the first place. This is called the free-rider effect. Other insurers can obtain a free ride on the cost-control efforts of more active firms. Clearly, this is less of a problem for insurers with larger market shares. Such an insurer obtains most of the benefits of its cost-control efforts. So there is a tendency for a monopolistic insurance industry to have greater incentive for administrative cost controls.

The second effect supporting large insurers with market power is simpler. An insurer with market power can exploit physicians and hospitals by holding down the fees and utilization below the competitive level. Since the hospitals and physicians have some monopoly power themselves and complicated arrangements might ensue, it is not clear that the economic efficiency would be hurt by such insurer buying power, but I suspect that it would.

In any case, there are respectable theoretical reasons why the administrative cost containment efforts of the Blues with substantial market power might be more effective than that of the commercials.

On the other hand, the influence the providers have over the Blues makes this outcome less likely, as we have discussed above. And the experience of the original Oregon Blue Shield appears to be a counter-example.

It is also the case that the other activities of the Blues, recounted above, might overwhelm the effects of more active cost containment so that the net effect of Blue Cross/Blue Shield market value would still be higher medical costs.

Test of Net Effect

What we seek is a direct test of the impact of the Blues' market power on medical costs that includes all the possible effects and routes of causation discussed in this paper. Such a test has been done for Blue Cross by Frech and Ginsburg.[39] They found that states with higher Blue Cross market shares had substantially higher hospital prices and costs than the other states. Specifically, a virtual Blue Cross monopoly would raise hospital prices by from 22 to 40 percent and would raise hospital costs (including ancillary services) by a somewhat lower

---

[39] Frech and Ginsburg, "Competition Among Health Insurers," pp. 180–183.

percentage.[40] This indicates that greater Blue Cross market share leads to higher hospital prices, either in spite of more effective administrative cost controls or because the cost controls are, in fact, less effective than those of the competitive commercial firms. From this test, one can only determine the net effect of Blue Cross monopoly power, not the channels through which it operates.

Summary and Conclusions

The research examined here suggests several findings.

1. Blue Cross and Blue Shield health insurance is more complete than commercial insurance.

2. Where tax and regulatory advantages give the Blues more market power over the commercials, the result is more complete insurance, higher market shares for the Blues, and greater inefficiency. For Blue Shield, the work of Eisenstadt and Kennedy indicates that there is an important interaction between physician control and tax/regulatory advantages. Where physician control is more complete, physicians are presumably similar to the stockholders of a private firm. Empirically, Eisenstadt and Kennedy show that where physicians are in better control, costs are reduced. This is especially true where the Blue Shield plan has substantial market power.

3. There is a great deal of work going on concerning the effect of physician dominance of Blue Shield on fees allowed by Blue Shield. At the moment, most of the work is secret. Very preliminary work by Lynk suggests that physician domination leads to lower fees. But we have certainly not heard the last word on this issue. I suspect that future work will show that physician control leads to higher fees.

My reading of this economic evidence leads me to the belief that Blue Cross and Blue Shield market power causes higher medical costs and lower economic efficiency. There are many (economically) possible remedies:

- Differences in tax and regulatory treatment between the commercial insurers and Blue Cross/Blue Shield ought to be removed. This would reduce the market power of the Blues.
- The various Blue plans should be prohibited from colluding on market areas and product lines. Ideally, several Blue Cross and

---

[40] These results are based on reduced-form regressions of hospital prices (daily charges for semiprivate rooms) and cost per bed-day on demand variables for hospital care and also insurance demand variables, along with Blue Cross market share. Blue Cross market share was treated as exogeneous because early work by Frech, "The Regulation of Health Insurance," indicated that the price of hospital care has little influence on insurance demand. Observations were for 1969 by states.

Blue Shield plans would compete for both hospital and medical insurance customers in the same area.

- The influence of medical providers over the Blues might have to be eliminated. This measure would only be necessary if one judged that above measures were insufficient to remove most of the monopoly power from most of the Blue plans.

Eliminating provider influence but otherwise leaving the system unchanged, as the Federal Trade Commission's Bureau of Competition suggests for Blue Shield, is fraught with problems. First, it is likely to lead to less efficient management, as shown by the work of Eisenstadt and Kennedy. After the change, the Blues may pay the physicians lower fees, but simply dissipate the savings through less efficient management or more complete insurance or both. From the viewpoint of economic efficiency, this might be a retrograde step. Second, the providers may be replaced with citizens who share the providers' philosophical or ideological preference for relatively complete insurance. Particularly for Blue Cross, the result would be essentially no change in the overly complete insurance sold.

My recommendation would be to remove the special tax and regulatory status of the Blues first and to stop them from colluding. If that seemed insufficient, I would require that the Blues be converted into ordinary profit-seeking firms, with physicians and hospital representatives prohibited from owning the stock, at least for a time.

The final outcome of such a policy would be less complete insurance, greater insurer efficiency, and lower health-care costs.

Commentaries

Jeffrey E. Harris

As I have argued in a recent manuscript,[1] the main issue in the benefit-cost analysis of health insurance is the relationship between the extent of insurance coverage and the rate and direction of technological change in the health-care sector. The prevailing argument that Americans are overinsured, I showed, is based on two critical assumptions: first, that the recent growth of public and private insurance has been the main cause of rapid changes in the technological sophistication of medical care; second, that the costs of technological changes caused by increased insurance have exceeded their benefits. To the extent that technical progress has occurred independently of the growth in insurance, the welfare gains or losses from further increments in coverage are likely to be relatively small. Moreover, the evaluation of innovations that result from increased insurance will require a benefit-cost calculus quite different from the conventional consumer surplus methodology.

Although Professor Pauly's paper is sympathetic to these views, he nevertheless concludes that "the overinsurance option is by far the better bet." For the most part, his conclusion is based on the simple paradigm that insurance coverage directly subsidizes the "demand for quality."

My task here is to outline why this conclusion is based on an incorrect characterization of technological progress in the health-care sector. The assertion that Americans have too much insurance is at best premature and at worst a poor guide to public policy.

During the past two decades, we have witnessed enormous advances in the state of the art of clinical medical practice. Take the case of coronary heart disease. In the late 1950s, the principles of closed chest cardiopulmonary resuscitation had not yet fully replaced the practice of emergency thoracotomy and open cardiac massage. The concept

---

[1] J. E. Harris, "The Aggregate Coinsurance Rate and the Supply of Innovations in the Hospital Sector," unpublished paper, Department of Economics, Massachusetts Institute of Technology, July 1979.

of clustering high-risk hospital patients in a special monitoring unit was only in the formative stage. The revelation in 1963 that the early deaths of apparently uncomplicated heart attack patients were due to sudden ventricular fibrillation was dramatic and shocking. The subsequent training and authorization of nurses to initiate immediate treatment, including intravenous lidocaine and defibrillation, resulted in a marked improvement in in-hospital heart attack mortality. These events were followed rapidly by fundamental advances in our understanding of the dynamics of coronary blood flow and their relation to the atrioventricular conduction pathways, and even more recently by experimental therapeutic interventions to limit the size of myocardial infarction.

Many of these advances were embodied in new diagnostic and therapeutic equipment and procedures, including pacemakers; cardiac catherization; Holter monitoring; exercise electrocardiographic testing; Swan-Ganz pulmonary artery wedge pressure monitoring; intra-aortic balloon counterpulsation; His-bundle electrocardiography; coronary artery surgery; positive end-expiratory pressure ventilation; antiarrhythmic, cardiac inotropic, and beta-blocking agents; and gated thallium scans, to name only a few developments. This increased use of new technology resulted in a complementary expansion of the range of application of conventional laboratory and X-ray studies. Insertion of an intra-aortic balloon pump, for example, inevitably requires intravenous anticoagulation, partial thromboplastin time measurements, repeated blood counts, cultures, transfusions, portable X-rays, special nursing, physician consultations, and so forth. Without doubt, this massive intensification of resource use has been the basic substrate for rapidly rising hospital costs.

Despite all this impressive hardware, these technical improvements reflected the continual redefinition of what constitutes appropriate cardiac diagnosis and treatment. Many advances reflected learning by doing, such as the decline in aorto-coronary bypass operative mortality resulting from improvements in microsurgical techniques and the increased experience with induction of general anesthesia in patients with high-grade left coronary artery occlusions. In other instances, they reflected novel applications of a conventional therapeutic modality, such as the use of vasodilators to reduce afterload impedance in congestive heart failure. A substantial part of the current conventional management of less acutely ill cardiac patients derives directly from the early experience of the coronary care unit.

It is implicit in Professor Pauly's hypothesis C that these quality improvements are selected à la carte from a known, fixed menu of technological possibilities. In this view, more extensively insured patients are willing to let their doctors choose the more expensive entrées on this menu. But this is hardly an accurate description of the process of technological change. What is actually happening is that the menu itself is expanding.

Let me pursue this critical point more carefully. At any one instant, there will be a given set of available diagnostic and therapeutic modalities directed toward a specific disease process. Some suppliers of health care may offer all of these modalities, while others will provide only a subset. If there is sufficient diversity in the extent of consumers' insurance coverage, then we can imagine that different consumers will sort themselves among different suppliers according to their willingness to pay for various levels of technological sophistication. Moreover, if we provided at least some of these consumers with more insurance, then they would shift over to the more technologically sophisticated suppliers. This is exactly the "market for quality" required in hypothesis C. Of course, such a scenario can be rightly criticized for making too many untested assumptions about the operation of health-care markets. The real problem, however, is that it tells us nothing about the mechanism of emergence of new concepts and techniques.

We can now see why empirical, cross-sectional studies are unlikely to shed light on the phenomenon of quality change. We could test whether hospitals in localities with more extensive coverage were more likely to offer, say, noninvasive tests for diagnosing occlusive lesions of the common and internal carotid arteries. But the important question is not why some hospitals in the 1960s adopted radionuclide angiography, while others retained only ophthalmodynamometry. What we really want to know is the origin of directional Doppler ultrasonography in the early 1970s and real-time B-scan imaging in the late 1970s, and whether we will better understand the significance of asymptomatic ulcerative plaques in the 1980s.

It is not clear exactly how more extensive insurance could result in the expansion of these technological frontiers. Nor is it obvious that increased insurance coverage is really the most important factor. Far upstream from doctors and patients are the basic research laboratories and biomedical instrumentation companies, with their complex relationships to academic medical centers, the federal research support establishment, and the private capital market. The pace at which new ideas are implemented at certain focal hospitals might be more heavily influenced by the extent of federal research support, changes in financing of hospital capital expenditures (including government subsidy of the cost of capital), or various regulatory controls. To a certain extent, the increased insurance coverage that has accompanied these technological changes has been a response to more sophisticated medical care.

Even the expansion of Medicare to cover renal dialysis can be interpreted as an instance where certain technological improvements recruited a sufficiently large political constituency to influence government policy. My motivation behind formulating hypothesis A was to focus sharply on the real possibility that factors other than the extent of insurance coverage might be the main cause of these technological changes.

Despite such empirical uncertainties, most economists would still maintain that the growth of insurance coverage was the primary cause of the rapid expansion of the technological frontier of the health-care sector. It should be clear, however, that this conclusion cannot rest on a simple demand-subsidy mechanism. What matters instead is the supply response to the insurance-induced increase in demand.

One possible story behind such a supply response—and my motivation for formulating hypothesis B—is the following. In the short run, an insurance-induced increase in demand will generate financial surpluses. If the health-care sector were typical of other capitalist markets, these economic rents would be distributed as profits to equity shareholders. And if such a market were competitive, the presence of these short-run profits would stimulate the entry of new firms, and the resulting expansion of supply would erode these short-run profit margins. But this is not the characteristic response of the market for health care, particularly the hospital sector. Instead, these surpluses are exhausted by the entry of new, cost-enhancing technologies.

As I have suggested elsewhere,[2] the critical institutional fact underlying this supply response is the organizational separation of medical staff and administration found in virtually all hospitals in the United States. What we observe as the burning up of economic rents is actually the outcome of a complicated allocative battle for internal control of the firm's resources. Such an organization has an inherent tendency to search out from the periphery of its technological opportunities whenever its budget constraint is relaxed.

This story does not invoke any arguments about willingness of the consumer to pay. The short-run surplus derived from an increase in insurance is merely the fuel for a widening of the hospital's technological opportunities. Hence, as Professor Pauly explains in his Figure 1, we have no a priori reason to conclude that hospitals have pushed technology beyond what consumers would be willing to pay.

But the theoretical story goes deeper than this logical nicety. The

[2] J. E. Harris, "The Internal Organization of Hospitals: Some Economic Implications," *Bell Journal of Economics*, 8 (Autumn 1977), pp. 467–482; and J. E. Harris, "Regulation and Internal Control in Hospitals," *Bulletin of the New York Academy of Medicine*, vol. 55, no. 1 (January 1979), pp. 88–103.

state of the art of clinical medicine, as I have characterized it, is really a collective good. Economists have long recognized that there are fundamental reasons why such a collective good might be undersupplied in a competitive world. Although this conclusion might apply to research and development in all sectors of our economy, it is the linkage between insurance and technical change that makes the health-care sector unique. Each consumer, in purchasing his insurance, necessarily takes the state of technology as given. Yet by increasing his insurance coverage, he is really buying more technology for himself and everyone else. The rapid expansion of public and private insurance coverage in the last twenty years could be viewed as a mechanism to correct for an undersupply of innovations in the health-care sector.

Nevertheless, Professor Pauly suggests that hospitals have now pushed technology to the point where its incremental benefits are zero. Although many current technologies may not be cost effective, nevertheless such an assertion oversimplifies some complicated research questions. The main issue is not whether a patient with tension headaches will benefit from the marginal unit of service of a CAT scanner. It is really whether the transition to faster, second-generation scanners, or third-generation gated scanners are worth their costs. Similarly, the issue is not whether the marginal heart attack patient will benefit from a marginal hour in the coronary care unit. It is whether the addition of a full-time director to these coronary care units would improve survival. I would like to know how we are to value the new concepts engendered by the origin of coronary care units, including the resulting growth in roving ambulances and early resuscitation. Even if coronary care units do no more than prolong an inevitable cardiac death, I want to know why this is presumed to have so little value. Underlying these questions are basic problems in the benefit-cost evaluation of public goods. Even if the marginal benefit of the intra-aortic balloon pump is small for the average heart attack patient, we might be willing to pay a considerable amount for its availability in certain cases.

For the sake of argument, let us assume that the growth of insurance has in fact been the main cause of increasing technological intensity, and that the benefits of such technologies do not match their costs. Do we now want to reduce the extent of insurance coverage to compensate for this distortion? Equity considerations aside, one wonders whether such simple policy instruments as deductibles and coinsurance rates are not far too crude for the task of fine tuning the rate and direction of technological change. Can we not influence the pace of innovation with policy instruments other than insurance coverage? Even if an increase in insurance coverage pushes out the technological frontier, do we know that this relationship holds in reverse?

268

I am also skeptical that the elimination of first-dollar coverage and the expansion of catastrophic coverage would have their purported effect on technology. The recent explosion of hospital costs has been accompanied, in fact, by substantial increases in major medical and catastrophic coverage as well as basic coverage.[3] How can we be sure that coverage for large expenses was not the critical force driving up the rate of technological change? Can we be certain that shoring up first-dollar coverage will not stifle some fundamental innovation in preventive health care, while expansion of coverage at the catastrophic end will not breed more ineffective maneuvers for inevitably terminal patients?

I am not certain how a system of specific indemnities can improve the discriminatory powers of the insurance system. The difficulty with setting a fixed, "reasonable" reimbursement for a specific illness is that the technology underlying its treatment keeps changing. As long as payments are somehow tied to costs, we will end up in the classic regulatory problem of shooting at a moving target. I am equally uncertain how well a scheme of reimbursements that are contingent on applications of specific technologies is likely to function. It is dubious that a third-party payer can enforce a benefit schedule that requires that physicians, say, use ultrasound imaging in the "old way" but not the "new way."

The sounder approach, it seems to me, is first to determine what factors have been the most important determinants of technological change in the last twenty years. If the growth of insurance was not the critical factor (hypothesis A), then we might as well cover the remainder of the uninsured population on equity grounds and focus on the other determinants of technical change. On the other hand, if the main issue is the health-care sector's supply response to an increase in insurance coverage (hypothesis B), then we ought to concentrate on those institutional conditions that fostered this supply response. In that case, as I have suggested, the internal organization of hospitals may be the main policy target. But that is a topic for another conference.

Robert Glen Beck

Professor Vogel's paper presents a combnied a priori and empirical argument that the current tax treatment of health insurance premiums in the United States leads to "overinsurance." From there it is argued that "overinsurance" leads to inflation of health costs. Neither the argu-

---

[3] J. E. Harris, "The Aggregate Coinsurance Rate."

ment nor the evidence is new, and indeed the argument, because of the criterion and model adopted, is tautological.

Vogel begins with a history of tax incentives for employer based health insurance in the United States. The history is for the most part a catalog of the tax provisions and the changes in legislation since 1942. Not only does the history precede the theoretical discussion of why there might be a relationship between insurance and tax treatment, but also the history is not later linked to changes in levels of insurance and health spending. If one wanted to make a case about levels of insurance and the tax incentives, it would be useful to compare the legislative changes with the levels of insurance. Vogel's conclusion that tax treatment has led to overinsurance is made largely by reference to another study,[1] which asserts this by referring to post-1950 data. Vogel argues that before 1960 tax treatment was not a "problem," one reason being that health insurance was not yet important in the insurance industry or economy. But the subsidy began in 1942 not 1960. The fact that the "problem" took so long to become a problem suggests that there may be other reasons for the post-1960 growth of health insurance than the mere presence of a tax subsidy. The history discussion is concluded with a "simple model" illustrating that employers would be indifferent to paying wages as money income or income in kind if both types of payment are identically expensed against income tax. This discussion yields the proposition that the employee has an incentive to channel income from money income to income in kind, which is a restatement of the definition of the income tax subsidy. The author argues that because the employer is indifferent he "bends to the incentives presented to his employees by government and pays what they ask in the form of (income in kind)"—at least after 1960. The extent to which employees actually react to this incentive depends upon their preferences for purchasing power in general versus earmarked purchasing power. It is conceivable that there has been a shift in these preferences, particularly in recent years. This possibility, of course, makes it difficult to separate out the effects of the tax scheme.

The next section of the paper restates a theme now familiar in some quarters of the U.S. literature. The demand for health services is assumed to be like that of any other commodity. The fully informed consumer is presumed to respond to price, balancing the welfare gain from consuming incremental health services against the price of obtaining them. Because the presence of health insurance reduces the price to the consumer, he will take more of it. How much more the consumer

---

[1] Martin S. Feldstein and Bernard Friedman, "Tax Subsidies, the Rational Demand for Insurance and the Health Care Crisis," *Journal of Public Economics*, vol. 7 (April 1977), pp. 155–178.

will take is critically important to establishing the magnitude of the "problem." Reliable estimates of this parameter are sufficiently scarce as to accommodate a wide range of opinion and debate.[2]

That the consumer-patient may consume more in the face of a price reduction means that the expected benefit from insurance is greater once insurance is obtained. Thus an individual may be confronted with a premium that is greater when evaluated on the postinsurance benefit distribution than when evaluated on the preinsurance benefit distribution. The theory has it then that a utility maximizing individual would reduce his insurance (cover himself through coinsurance) to bring his expected (postinsurance) benefit to equality with the premium he must pay. Therefore, Vogel concludes "most individuals are willing to pay coinsurance." Students of the Canadian setting would find this empirical observation surprising.[3]

There are a number of difficulties with this paradigm that might be explored. First, it is now well known that there is an interdependence between the demand and supply functions for health services. The consumer-patient is not in a supermarket where he chooses things off the shelf according to his inner hunger. The patient chooses to visit a physician; after that the choice decision is substantially the physician's. If the utilization response to insurance, typically referred to as moral hazard, could be partitioned into demand and supply influences, their comparative magnitudes might indicate policies targeted upon the supplier rather than "problem" levels of insurance.

Second, there is the question of the appropriateness of this specification of the demand curve. To be sure, the author does refer to the possibility that health services might be a "merit good," that there may be a community preference function for health services. In the context of this discussion, the presence of a community demand function would change the question to one of whether the tax subsidies varied appropriately with income.[4] The distributional data presented by Vogel would

---

[2] For a good review of the empirical attempts to estimate the demand for health services see J. M. Horne, "Copayment and Utilization of Publicly Insured Hospital Services in Saskatchewan: An Empirical Analysis," Ph.D. dissertation, Carleton University, 1977. As Horne observes, "faulty theoretical formulations, inappropriate methodologies, and inadequate data have all too often been the rule rather than the exception."

[3] In the most recent federal election, all political parties were careful to avoid advocating coinsurance since the electorate appears unwilling to accept such provisions.

[4] Mark Pauly has examined the case where the community demand curve evaluates care equally for all persons, and he shows that subsidies should vary inversely with income. See Mark V. Pauly, *Medical Care at Public Expense* (New York: Praeger Publishers, 1971), chap. 2.

suggest that the present tax subsidy does not. But the recommended action would be to adjust the subsidies so that they vary with income. The criterion for determining the existence of overinsurance would be different and the simple theory would have a message with a different ring. By effectively ignoring the possibility of a community demand curve for health services, this paper may be ignoring the basis of the original preference for a tax subsidy—regardless of whether the subsidy was, or is, appropriately structured.

There is another aspect of the argument that makes it tautological, namely the definition of overinsurance and the context to which it is applied. Vogel defines overinsurance as "the quantity of health insurance over and above that amount of health insurance which the consumer would buy in the absence of tax subsidies." Thus by definition tax subsidies result in distortion or resource misallocation.

The choice of the word "distortion" is rooted in the assumptions about the nature of the world within which the tax subsidies occur—perfectly competitive suppliers, fully informed consumers, independence of demand and supply relations, etc. But suppose we relax these assumptions so that the world in the absence of government policy reflects something less than the competitive ideal.[5] Let us define the optimum amount of insurance as the amount existing in an ideal world where there are no loading charges and where providers are unable to influence demand. Now we introduce an insurance-induced utilization effect that includes a supplier effect; we also introduce loading charges with the assumption that they are excessive in the market as it is. In these circumstances, in the absence of intervention we would have "underinsurance."

What form might intervention take? One might argue that certain forms of insurance, such as public medical care insurance, are more effective in policing demand generation. Horne's finding of no copayment effect on hospital services in Saskatchewan may reflect not only the fact that such decisions are nondiscretionary to the patient, but also that the institutional framework maintains fairly strict surveillance on bed utilization by physicians.[6] One might also hypothesize that certain forms of insurance may, for a number of reasons, be more

---

[5] Bob Evans sets this case out graphically in appendix A of R. G. Evans and M. F. Williamson, *Extending Canadian Health Insurance: Options for Pharmacare and Denticare*, Ontario Economic Council Research Study (Toronto: University of Toronto Press, 1978).

[6] R. G. Beck and J. M. Horne, "An Analytical Overview of the Saskatchewan Copayment Experiment in the Hospital and Ambulatory Care Settings," Ontario Council of Health Study, mimeographed (1978).

efficient and therefore involve smaller loading charges than private insurance. There is some evidence that public medical care insurance involves substantially smaller loading charges than private insurance.[7] In any event, if we model the world slightly differently the analysis yields a world with technical underinsurance. In such a world public policy might be directed to trying to encourage the consumption of more health insurance, perhaps in a 1942 setting by providing a subsidy at the workplace.

The issue of the relationships among health insurance, the demand for health services, and inflation is also conveniently finessed with the assumption of perfectly competitive suppliers. Prices only go up because of rising consumer demands in the presence of less than perfectly elastic supply, or because an ever-widening range of specific services falls into the generic commodity, "health care." In the absence of this assumption, the "how" question becomes more important.

In Canada, judicious adjustment of physician fee schedules took place in some provinces on the eve of medicare; in addition, there were generous increases in the honeymoon period following the introduction of medicare. Hospital cost increases are contingent upon developments in the labor market, particularly for public nonprofit hospitals. But in the Canadian setting the institutional framework provides machinery for cost control. Indeed, the comparative figures for the share of GNP spent on health care would suggest that public medicare is more successful in containing costs than the private markets in the United States. As Table 1 indicates, Canadian performance began to improve relative to the United States after medicare was in place.

In any event, Vogel presents little evidence to support rejection of health insurance on stabilization grounds. Even if one turns to the Feldstein and Friedman study that the author cites, the thesis is essentially an assertion. The relevant section of that paper virtually begins with the statement, "Because the growth of insurance has been the primary cause of the exceptional rise in health care prices, it can with justice be said that the tax subsidy has been responsible for much of the health care crisis of the past decade [p. 172]." The lag from 1942 to 1967 begs some explanation, as does the comparative performance in Canada.

In summary, Vogel's chapter addresses interesting and important issues in the current debates over U.S. health policy. There are some qualifications to the analysis, however. The "overinsurance" that is demonstrated to exist is "technical overinsurance" appropriate to a

---

[7] In a study currently under way by the author and J. M. Horne, Saskatchewan's medicare plan records administrative costs of sixty-one cents per claim or about 3.5 percent of program costs. This may be contrasted with costs in the order of 12 percent in the United States and 17 percent in pre-medicare Canada.

TABLE 1

U.S. and Canadian Health Expenditures as a Percentage of GNP

Year	Canada	United States
1950	—	4.5
1955	—	4.5
1960	5.6	5.2
1961	5.9	—
1962	5.9	—
1963	6.0	—
1964	6.0	—
1965	6.1	5.9
1966	6.1	5.8
1967	6.4	6.2
1968	6.6	6.5
1969	6.8	6.7
1970	7.1	7.2
1971	7.4	7.6
1972	7.2	7.8
1973	6.8	7.7
1974	6.7	7.8
1975	7.1	8.5
1976	7.1	8.7
1977	—	9.0
1978	—	9.1

Source: Canada: Barer, Evans, Stoddart, *Controlling Health Care Costs by Direct Charges to Patients*, Ontario Economic Council, p. 6. United States: R. J. Vogel, "The Tax Treatment of Health Insurance Premiums as a Cause of Overinsurance," published in this volume.

rabbits and berries world. The case against health insurance on stabilization grounds balances precariously on the assumption of an unrealistic work on the supply side. Moreover, it begs explanation of the Canadian cost experience. On equity grounds it has been argued that the tax subsidies to health insurance are regressive. But to jump from this conclusion to the advocacy of health insurance with extremely high deductibles and high coinsurance seems unwarranted. In the Saskatchewan setting, examination of postinsurance benefit distributions suggests that deductibles in the order of $100 would shift over half of program costs of medicare to the patient.[8]

---

[8] R. G. Beck and J. M. Horne, "Economic Class and Risk Avoidance: Experience under Public Medical Care Insurance," *Journal of Risk and Insurance*, vol. 43, no. 1 (March 1976), pp. 73–86.

Louise B. Russell

The research Professor Frech reviews in his paper starts from the facts that Blue Cross and Blue Shield have been granted a number of tax exemptions and regulatory advantages by the government, and that the two organizations write about 45 percent of all private health insurance policies, giving them a larger share of the market than any commercial insurer. In some states their share is over 80 percent.

The logical link between the two facts seems obvious. Other things equal, the Blues' advantages mean they can offer a lower price for a given level of coverage, or better services and coverage for a given price. By beating their competitors—the commercial insurers—on price, the Blues can capture a larger share of the market. But the studies Frech reviews do not try to show that the Blues' premiums are lower; they do not examine relative premiums at all. At the same time, they offer a number of reasons to think the Blues' premiums should be the same as or higher than those of the commercial insurers, and without any attendant advantages that would be apparent to the buyer. The buyers in this market are conceded to be well informed.

The size, in dollar terms, of the Blues' advantages is not spelled out precisely. The Blues are often exempted from state premium taxes, which are usually about 2 percent of the premium. They are exempted from federal corporate taxes and, in many states, from state corporate and property taxes.[1] But Law cautions that these exemptions from tax may not be that important. She writes: "Because commercial insurance companies may be able to allocate funds to policy reserves, and thereby avoid payment of substantial income tax, this difference between Blue Cross and the commercial companies may not be of great practical importance. More research is needed to evaluate the actual relative tax burdens of Blue Cross and commercial insurers."[2]

But whatever the value of these other tax exemptions, we know that the Blues often start with an initial advantage that is at least 2 percent of the premium price, and may be more. The research reviewed by Frech argues that they do two things with this differential: indulge in higher administrative costs and pay higher prices to providers, because they have the providers' interests at heart. The higher prices together with the more comprehensive policies written by the Blues make it possible for providers to give more services and invest in more technology. To the extent that the buyer perceives a higher premium as bringing him more of what he wants, and more than he could get else-

---

[1] Sylvia A. Law, *Blue Cross: What Went Wrong?*, second edition (New Haven: Yale University Press, 1976), pp. 8–10.

[2] Ibid., p. 10.

where, there is no difficulty here. But the implications of the research are that the Blues probably charge more than their competitors for a given level of service.

Consider administrative costs first. In general, the studies reviewed show that the Blues' administrative costs are higher. In fact, Frech finds that, when the Blues are compared with other insurers on the costs of administering Medicaid claims, their costs are about 20 percent higher than those of mutual insurers and about 40 percent higher than those of profit-seeking firms. If these differences carry over into their private insurance business, they would go a long way toward eliminating a 2 percent advantage on premiums. In fact, Frech's calculations showing the 2 percent tax as a fraction of administrative costs indicate that a 40 percent difference in costs would more than eliminate the tax advantage.

A minor point here. In his paper, Mark Pauly states that administrative costs average 12 to 14 percent of health insurance premiums. Frech states that Blue Cross averages 5 percent of premiums for administrative costs, and Blue Cross and Blue Shield together average 8 percent, and argues further that the Blues' expenses are higher than those of other insurers. This apparent contradiction may have a reasonable explanation, such as that the conflicting cost estimates include different things, but not enough information is given about the data in the papers to tell whether this is the case.

The second line of argument is that the Blues use their initial advantage to pay providers more generously. To the extent that this means higher fees for the same service, premiums will be higher; but unless this means that providers treat Blues' subscribers differently from other subscribers—by refusing service to the latter, for example—the higher premiums will not bring any apparent difference in benefits. No evidence is presented that the subscribers of the Blues and of commercial insurers are treated differently. Further, although the more comprehensive coverage and allegedly more generous payments of the Blues should make it possible for providers to invest in more technology, once purchased, this technology is available to everyone. If Blue Cross ran its own hospitals, it could make it clear that these investments were an advantage of being a Blue Cross subscriber, but it does not.

I am left with the impression then that this research shows that the Blues fritter away their initial advantage on things of little or no interest to health insurance buyers. How do they maintain large market shares in the face of such behavior? There are two points to consider.

First, the market share of Blue Cross has been declining. Law states that Blue Cross had 61 percent of the market in 1945, but only

37 percent in 1969.[3] She defines the 1969 market as the civilian population under sixty-five, thus excluding the supplementary coverage insurers write for Medicare enrollees.

Second, none of the research reviewed by Frech mentions the Blue Cross discount. (I am less certain whether Blue Shield also receives discounts.) In many states the Blues have negotiated special rates for themselves with hospitals, and contrary to the argument set out in Frech's paper, these rates are lower than the ones paid by commercial insurers. Two recent items of evidence indicate that this discount, where it exists, is not only important, but may be more important than ever. The first is a recent advertisement in the *Wall Street Journal* in which the newly merged national organization explicitly states that the Blues are often able to arrange payments lower than those paid by other carriers, and argues that insurance buyers will get more for their money as a result.[4] The second item occurred at a meeting I recently attended in Chicago. The representative of one Chicago hospital raised what the hospitals see as a serious problem. Blue Cross, Medicare, and in most states Medicaid reimburse hospitals on the basis of costs while other carriers pay charges.[5] Cost reimbursers pay a lower rate, and when this does not provide the hospital with enough revenue, the difference is loaded onto charge payers. At this hospital the difference between the two rates has grown until, currently, charges are ninety dollars higher per day than the rate paid by cost reimbursers. A 2 percent premium tax exemption pales in comparison.

In fact, the discounts together with cost reimbursement could explain several things. The discount could give Blue Cross a substantial premium advantage, substantial enough to outweigh higher administrative and other costs, and cost reimbursement could explain the higher administrative costs. The process of negotiating costs and discounts may be more expensive than administering a charge system. There is some evidence for this in the complaints from providers about how long it takes to settle the bills under cost reimbursement. Thus cost reimbursement, high Blue Cross discounts, and high Blue Cross market share and administrative costs might go together. The study by Frech and Ginsburg, "Competition Among Health Insurers," is consistent with this view. Frech and Ginsburg found that states with higher Blue Cross market shares had higher hospital charges. Costs were also higher, but not by as much. This makes sense because charges measure what commercial insurers pay; where the difference between the Blue Cross

---

[3] Ibid., p. 11. I have no information about the market share of Blue Shield.

[4] *Wall Street Journal*, September 27, 1979, p. 13.

[5] Some Blue Cross organizations pay on the basis of charges. I do not know whether they too negotiate discounts.

rate and the charge is higher, Blue Cross could be expected to have a larger share of the market.

But I find myself wondering, regardless of what the Blues do or do not accomplish with their tax and regulatory advantages, what justification is there for giving them the advantages in the first place? The justification might once have been the Blues' policy of community rating. They did this to make the cost of insurance lower for high-risk groups, and as a result could not offer low-risk people as good a bargain as the commercials could. But a lot of high-risk people are now insured by the government—people sixty-five and older, the disabled, and many of the poor. And even for the rest the Blues do not do much community rating anymore. Most of them now experience rate group plans in order to be able to compete more effectively with the commercial insurers.[6]

It seems as though one could make a strong case for removing these advantages without even knowing what the Blues had done to administrative or total medical care costs. And indeed, in the states where the Blues' tax exemptions have been challenged, the courts have usually been unable to find compelling reasons for allowing the exemptions to continue.[7]

I would like to make one final point about the three papers as a group. I agree completely with the reasoning that insurance increases the demand for care—with the additional units demanded returning benefits that are in some sense less than their costs—and that tax advantages, whether to the buyers or the sellers of insurance, increase the demand for insurance and thus, again, for medical care. But I think we make a mistake if we look upon these mechanisms as the "cause" of many of the difficulties—especially rising costs—in medical care. These mechanisms were chosen *because* they reduce cost as a consideration in medical care, not in ignorance of that fact. The proponents were, I think, ignorant of just how far things would go once the mechanisms were in place, but it was the desire to base medical care on need, not on benefit-cost, that led to their introduction. Evidence for the strength of this philosophy can be found in the experience of other countries. We have taken many different roads to end up, most of us, in much the same place.[8]

In fact, the philosophy and its attendant problems are so pervasive and so persistent that I hesitate to accept a diagnosis that they are the result of irrational or undesirable behavior—"overinsurance," "moral hazard," and the like. Our models may omit some force critical to medi-

---

[6] Law, *Blue Cross*, p. 12.

[7] Ibid., p. 9.

[8] Louise B. Russell, *Technology in Hospitals: Medical Advances and Their Diffusion* (Washington, D.C.: The Brookings Institution, 1979), chap. 6.

cal care that makes the observed behavior more rational than we realize, and that would point to policies different from those we now prescribe.

It is worthwhile to point out the consequences of various insurance and tax mechanisms, and to estimate their costs. But I think we should not be surprised to find that this does them less damage than we expected, and that they, or something like them, are kept in place.

Part Four

Cost Containment: Long- and Short-Run Strategies

Health Maintenance Organizations, Competition, Cost Containment, and National Health Insurance

Harold S. Luft

Various forms of health maintenance organizations, or HMOs, have been providing medical services to a small segment of the population for a half century; some HMO precursors date back to the mid-1880s. The current interest in HMOs, however, stems not from their history, but from their potential role in cost containment—especially under national health insurance.

HMOs, or the more broadly defined "alternative delivery systems," are perceived as having both a direct and an indirect impact on health care expenditures. The direct effect is attributed to the lower costs of care for HMO enrollees when compared to those who have conventional health insurance, which reimburses hospitals on the basis of costs and physicians on the basis of fee for service. The indirect effect is believed to be an outgrowth of the competition between HMOs and conventional providers, with the fee-for-service sector adopting cost-saving techniques to ensure economic viability.

This paper will explore available evidence concerning HMO performance in both direct and indirect cost containment. Much more is known about the experience of HMO enrollees than about the indirect competitive impact of HMOs. Yet, it will be argued that we still know far too little about HMOs to explain adequately their current performance, let alone predict accurately the outcome of HMO competition in a radically restructured market environment. To lay a foundation for the discussion, the first section will define briefly what is and what is not incorporated in the generic concept of an HMO. The second section will summarize critical findings concerning HMO performance in rela-

NOTE: The author is indebted to Patricia E. Franks, Philip R. Lee, Susan C. Maerki, Lois Myers, Paul Newacheck, Steven A. Schroeder, Jonathan A. Showstack, and Joan B. Trauner for their valuable comments. This research was supported, in part, by grant number 18-P-97127/9-01, "The Competitive and Selection Effects of HMOs," from the Health Care Financing Administration, and grant number P50 HS02975-02 for the Health Services Policy Analysis Center from the National Center for Health Services Research.

tion to their own enrollees.[1] The third section will explore the importance of the indirect impact of HMO competition. A final section will suggest some implications for national health insurance proposals.

Definition of the Health Maintenance Organization

Although some HMOs are fifty years old, the term itself is less than a decade old. It was coined by health policy activist Paul Ellwood in 1970 to gain the Nixon administration's support for changing the delivery system by encouraging prepaid, fixed-budget medical care. Reflecting its political origins, the term "health maintenance organization" has been used to refer to a variety of organizational forms. Some limit its use to the prepaid group practices that have existed for decades, such as the Kaiser-Permanente plan. In contrast, the federal HMO Act defines them as organizations that comply with an extensive array of requirements. Associations of individual physicians as well as group practices can qualify as HMOs under the act. Some well-established prepaid group practices, however, have chosen not to seek federal designation.

Each of these definitions is too narrow to permit comprehensive analysis of health maintenance organizations' potential role in the health care delivery system and in a national health insurance program. In 1978, more than 200 HMOs of different types existed, and 7.4 million people were enrolled, most of them in group practice plans.[2] For purposes of this analysis, HMOs will be defined in terms of their essential behavioral characteristics. The critical features are as follows:

1. The HMO assumes a *contractual responsibility* to provide or assure the delivery of a stated range of health services, including at least physician and hospital services.
2. The HMO serves an enrolled, *defined population*.
3. The HMO has *voluntary enrollment* of subscribers.
4. The HMO receives a *fixed periodic payment* that is independent of use of services.
5. The HMO assumes at least part of the *financial risk* or *gain* in the provision of services.

Contractual responsibility implies that an HMO member has the legal right to medical care provided by the HMO. This contrasts with

---

[1] This summary is drawn from the analyses presented in Harold S. Luft, *Health Maintenance Organizations: Dimensions of Performance* (New York: Wiley-Interscience, forthcoming 1980).

[2] U.S. Department of Health, Education, and Welfare, Office of Health Maintenance Organizations, *Fourth Annual Report to the Congress* (draft), Washington, D.C., 1978.

the conventional situation in which the medical care provider has the right to decide whether to accept the patient and is under no obligation, other than an ethical one, to provide treatment to a new patient.

The existence of an enrolled, *defined population* means that the health maintenance organization knows its obligations and can estimate the probable demand for its services. The population is usually limited to a specified geographic area.

Voluntary enrollment implies that consumers can choose not to participate in a health maintenance organization; mandatory enrollment would violate the assumption of responsiveness to consumers—a factor that enhances the desirability of HMOs.

The *fixed periodic payment*, independent of the quantity of services provided, implies that, for a given enrollee, the health maintenance organization does not gain any substantial revenue by providing more services. In fact, the fewer services the HMO provides, the more the HMO will increase its net revenue after expenses. In the long run, of course, the HMO may gain more enrollees by offering more services, and it will lose members if it noticeably underserves them. At times patients may be required to make small copayments related to utilization, but these copayments are usually a small fraction of the cost of services and the charges exist primarily to reduce the monthly premium.

Finally, *financial risk* implies that the HMO will suffer or benefit financially from its decisions to provide services. The presence of risk creates the incentives for cost containment that have made HMOs so attractive.

This definition purposefully allows for considerable latitude in organizational characteristics. The definition does not specify two characteristics that define the two major types of HMOs—prepaid group practices (PGPs) and individual practice associations (IPAs). IPAs, often called foundations for medical care, sponsor prepaid programs and conduct peer review of physicians in independent practice. The definition of an HMO excludes any restrictions on method of payment of individual physicians or organization of services—for example, whether they are offered in a single group setting or dispersed over a large number of practitioners' offices. Although there are many important exceptions, most PGPs pay their physicians on a salary basis, and most IPAs are composed of physicians in private offices who are paid on a fee-for-service basis by the health maintenance organization.

The definition of an HMO also allows for variability in other organizational characteristics, such as reliance on part-time versus full-time physicians, profit versus nonprofit orientation, extent of consumer

participation and control, centralization of administration, and ownership and control of facilities.

Even broader than the concept of an HMO is the alternative
delivery system (ADS) proposed by Ellwood and his associates.[3] The
ADS allows more flexibility in the organization and delivery of services
and in the determination of which entities bear the financial risk for
the costs of care. For instance, coinsurance and deductibles can play
a much larger role within an ADS than an HMO. The physician in an
ADS may bear no financial risk; instead, the organization may select
physicians on the basis of their ability to control patient costs. Both an
HMO and an ADS, however, operate within budget constraints, in
contrast to the conventional system of open-ended third-party reimbursement of fee-for-service providers. Although future NHI strategies may
consider the more inclusive ADS, the available evidence on performance
is almost entirely on HMOs or HMO-type plans. This discussion will
take into account that limitation.

A Review of HMO Performance

With respect to NHI, HMOs are attractive primarily for their potential
to contain costs. It would be inappropriate, however, to focus only on
the cost side and ignore other measures of performance, such as quality
of care and consumer satisfaction. If HMOs achieved cost savings by
lowering quality of care, they would hardly be politically attractive.
Similarly, it would be fruitless to encourage plans that are unattractive
to potential enrollees.

As we evaluate the HMO experience, two important caveats must
be kept in mind. The first holds throughout this paper: There have
been no randomized, controlled experiments that involve the assignment of a representative group of people to a wide range of health
insurance plans and health maintenance organizations. (The Rand
Health Insurance Experiment involves only one HMO, and results will
not be available for some time.) Therefore, while we can speak of costs
(or utilization, or satisfaction) being lower in one situation than in
another, we cannot really determine whether differences are attributable
to general characteristics of the plans, to unique features of providers
and administrators, or to subtle differences among people selecting each
plan. This last aspect, self-selection, has been largely overlooked. For
some purposes, self-selection under national health insurance can be
an advantage; for other purposes, a disadvantage.

---

[3] Walter McClure, "On Broadening the Definition of and Removing Regulatory
Barriers to a Competitive Health Care System," *Journal of Health Politics, Policy,
and Law* (Fall 1978), pp. 303–327.

The second caveat concerns the availability of data. A recent comprehensive review of the published evidence on HMO performance indicates great variation in the depth, breadth, and quality of the data.[4] For example, there are more than fifty comparisons of hospitalization, but evaluation of some performance dimensions—such as savings due to ownership of a hospital or long-term trends in performance—relies on a single study. Furthermore, studies frequently concentrate on a single HMO, thus limiting applicability to other HMOs and to NHI policy making. This dictates the use of caution in making definitive conclusions.

HMO Costs. Health maintenance organizations are intuitively attractive as a means for cost control because they alter the usual economic incentives in medical care and give providers a stake in holding down costs. The evidence supports this theory, particularly when the response to HMO incentives is compared with a system of extensive third-party reimbursement for providers. In all instances, the total cost of medical care (premium plus out-of-pocket costs) for HMO enrollees is lower than for apparently comparable people with conventional insurance coverage.[5] The lower costs are clearest for enrollees in prepaid group practices, whose total costs range from 10 to 40 percent below costs for conventional insurance enrollees. Although the difference is smaller, costs for enrollees in individual practice associations also appear somewhat lower than for enrollees in conventional plans.

While there is substantial evidence of lower costs for HMO enrollees, there is little evidence that costs in HMOs are growing less rapidly than in the overall medical care sector.[6] This is not to belittle the importance of a 10-to-40-percent cost difference, but it suggests that HMOs may not have the solution to the dynamic of escalating medical costs within a predominantly third-party, cost-reimbursement medical system.

Knowing that costs are lower for HMO enrollees is only the first step. Before deciding upon the role of HMOs under NHI, we must try to understand how these cost differences are achieved. Total costs can be divided into the cost per unit of service and the number of units of each type of service provided by the system. Differences in total cost, then, theoretically can reflect differences in each of these elements. If

---

[4] Luft, *Health Maintenance Organizations.*

[5] Harold S. Luft, "How Do Health Maintenance Organizations Achieve Their 'Savings'?: Rhetoric and Evidence," *New England Journal of Medicine,* vol. 298 (June 15, 1978), pp. 1336–1343.

[6] Harold S. Luft, "Trends in Medical Care Costs: Do HMOs Lower the Rate of Growth?" *Medical Care,* vol. 18, no. 1 (January 1980), pp. 1–16.

lower HMO costs reflect lower costs per unit, HMO input prices must be lower, or HMO production more efficient. Because HMOs generally pay competitive salaries for the people they hire, and their physicians have earnings comparable to those in fee-for-service practice, we direct our attention to efficiencies in production.

The question of whether group practice leads to economies of scale has long been a subject of debate.[7] It is important to recognize that the issue here has little to do with the performance of HMOs as a unique organizational form; whatever economies of scale exist should be equally obtainable by both fee-for-service and prepaid medical groups. Although most studies agree that economies of scale may occur as practice size increases, these economies peak at a relatively low scale, between two and five practitioners.[8] Whether productivity per physician remains constant or even declines beyond that point is hard to evaluate. Thus, there is no real support for the claim that large prepaid group practices realize substantial economies of scale in ambulatory care.

Because the expensive part of medical care occurs in the hospital, more efficient production of hospital services by health maintenance organizations could have a significant impact on total costs. Until recently, however, only the Kaiser plans and Group Health Cooperative of Puget Sound controlled their own hospitals. The available data show no consistent differences in cost per patient day, although lengths of stay are shorter, and thus, costs per case are lower in the HMO-controlled hospitals.[9] A detailed examination of hospital costs for people in Group Health Cooperative of Puget Sound and those in a comprehensive Blue Cross-Blue Shield plan in Seattle indicates hospital

[7] See, for instance, Rashi Fein, *The Doctor Shortage: An Economic Diagnosis* (Washington, D.C.: The Brookings Institution, 1967); Herbert E. Klarman, "Economic Research in Group Medicine," in *New Horizons in Health Care*, proceedings of the First International Congress on Group Medicine, Winnipeg, Manitoba, April 26–30, 1970, pp. 178–193; Donald E. Yett, "An Evaluation of Alternative Methods of Estimating Physicians' Expenses Relative to Output," *Inquiry*, vol. 4, no. 1 (March 1967), pp. 3–27; Uwe E. Reinhardt, "A Production Function for Physician Services," *Review of Economics and Statistics*, vol. 54, no. 1 (February 1972), pp. 55–66; Richard M. Bailey, "Economies of Scale in Medical Practice," in Herbert Klarman, ed., *Empirical Studies in Health Economics* (Baltimore: Johns Hopkins University Press, 1970), pp. 255–273; John H. Lorant and Larry J. Kimbell, "Determinants of Output in Group and Solo Medical Practice," *Health Services Research*, vol. 11, no. 1 (Spring 1976), pp. 6–20.

[8] Lorant and Kimbell, "Determinants of Output"; Reinhardt, "Production Function"; John B. MacFarland and Richard J. Odem, "Income and Expenses of Group Practices and the Role of the Business Manager," in Judith Warner and Phil Aherne, eds., *Profile of Medical Practice* (Chicago: American Medical Association, 1974), pp. 66–79.

[9] Luft, *Health Maintenance Organizations*, chapter 7.

costs in the HMO were about 25 percent lower. Almost all of this difference, however, was attributable to lower utilization rates; the unit costs for drugs, X-rays, laboratory, and other services were comparable.[10]

HMOs also may increase their relative efficiency by avoiding duplication of facilities. Critics have often observed that community hospitals compete for physicians by purchasing special equipment that subsequently is used at far less than capacity. Because HMO-controlled hospitals can plan for a defined population, they should not face this problem. For example, Kaiser appears to centralize its services and to have less duplication of facilities than do conventional hospitals.[11] This is in addition to its use of highly specialized facilities available at other hospitals. Occupancy rates are difficult to compare because of the charge that conventional hospitals sometimes admit or retain patients unnecessarily when they have excess capacity.

To summarize the evidence on costs, existing prepaid group practices clearly have been able to provide medical care for their enrollees at costs 10 to 40 percent lower than costs for enrollees in conventional plans. Individual practice associations have experienced smaller differentials. The lower costs appear to stem from lower utilization rates, rather than from lower costs per unit of service. Finally, there are few economies of scale, but large systems that control their own hospitals, such as Kaiser, do appear to reduce duplication of facilities.

Utilization of Services. In contrast to the relative paucity of data on costs, there is ample evidence on both inpatient and ambulatory care utilization by enrollees in HMOs and in conventional plans. Differences are likely to be concentrated in hospital rather than in ambulatory care services because hospital use is easier to control. The consumer can initiate directly an ambulatory visit, but only a physician can authorize a patient's admission to a hospital. Furthermore, HMOs typically lower financial barriers to ambulatory care use and may attempt to substitute ambulatory for inpatient care.

The evidence supports the expectation of greater differences in hospital use than in ambulatory care visits.[12] A review of more than two

---

[10] K. M. McCaffree et al., "Comparative Costs of Services," in *The Seattle Prepaid Health Care Project: Comparison of Health Services Delivery*, chapter 3, W. C. Richardson et al., eds., National Technical Information Service, PB #267488-SET, 1976.

[11] Harold S. Luft and Steven Crane, "Regionalization of Services within a Multihospital Health Maintenance Organization," *Health Services Research*, Fall 1980.

[12] Luft, "How Do HMOs Achieve Savings?"

dozen studies indicates somewhat more ambulatory visits for HMO enrollees, particularly those in individual practice associations, than for patients in the fee-for-service system.

Differences are larger and the direction is reversed when hospitalization studies are reviewed. Based on more than fifty observations over a twenty-five-year period, those studies with good data almost unanimously support the claim that enrollees in prepaid group practices have lower hospitalization rates than do people with conventional insurance. Results for IPA enrollees are less conclusive.

Average differences in utilization between enrollees in HMOs and people who rely on fee-for-service medical care are substantial, with about 30 percent fewer hospital days for enrollees in prepaid group practices and 20 percent fewer days for enrollees in individual practice associations. The number of hospital days per enrollee is the product of admissions per enrollee and length of stay per admission. HMO enrollees have somewhat shorter stays than do people in conventional plans, but most of the overall utilization difference stems from lower admission rates.

Explaining these lower admission rates is critical to evaluating the performance of HMOs. There are two alternative explanations: (1) HMOs identify and screen out cases that really do not require hospitalization—the discretionary or "unnecessary" cases; or (2) HMOs achieve a lower hospitalization rate without any apparent discrimination among cases according to obvious "necessity." If the first explanation holds, HMO desirability is confirmed both on cost and on quality grounds. If the second explanation holds, HMO experience must be assessed cautiously to make sure that lower costs are not the result of lower quality or a different patient mix, and then to investigate further other factors that may potentially explain the lower hospitalization rates in HMOs.

A survey of the best available data from a broad range of HMOs tends to support the second explanation rather than the first. HMO admissions are not disproportionately lower among surgical as opposed to medical cases; instead, admissions seem to be lower across the board.[13] Similarly, although admissions for certain "discretionary procedures," such as hernia repair and hysterectomy, are lower in HMOs than in matched conventional plans, figures for discretionary procedures are not disproportionately lower than figures for all surgery. Unfortunately, categories of "discretionary" care are rough approximations that mask fine distinctions in patient care. It is very likely both that

---

[13] Ibid.

many so-called discretionary admissions are actually essential, and that many "nondiscretionary" admissions are actually optional.

Recognizing the complexities of evaluating admissions and assuming a scattering of discretionary cases in all patient categories, we find four possible, but not mutually exclusive, explanations for lower hospital admissions in HMOs:

1. Rather than reducing admissions for categories of cases the literature has identified as "discretionary," an effective HMO can still avoid individual discretionary admissions. A good physician can, if pressed, triage patients on a one-by-one basis and decide who really needs admission and who can be treated on an ambulatory basis.

2. HMOs may undertreat, or traditional providers overtreat, nondiscretionary cases. This will lead to our discussion of quality of care in HMOs.

3. HMOs may provide preventive care that reduces the occurrence of health problems that require hospital admissions.

4. Self-selection among HMO enrollees may be critical to lower admission rates; that is, better health or greater aversion to hospital admissions among HMO enrollees may contribute to the differential between HMO and fee-for-service age-sex adjusted admission rates in so-called nondiscretionary categories.

Sufficient evidence is not yet available to allow for a comprehensive evaluation of these hypotheses, but some evidence does exist with respect to quality, preventive care, and self-selection.

Quality of Care. Improved health status or outcome is a major objective of medical care, but outcomes are very difficult to measure. Health services researchers often rely on other measures of medical care quality, such as the presence of "appropriate" resources (structural measures) and the use of "appropriate" procedures for given cases (process measures).[14] There is little evidence, however, that structure, process, and outcome measures correlate well with each other or with what people might recognize as "quality."[15] Despite these limitations, all three measures are used here to review the quality of care in HMOs.

---

[14] Avedis Donabedian, "Evaluating the Quality of Medical Care," *Milbank Memorial Fund Quarterly*, vol. 44, no. 3 (July 1966, part 2), pp. 166–203.

[15] Robert H. Brook, "Critical Issues in the Assessment of Quality of Care and Their Relationship to HMOs," *Journal of Medical Education*, vol. 48, no. 4 (April 1973, part 2), pp. 114–134; William E. McAuliffe, "Studies of Process-Outcome Correlations in Medical Care Evaluations: A Critique," *Medical Care*, vol. 16, no. 11 (November 1978), pp. 907–930.

Although furthest removed from outcomes, structural measures are the most visible indexes of quality of care. The available data generally support the argument that HMOs have resources at least as good as resources of the conventional system.[16] HMOs tend to have higher proportions of more highly trained physicians and are more likely to use accredited hospitals. There are, however, a number of important exceptions. Some HMOs have not been able to obtain ready access to the "better" hospitals, and others apparently have chosen not to emphasize specialists and use of accredited, nonprofit facilities. Although many HMOs have excellent resources, there is nothing in a health maintenance organization's direct financial incentives to promote structural quality, other than the possible advantages structural quality offers in attracting physicians or enrollees.

With respect to organizational factors, there is little evidence that HMO characteristics, in contrast to specific HMOs, lead to quality of care above or below that in the fee-for-service sector. Despite frequent claims, there is no convincing evidence that group practice really leads to more informal consultations among physicians.[17] Group practice does seem to encourage more time for continuing education, but there is little evidence that such programs make a difference in the delivery of care; they may well be just a fringe benefit. Finally, group practice is not essential to peer review; physicians in group practice have the advantage of physical proximity, but individual practice associations and fee-for-service practice allow for the development and use of practice profiles to evaluate physician care.

The available evidence supports the view that the average HMO offers care comparable or somewhat superior to the "average" fee-for-service practitioner, but there is no evidence it is superior to that of the "better" conventional settings. Although HMO physicians tend to receive higher ratings on process measures based on laboratory tests than do conventional practitioners, this differential appears to reflect comprehensiveness of coverage rather than organizational characteristics. Large prepaid group practices often exhibit higher quality than do average fee-for-service providers, but the quality is not higher than that of large fee-for-service multispecialty group practices.[18] The HMO financial

---

[16] Luft, *Health Maintenance Organizations*, chapter 11.

[17] Paul B. Guptill and Fred E. Graham, II, "Continuing Education Activities of Physicians in Solo and Group Practice: Report on a Pilot Study," *Medical Care*, vol. 14, no. 2 (February 1976), pp. 173–180.

[18] Beverly C. Payne and Thomas F. Lyons, *Detailed Statistics and Methodologies for Studies of Personal Medical Care in Hawaii* (Ann Arbor: University of Michigan School of Medicine, 1972). (Available through University Microfilms, LD 00039.)

structure, therefore, does not appear to be as critical to performance as is multispecialty group practice.

Outcome measures are expected in quality evaluation, but most studies focus on narrowly defined mortality-morbidity measures or on broad outcomes such as disability days. The early Health Insurance Plan studies showed lower prematurity and mortality rates for HMO enrollees. Few subsequent studies offer as conclusive evidence in any direction. In general, the available data suggest that outcomes in HMOs are much the same as or slightly better than those in conventional practice.

Use of Preventive Services. Studies of the provision of preventive services can be divided into two groups that appear to have contradictory findings.[19] The first group supports the hypothesis that HMO enrollees receive more preventive services than do people with conventional health insurance. The second group suggests that there are no differences in the use of preventive services or that the HMO enrollees receive even fewer services than do people with conventional coverage. In fact, the two sets of studies are not really in conflict. With a few exceptions, the different results can be explained by focusing not on the distinction between HMO versus other coverage, but on the presence or absence of coverage for preventive visits. Such coverage is almost universal with HMOs, but it is rare with conventional insurance. In fact, studies comparing HMO enrollees with people having conventional coverage for preventive services typically have ambiguous results; the HMOs provide more preventive care of some types and less of others.

These results may reflect recent skepticism in the medical community concerning the efficacy of many "preventive services," such as tests, screenings, and checkups.[20] More importantly, even if the better coverage in HMOs leads to more use of certain preventive services, this does not account for the lower hospitalization rates. As was mentioned, the efficacy of many of these services is questionable. Furthermore, many new HMOs have started with low hospitalization

---

[19] Harold S. Luft, "Why Do HMOs Seem to Provide More Health Maintenance Services?" *Milbank Memorial Fund Quarterly/Health and Society*, vol. 56, no. 2 (Spring 1978), pp. 140–168.

[20] Anne-Marie Foltz and Jennifer L. Kelsey, "The Annual Pap Test: A Dubious Policy Success," *Milbank Memorial Fund Quarterly/Health and Society*, vol. 56, no. 4 (1978), pp. 426–462; Herbert L. Abrams, "The Overutilization of X-Rays," *New England Journal of Medicine*, vol. 300, no. 21 (May 24, 1979), pp. 1213–1216; Jocelyn Chamberlain, "Screening for the Early Detection of Diseases in Great Britain," *Preventive Medicine*, vol. 4 (1975), p. 268; David L. Sackett, "Screening for Early Detection of Disease: To What Purpose?" *Bulletin of the New York Academy of Medicine*, vol. 51, no. 1 (January 1975), pp. 39–52.

rates on day 1, with no chance for their preventive services to have an effect.[21]

The Impact of Self-Selection. The immediate appearance of lower hospitalization rates suggests two different explanations: (1) HMO physicians have different practice patterns, so new enrollees immediately experience less hospitalization; or (2) people joining HMOs are less likely to use hospital services. The definition of an HMO implies voluntary enrollment, so people in an HMO have had an option to select the plan most suitable for their needs. This option of HMO coverage is not available to most people, who are offered typically a single type of health insurance coverage by their employer or union.

The literature about self-selection in HMOs is somewhat ambivalent. The theory of consumer preference, often identified in this instance as the "risk-vulnerability hypothesis," argues that people most concerned about the expected costs of medical care will choose the HMO option with its more comprehensive coverage. In fact, HMOs have been concerned that such self-selection during open enrollment periods will leave them with a high proportion of people needing immediate care. This has often been the case with maternity services, because of better HMO coverage.[22] Conversely, it has been argued that HMOs attract healthier people and that this is the basis of their low utilization rates.

Until very recently, the self-selection issue had been addressed only indirectly, by examining the age, sex, marital status, income, or employment characteristics of HMO members and enrollees in conventional plans. Some comparisons have been more direct, and plan members have been asked about their health status, including chronic conditions. In general these studies have shown few differences between people enrolling in HMOs and in conventional plans.[23] Unfortunately, a great many factors influence medical care utilization and, even in the best of studies, the variables that have been examined explain only a small fraction of the variation in use.

In the last few years, however, new data have become available that allow for a more direct test of self-selection.[24] The approach is

---

[21] Office of Health Maintenance Organizations, *Fourth Annual Report.*

[22] Jack Hudes, et al., "Are HMO Enrollees Being Attracted by a Liberal Maternity Benefit?" a paper presented at the Joint National Meeting of the Institute of Management Sciences/Operations Research Society of America, New Orleans, La., May 1, 1979.

[23] Luft, *Health Maintenance Organizations,* chapter 3.

[24] Klaus Roghmann, Andrew Sorensen, and Sandra Wells, "Hospitalizations in Three Competing Health Maintenance Organizations during Their First Two Years: A Cohort Study of the Rochester Experience," *Group Health Journal,* vol. 1, no. 1 (Winter 1980), pp. 26–33; William C. Richardson et al., *The Seattle Pre-*

simple: First, measure the medical care utilization of a group of people with conventional insurance coverage. Then, after this group has been offered an HMO option, measure the use of both those who choose the HMO and those who remain in the conventional plan. This before-and-after design provides direct estimates of whether people joining HMOs are high or low utilizers.

These direct estimates indicate that self-selection can be an important factor. Furthermore, the type of selection depends upon the type of HMO being offered and the net premium cost to potential enrollee. When offered an IPA or an HMO option that allows a person to retain his or her original physician, those joining the HMO were relatively high utilizers. People joining PGPs tended to be substantially lower utilizers of hospital care before enrolling. In fact, some groups of new PGP enrollees had hospitalization rates while in Blue Cross that were as low as their subsequent utilization rates in the HMO, implying no reduction in utilization, or no HMO effect. (This is probably an extreme example.)

The figures for ambulatory use are different. Except for maternity coverage, relative to conventional insurance, the HMOs' comprehensive coverage is much more of an advantage for ambulatory than for in-patient services. Those who were faced with a substantial extra premium for joining the HMO would make that choice only if previously they had been relatively high users of ambulatory care. But, as noted above, from the HMOs' perspective, ambulatory care use is a small cost relative to the cost of hospital care. People who faced no additional premium for the HMO seem to view it as a convenient, new one-stop source of care, should they need it. An existing relationship with a physician, however, would influence their decision not to join an HMO.[25]

Although these self-selection findings are important, one should use them with care. By design, the studies measure only differences in utilization during the first year or so of membership, when the new enrollees have not yet established a relationship with a physician. Over time, that situation will change, and these relatively low utilizers are likely to become greater consumers of services. Thus, although the selection effect may account for part of the utilization differences among

paid Health Care Project: Comparison of Health Services Delivery, final report for Grant No. R18 HS 00694, National Center for Health Services Research, National Technical Information Service, PB #267488-SET, 1976.

25 Anne A. Scitovsky, Nelda McCall, and Lee Benham, "Factors Affecting the Choice between Two Prepaid Plans," *Medical Care*, vol. 16, no. 8 (August 1978), pp. 660–681; S. E. Berki et al., "Enrollment Choices in Different Types of HMOs: A Multivariate Analysis," *Medical Care*, vol. 16, no. 8 (August 1978), pp. 687–697.

new enrollees, it is unlikely that self-selection fully explains the performance of mature HMOs.

The second important lesson is that enrollment in an HMO can be influenced substantially by the details of the benefit package, the premium, and the enrollee contribution. We will return to this point later when we consider the role of the competitive environment in HMO performance.

Consumer Satisfaction

The self-selection issue bears directly on the question of consumer satisfaction with HMOs. Aside from the common, but unrepresentative anecdotal story about a particular HMO, there are two different approaches to measuring satisfaction.[26] One approach focuses on feelings that people have about various aspects of medical care, such as access, cost, information transfer, quality, and humaneness. Each aspect is treated as a separate dimension and no effort is made to combine them. Another approach identifies and measures the behavioral correlates of satisfaction or dissatisfaction, such as use of services out-of-plan and withdrawal from the HMO.

Among a broad range of access measures, prepaid group practices offer shorter office waiting times, but longer waiting periods to obtain an appointment. The relative importance of these two measures varies among individuals. The PGP pattern is probably best for people with routine problems that can be scheduled, such as for checkups and periodic visits for chronic conditions. People with "semi-urgent" acute problems who can afford the time to wait in the office are more likely to prefer fee-for-service practitioners and the guarantee of eventually seeing one's own physician.

It is not surprising that financial coverage is the feature of health maintenance organizations that members like most. HMO members almost universally express greater satisfaction with financial coverage provided by their HMOs than do people with other insurance coverage.

HMOs and fee-for-service arrangements also seem to differ with respect to physician-patient relationships.[27] Prepaid group practices appear to offer less consumer identification with a single physician, but more continuity within a system having the patient's records. In medical care, communication between physician and patient is vital. Overall, people enrolled in prepaid group practices seem less happy with their communication with physicians than do fee-for-service patients

---

[26] Luft, *Health Maintenance Organizations*, chap. 11.

[27] David Mechanic, *The Growth of Bureaucratic Medicine* (New York: John Wiley and Sons, 1976).

or people enrolled in individual practice associations. The general view is that PGP physicians are less willing than individual practitioners to spend time with patients. Physicians in prepaid group practice also are reported to be dissatisfied with the degree of communication that they have with their patients.[28]

The second approach to measuring consumer satisfaction assumes, logically enough, that an "important indicator of consumer satisfaction might be the extent to which PGP subscribers continue to use services outside the plans in preference to the corresponding services available to them within the plans."[29] In fact, there is substantial evidence of a negative correlation between outside utilization and expressed satisfaction. The data on outside utilization reflect a reasonably consistent pattern; between 5 percent and 10 percent of prepaid group practice members are regular outside users, while a comparable proportion of different members each year use an occasional service outside the plan.[30] Why people continue to use outside services yet remain enrolled is an unsolved issue.

The dual-choice arrangements available to most HMO members offer what may be the best single *objective* measure to overall satisfaction. The impressive record of long-term growth in the HMO share of given enrollee groups implies that the levels of dissatisfaction are relatively low and have an insignificant effect on membership growth. Among every group of new enrollees, a small portion, perhaps 5 percent to 10 percent, finds that they really do not like the HMO. Such people probably become dissatisfied for one reason or another and leave. These withdrawals, however, are more than offset by withdrawals of people from conventional plans who join health maintenance organizations.

The coexistence of dissatisfaction and continued and growing HMO membership reflect the multiple factors affecting the choice of a health care plan. In the dual-choice setting, people who joined a health maintenance organization obviously felt that it was the best option

---

[28] David Mechanic, "The Organization of Medical Practice and Practice Orientations among Physicians in Prepaid and Nonprepaid Primary Care Settings," *Medical Care*, vol. 13, no. 3 (March 1975), pp. 189–204.

[29] Avedis Donabedian, "An Evaluation of Prepaid Group Practice," *Inquiry*, vol. 6, no. 3 (September 1969), p. 9.

[30] Eliot Freidson, *Patients' Views of Medical Practice: A Study of Subscribers to a Prepaid Medical Plan in the Bronx* (New York: Russell Sage Foundation, 1961); John G. Smillie, "Testimony" in U.S. Congress, House of Representatives, Subcommittee on Public Health and Environment of the Committee on Interstate and Foreign Commerce, *Hearings on Health Maintenance Organizations*, 92nd Congress, 2nd session, April 1972, p. 290; Anne A. Scitovsky, Nelda McCall, and Lee Benham, "Use of Out-of-Plan Services under Two Prepaid Plans" (Palo Alto, Calif.: Palo Alto Medical Research Foundation, 1979).

available to them. In making that decision, they weighed various factors, such as financial coverage, premiums, perceived quality, and access. For some people, the benefits of the HMO option outweighed the possible costs in terms of doctor-patient relations or scheduling visits.

The costs nevertheless continued to exist and, when opinions are solicited, dissatisfaction is likely to be expressed. Hence HMO members like the short waits and financial coverage, but are dissatisfied with the amount of time it takes to get an appointment, their inability to see their usual physician for urgent visits, and the limited communication and warmth in their patient-physician relationship. People would like the plan to improve all the characteristics that bother them but at the same time to maintain its low costs. However, when people are offered, through open enrollment periods, the alternative of improved access and physician-patient interaction versus the price differential associated with conventional coverage, most choose to stay in the HMO.

This summary has been necessarily brief, condensing the major findings of a long book into a section of a paper. The difficulty with a summary is that it omits the qualifications, interpretations, and hesitations, leaving only conclusions that appear certain. In reality, although the lower costs and utilization experienced by HMO enrollees are well documented, we still do not really know how these effects are achieved. It is important to consider two alternative explanations, or scenarios, because they imply markedly different roles for HMOs in terms of their ability to contain costs under NHI.

In one scenario, HMOs attract certain types of physicians and provide incentives for them to practice cost-conscious medicine. This results in marked reductions in hospital use and in substitution of ambulatory for inpatient services. These changes are possible without a measurable sacrifice in quality because current medical practice is "on the flat of the curve," where additional services at the margin have little effect on outcomes. There may be some consumer dissatisfaction with the ambience of care in HMOs, but as for customers at self-serve gasoline stations, the cost savings are worth lack of attention. This scenario is rather encouraging in terms of the potential for cost containment. If the competitive effects of HMOs (discussed in the next section) also exist, then an NHI proposal might use HMOs as its cornerstone.

The second scenario is quite different. In it, much of the lower costs and utilization of HMO enrollees is due to the selective enrollment in PGPs of people less desirous of medical care. To some extent, they need less care because they are younger, employed, mobile, et cetera. More importantly, they may differ from other people, even after adjusting for age, sex, and employment, in subtle preferences for medical care. As already mentioned, beyond the basic level of medical care provided by all reputable HMOs, additional services are generally nonemergency and nonlifesaving. Instead, they serve to improve the "quality of life" and "peace of mind."

But the importance of such quality-of-life or peace-of-mind medical services varies with the individual. One person may choose to undergo a series of surgical treatments for a back problem while another may exercise. Similarly, some people run to a physician for treatment of a cold, while others ignore it and continue to work. There is substantial evidence that the people most likely to join a PGP are those who have no longstanding relationship with a physician. Such people are also lower users of medical care before joining the PGP than are people of the same age, sex, and employment status who choose to remain in a conventional reimbursement plan.

Furthermore, after joining an HMO, a prime determinant of low use is not having a regular physician.[31] Although the structure of many PGPs is not designed to encourage the development of such relationships, those people who join also may not value these relationships highly. This is consistent with the findings of complaints about doctor-patient relationships and low, but significant levels of outside use combined with enough overall satisfaction for increasing enrollment levels. The wide range of discretion in medical care also implies that those people less desirous of care may still have the same outcomes as those in the conventional system.[32]

If this second scenario is close to reality, then the apparent HMO savings are illusory and merely result from isolating the low-cost people in HMOs. A major increase in HMO enrollment would have little direct effect on overall costs.

The true situation probably lies somewhere between these two scenarios, but our ignorance of the real potential for HMO cost containment should give us pause in designing NHI. However, even if HMOs have no direct effects on their enrollees, they may have a beneficial indirect effect through competition with conventional providers.

---

[31] Anne A. Scitovsky, Lee Benham, and Nelda McCall, "Use of Physician Services Under Two Prepaid Plans," *Medical Care*, vol. 17, no. 5 (May 1979), pp. 441–460.

[32] It is noteworthy that in the most carefully studied comparison of HMO and non-HMO care, one of the few instances in which the outcomes were worse for HMO members involved *patient* delays in presenting symptoms of appendicitis. See J. P. LoGerfo et al., "Quality of Care," in William C. Richardson, ed., *The Seattle Prepaid Health Care Project: Comparison of Health Services Delivery*, National Technical Information Service, PB #267488-SET, 1976.

The Competitive Impact of HMOs

Perhaps the most important potential role for HMOs under NHI is their indirect effect as a catalyst for cost containment by conventional providers responding to competition for enrollees. Alain Enthoven's "Consumer-Choice Health Plan" is based on this premise, as are several recent legislative initiatives.[33] Unfortunately, only a handful of studies address this crucial problem and the available evidence is often conflicting.

A 1977 Federal Trade Commission study argues that the entry of HMOs is responsible for lowering the hospital utilization of people in conventional plans.[34] These investigators rest their case on two types of analysis: (1) regressions of hospital utilization by Blue Cross members as a function of HMO market share and other variables; and (2) interviews in various HMO market areas. Unfortunately, the regressions are dominated by four states on the West Coast—California, Washington, Oregon, and Hawaii—all of which have both high HMO market shares and low utilization rates. If these four states are omitted, the negative relationship is no longer significant.[35] The interviews indicate clear competitive reactions by Blue Cross of Northern California to Kaiser's growth, but little supporting evidence in other areas.

A historical perspective supports the notion of a competitive response in Northern California. The San Joaquin Foundation for Medical Care was founded to prevent Kaiser from expanding into the Stockton area.[36] Reactions by fee-for-service physicians to Kaiser in the early 1950s included picketing and leafleting.[37] Numerous articles

---

[33] Alain C. Enthoven, "Consumer-Choice Health Plan," *New England Journal of Medicine*, vol. 298, nos. 12 and 13 (March 23 and March 30, 1978), pp. 650–658 and 709–720; Al Ullman, "Address by the Honorable Al Ullman, Chairman of the House Committee on Ways and Means," a paper presented at the *National Journal* Conference on Health Policy, Washington, D.C., June 7, 1979; David Durenberger, "Health Incentives Reform Act of 1979," Senate Bill 1485, 96th Congress, 1st session, July 12, 1979; Dave Stockman, "Rethinking Federal Health Policy: Unshackle the Health Care Consumer," *National Journal*, vol. 11, no. 22 (June 2, 1979), pp. 934–936.

[34] Lawrence G. Goldberg and Warren Greenberg, *The HMO and Its Effects on Competition* (Washington, D.C.: Federal Trade Commission, Bureau of Economics, 1977).

[35] Alain Enthoven, "Competition of Alternative Health Care Delivery Systems," in Warren Greenberg, ed., *Competition in the Health Care Sector: Past, Present and Future*, proceedings of U.S. Federal Trade Commission Conference, Bureau of Economics, Washington, D.C., June 1–2, 1977 (March 1978), p. 336.

[36] Richard Sasuly and Carl E. Hopkins, "A Medical Society-Sponsored Comprehensive Medical Care Plan: The Foundation for Medical Care of San Joaquin County, California," *Medical Care*, vol. 5, no. 4 (July/August 1967), pp. 234–248.

[37] Joseph W. Garbarino, *Health Plans and Collective Bargaining* (Berkeley: University of California Press, 1960).

appeared in local medical society journals decrying rising hospital utilization and predicting the demise of voluntary Blue Cross and Blue Shield plans. Calls for shorter stays, more outpatient care, and the like appear with clear references to the dangers that increasing premiums posed to the continued existence of such health insurance programs.[38] Thus, the historical situation was consistent with the hypothesis that conventional providers saw the threat posed by the new HMOs and began to change their practice patterns to prevent further competitive losses.

Long-term trends in hospital utilization also lend support to a desirable competitive response by conventional providers. One of the major weaknesses in the Goldberg-Greenberg study is that the regressions primarily reflect the lower utilization rates on the West Coast. These geographic patterns appear in all population groups—Medicare beneficiaries, Blue Cross members, federal employees, the National Health Survey, and total hospitalization statistics.[39] But this well-known pattern of lower utilization first appeared between 1950 and 1955, precisely the period of substantial HMO growth on the West Coast. Although this evidence supports the notion of a competitive response, it could also be attributable to a wide variety of other factors, such as a rapidly growing and a young population, or pressures on available medical resources.

At first glance, additional support for the competitive model comes from Rochester, New York, where there has been intense competition between several HMOs and the local Blue Cross-Blue Shield plan. The

[38] John W. Sherrick, "Blue Cross Blues: Doctor's Use or Abuse of Voluntary Health Insurance Plans Determines Their Success," *Alameda-Contra Costa Medical Association Bulletin*, vol. 7, no. 4 (April 1951), pp. 8–11; John W. Sherrick, "A Further Report on Blue Cross," *Alameda-Contra Costa Medical Association Bulletin*, vol. 8, no. 12 (December 1952), pp. 11–14; Robert L. Thomas, "Letter to the Editor," *San Francisco Medical Society Bulletin*, vol. 24, no. 10 (October 1951), pp. 4, 42; Herbert C. Moffitt, Jr., "Use and Abuse of Hospital Insurance— Editorial," *San Francisco Medical Society Bulletin*, vol. 24, no. 10 (October 1951); Garnett Cheney, "President's Page: Physician Responsibility in Medical Welfare Plans," *San Francisco Medical Society Bulletin*, vol. 24, no. 11 (December 1951), pp. 17, 42.

[39] Marian Gornick, "Medicare Patients: Geographic Differences in Hospital Discharge Rates and Multiple Stays," *Social Security Bulletin*, vol. 40, no. 6 (June 1977), pp. 22–41; Blue Cross Association, "The Use of Hospitals by Blue Cross Members in 1972," Research Series 12 (Chicago, March 1974); U.S. Civil Service Commission, *Blue Cross/Blue Shield Utilization Reports*, Washington, D.C. (annual); U.S. National Center for Health Statistics, "Persons Hospitalized by Number of Episodes and Days Hospitalized in a Year: United States—1972," *Vital and Health Statistics*, series 10, no. 116, DHEW Publication No. (HRA) 77-1544, Washington, D.C., 1977; American Hospital Association, *Hospital Statistics—1974 Edition* (Chicago, 1974).

inpatient medical-surgical utilization rate for BC-BS members under 65 years of age was relatively constant until 1975 when it dropped from 512 days to 408 days in 1978, a decline much larger than for any other Blue Cross plan in the East. Much of this decline is attributed to a competitive effect.[40]

There are a number of alternative explanations, however. First, Rochester has had aggressive health planning since the late 1940s, and traditionally has had a very low ratio of beds per capita. It also has an actively interested group of large employers who are encouraging innovation and cost control.[41] An unusual regional budgeting strategy is being implemented.[42] Finally, changes in New York State policies towards nursing home reimbursement have made it more difficult to transfer Medicare and Medicaid recipients out of hospitals. Given the tight bed supply, this could force down the BC-BS utilization rate by limiting the number of beds available to the nonelderly, nonpoor population.[43]

In Hawaii there is very low hospital utilization in both Kaiser and the Hawaii Medical Service Association (HMSA). Although HMSA is nominally a Blue Shield plan, it exercises rather stringent controls over utilization and, thus, acts more like an IPA or an Ellwood-McClure-type alternative delivery system. But the history of HMSA, beginning with its founding by local social workers, the Hawaiian heritage of plantation-provided medical care, and Hawaii's unique ethnic mix, suggest that the HMSA behavior may have more to do with its special history than with competition with Kaiser.[44]

A study of premiums for federal employees enrolled in HMOs offers some support for the competition argument. It shows slower growth in premiums in markets with several HMOs than with a single HMO.[45] Unfortunately, there are only eight market areas and alternative explanations exist for much of the observed behavior.[46] Christianson

---

[40] Finger Lakes Health Services Agency Task Force on Prepaid Health Care, *Health Maintenance Organizations in Rochester, New York: History, Current Performance and Future Prospects*, January 1980.

[41] William G. Von Berg, "Experiments in the Development of Prepaid Group Practice," remarks to Group Health Institute, sponsored by Group Health Association of America, Detroit, May 16, 1972.

[42] Andrew Sorensen and Ernest Saward, "An Alternative Approach to Hospital Cost Control: The Rochester Project," *Public Health Reports*, vol. 93, no. 4 (July/August 1978), pp. 311–317.

[43] Richard Wersinger, personal communication, May 1, 1979.

[44] Richard M. Bailey, *Medical Care in Hawaii: 1970* (Berkeley: University of California, Institute of Business and Economic Research, February 1971).

[45] ICF, Inc., *Analysis of HMO Markets* (Washington, D.C., September 1976).

[46] Enthoven, "Competition of Alternative Systems," p. 456.

and McClure offer a detailed description of competition among seven HMOs in Minneapolis-St. Paul.[47] All but one of these HMOs was formed within the past five years, however, and the Christianson-McClure focus is primarily on the behavior of the HMOs, rather than on the long-term responses of conventional providers.

The Minneapolis situation has been highly publicized as an example of vigorous competition and rapid HMO growth. It therefore warrants further examination. The market share of HMOs grew from 2 percent in 1972 to 4 percent in 1975 to 10 percent in 1978. More importantly, this occurred through the establishment of six new HMOs, widespread dual choice among employers, and much visibility. The potential for savings was also present; the HMOs average about 500 hospital days per 1,000 enrollees, 42 percent below the Blue Cross group average of 860.

Yet, between 1975 and 1977, while HMO enrollment doubled, overall hospital utilization in the Minneapolis-St. Paul metropolitan area stayed constant or increased slightly.[48] Even ignoring a competitive effect, if the new HMO enrollees actually experienced a 42 percent reduction in hospital use, there should have been an areawide decline of 15 days per 1,000. Obviously, many factors could explain this result, but it is consistent with both the notions of no major competitive response and the selective enrollment of low utilizers in HMOs.

The previous discussion noted that the generally low hospital utilization on the West Coast might provide some support for the competitive model. A contrasting approach would examine total expenditures on health care, because even if conventional providers constrained hospitalization in the face of HMO competition, they might maintain their incomes by increasing charges and by providing more physician services. In fact, one of the responses by Blue Cross of Northern California to Kaiser competition was to increase its coverage of ambulatory services and encourage efforts to reduce hospitalization.[49]

If competition between HMOs and conventional providers had an impact on overall costs, one might expect it to appear in California, with its massive Kaiser plans, competing HMOs in Southern California, and a documented history of Blue Cross concern. Although the most recent figures on state per-capita health expenditures are for 1969,

---

[47] Jon B. Christianson and Walter McClure, "Competition in the Delivery of Medical Care," *New England Journal of Medicine*, vol. 301, no. 15 (October 11, 1979), pp. 812–818.

[48] American Hospital Association, *Hospital Statistics*, 1975, 1976, 1977, 1978 editions (Chicago, 1975–1978).

[49] Goldberg and Greenberg, "HMO Effects."

these figures provide little support for the competitive model.[50] (More recent data for the Medicare population yield similar results.) California ranked third among the fifty states, even before adjusting for the lower cost of living.

But how could this happen when hospitalization in California is so low? The answer is that, although hospitalization is the largest single type of expenditure and is easily measurable, there are other pieces of the pie. Perhaps as a result of the improved ambulatory care coverage by conventional insurers, California ranked second in the share of per-capita expenditures for physicians' services. (Washington State, also with high HMO penetration, was first.) Consequently, California ranked forty-sixth in the share of expenditures for hospital care. Thus, by some standards the mix of medical services bought by Californians may be more efficient, but there is no evidence that even massive HMO enrollment has resulted in overall cost containment.

Most interest in the competitive environment has focused on the impact of HMOs on conventional providers, but it is also important to underscore the importance of the precise nature of the effect of market environment on HMO performance. A recent study of University of California employees demonstrates rather clear price sensitivity in enrollment choice.[51] In response to consistently higher Blue Cross premiums, Kaiser enrollment has more than doubled, from 7,500 in 1967 to 15,500 in 1978, while Blue Cross enrollment remained stable at about 9,200. But the more interesting issue is on the cost side. Between 1971 and 1978 the Kaiser premium rose 78 percent; the increase for Blue Cross was nearly twice that—146 percent. By 1978, the additional cost to the employee for choosing Blue Cross rather than Kaiser was $246 for single and $551 for family coverage.

One cannot translate the Kaiser premiums into expenditures because it is based on a community rate, representing the experience of all Northern California Kaiser members. The Blue Cross premium, however, reflects the University of California experience, and suggests the stable group of enrollees was increasingly composed of high utilizers. This conjecture is supported by what has occurred at Stanford during the same period. Enrollments in both Kaiser and Blue Cross grew at about the same rate, as did their premiums, suggesting that the widening differential at the University of California reflects a shifting enrollment

[50] Barbara S. Cooper, Nancy L. Worthington, and Paula A. Piro, *Personal Health Care Expenditures by State*, DHEW Pub. No. (SSA) 75-11906, Washington, D.C., 1975.

[51] Dyan Piontkowski and Lewis H. Butler, "Selection of Health Insurance By an Employee Group in Northern California," *American Journal of Public Health*, vol. 70, no. 3 (March 1980), pp. 274–276.

mix, rather than general cost increases faced by all BC enrollees. The reasons for the different patterns at the two universities is not yet clear, but probably relate to different patterns of employer contributions and their effects on net premium cost to the enrollee.

Implications for National Health Insurance Proposals

There are several implications in all this for the role of HMOs in promoting cost containment under NHI, but they must all be qualified by a single phrase—*proceed with caution*. Caution is warranted because we do not yet know enough about the effects of HMOs, either on their members or the conventional system, to predict accurately their performance under any but the most trivial NHI proposals. Care in the design of a proposal is particularly important because a poorly designed plan, such as the California experiment with prepaid health plans for the poor, could result in a political disaster that makes subsequent changes in any reasonable fashion exceedingly difficult.

Our ignorance about HMO performance is only partial. Costs are lower for HMO enrollees, and this is largely due to lower hospitalization rates. The quality of care is generally comparable to or better than that of the average provider. PGP enrollees are less satisfied with many aspects of HMO membership, such as the nature of the doctor-patient relationship, long appointment lead times, and the time spent with the physician, but the short waiting times and lower cost result in increasing enrollments. Thus, at one level, HMOs are effective in containing costs for their enrollees. The problem is that we cannot be sure whether the HMOs have actually lowered costs or whether a large part of the apparent cost difference is due to self-selection. The second major area of ignorance is the potential influence that HMOs may have on the conventional delivery system.

One thing seems to be certain: The specifics of the benefit package and the net premium cost to the enrollee have a crucial impact on the volume and composition of enrollment. For instance, the distinction between community and experience rating is complex, yet crucial for the prediction of HMO performance under NHI. In general, community rating means that costs are spread over all enrollees in the area; experience rating means that premiums reflect only the experience of a specific subgroup of enrollees. When one is comparing HMOs and conventional plans, the reality sometimes seems the reverse of the usual definition. Community rating for an HMO reflects its own membership, which may not represent the community at large. A simple example can be drawn from the Federal Employees Health Benefits Program, where Blue Cross-Blue Shield premiums are experience-rated and most

HMOs community-rated. There is a single premium for BC-BS enrollees, which, because they constitute 63 percent of all enrollees, may approximate a "community rate." The premium for each HMO reflects local experience, not just of federal employees, but of all members of that HMO. Thus, although the hospitalization rate for FEHBP members across HMOs does not vary much, the premiums range from $14.38 to $46.96, reflecting differences in the costs of medical services. In Washington, D.C., the Group Health Association's rate reflects local high-cost practice patterns, but federal employees with BC-BS coverage in Washington pay premiums based on the average national cost. Regional adjustments to the BC-BS premium would help to rectify this problem, but the problem can reoccur within small areas. Because a PGP can partially control its enrollment mix through the location of its facilities, one can easily imagine aggressive operators segmenting the market and subverting the intended competition of many NHI proposals.

Another lesson is that the health-care delivery market works in slow motion, in contrast to the textbook model of economics. This is especially true when changes must occur through periodic dual-choice periods. Premiums and benefits are set before the open enrollment period and must be held constant for a year. Miscalculation and mis-readings of the competitive situation can lead to painfully slow growth among PGPs or overkill by adverse selection in an IPA. Thus, we may find the analogue to the wild fluctuations of the corn-hog cycle with its built-in adjustment lags. Yet people may be less willing to accept such a market for their medical care.

Finally, there is a strong suggestion that consumer choices in medical care delivery may not be as rational as is often assumed, or at least consumers may not be very interested in cost containment. The continued enrollment of University of California employees in a Blue Cross plan with less comprehensive coverage than Kaiser and $551 extra per year in premiums bodes ill for a cost containment strategy through competition. Similarly, the fact that Californians are among the top medical spenders in spite of HMOs and low hospitalization rates suggests that potential savings may not be desired. Instead, medical care may be a luxury that people choose to buy more of as their incomes rise.

In fact, we may go back to square one and ask whether the interest in cost containment comes from consumers or from the government, whose costs reflect largely the exceptionally high expenses of the old and disabled, people who cannot really be insured in the true sense of the word. Perhaps cost containment and NHI are two separate issues. If so, even more work will be necessary to determine the appropriate future role of HMOs.

Income-Related Consumer Cost Sharing: A Strategy for the Health Sector

Laurence S. Seidman

Many health economists emphasize the importance of consumer cost sharing in promoting health-sector efficiency. At the same time, many believe public policy should assure that every household can afford the medical care it needs. This paper tries to reconcile these two concerns. It sets out the case for *income-related* consumer cost sharing in the health sector. I begin by contrasting the cost-sharing strategy with two alternative approaches: the laissez-faire strategy and the regulatory strategy. I then describe and analyze a consumer cost-sharing strategy which contains three elements: (1) a tax incentive to induce significant patient cost-sharing under private health insurance policies; (2) a medical tax credit on the federal personal income tax; and (3) a guaranteed medical loan program.[1] The tax credit plus loan would provide "insurance of last resort" for households inadequately covered, or completely uncovered, by private insurance.

The Laissez-Faire Strategy

Why is it not best for the government to leave the operations of the health sector completely to the private sector?

---

[1] A tax incentive to induce significant patient cost sharing under private policies has been advocated by several health economists, including Martin Feldstein and Mark Pauly, and has been recently proposed by Rep. Al Ullman, chairman of the House Ways and Means Committee, and by Sen. Richard Schweiker. To my knowledge, the use of the tax credit to implement income-related consumer cost sharing was first proposed by Bridger Mitchell and Ronald Vogel in "Health and Taxes: An Assessment of the Medical Deduction" (Rand Corporation, R-1220-OEO, August 1973). A medical tax credit bill has been introduced in Congress by Rep. Jim Martin, member of the Health Subcommittee of the Ways and Means Committee; the bill is a modification of the bill previously introduced by former Sen. William Brock. The use of guaranteed loans to supplement cost sharing was suggested by Martin Feldstein, "A New Approach to National Health Insurance," *The Public Interest*, vol. 23 (Spring 1971), pp. 93–105 and analyzed in detail by me in Laurence Seidman, "Medical Loans and Major-Risk National Health Insurance," *Health Services Research*, vol. 12 (Summer 1977), pp. 123–128. The importance of consumer cost sharing to promote efficiency has been emphasized by many health economists.

Although I believe the laissez-faire approach is desirable in many sectors of the economy, serious inefficiency and inequity would result from such a policy in the health sector.

There is broad agreement that complete insurance—the absence of cost-sharing for the average patient—is the driving engine of hospital inflation. The advocate of laissez-faire sometimes emphasizes the contribution of public insurance—Medicare and Medicaid—to the inflationary process. But private insurance has the identical effect. If an insurer pays 100 percent of the bill, the patient has no incentive to care about cost. It is irrelevant whether the insurer is private or public.

Today, over 90 percent of all hospital revenues for patient care come from a "third party," private or public.[2] Clearly, most private insurance policies require little or no patient cost sharing for a typical hospital stay. Physicians, choosing on behalf of their privately insured patients, have no reason to consider cost.

"Third-party" inefficiency can be easily understood by a familiar experience: restaurant bill splitting. When a group agrees in advance to split the bill, each person realizes that he will share the burden if others order extravagantly, but his own extravagant order will have little effect on his own burden. In a large group, each person would regard food as free when ordering. Of course, each person must then pay his share of the inflated total bill—his "premium." As long as he pays a premium based on what everyone orders, rather than what he alone orders, he will have no incentive to conserve.

Under private insurance, each person's share of the total bill is his insurance premium. Although that premium is often partly or fully paid by his employer, each employee in reality bears most of the burden, because the premium contribution reduces the employer's ability to pay cash wages. Under group insurance, provided at the workplace, each employee's premium is independent of his own use of medical care, just as under restaurant bill splitting.

In fairness to the laissez-faire approach, it must be recognized that governmental tax policy has encouraged complete private insurance. If an employer pays an employee $100 of cash wage, the employee must pay perhaps $30 of income and payroll tax, so his after-tax income is $70. If the employer instead buys $100 of additional insurance, no tax need be paid. If all compensation—cash or insurance—were taxed equally ("tax neutrality"), it is possible that most employees would prefer private insurance policies with lower premiums; such policies would require more patient cost sharing.

Nevertheless, most would not find the laissez-faire result satis-

[2] Robert Gibson, "National Health Expenditures, 1978," *Health Care Financing Review* (Summer 1979), p. 1.

factory, even with tax neutrality. Such a result would probably not lead to a pattern of coverage in which copayments for medical care varied with the social perception of ability to pay. Moreover, even if varying cost sharing with ability to pay were desired by the private sector, it would be difficult for it to do so. In practice, it is difficult, if not impossible, for private insurers to vary consumer cost sharing according to each employee's ability to pay. Some households have two earners; others, only one. Some have significant property income; others, little or none. Many employees would object to providing such data to private companies. Moreover, the problems of verification might well tempt employees to understate household income. Thus, if income-related cost sharing were attempted, honest employees might well bear larger burdens than dishonest ones, a result unlikely to breed satisfaction with the system. In fact, few private companies that use deductibles and coinsurance—patient cost sharing—have tried to vary them by household income.

If cost sharing must be uniform under private policies, then there are two possibilities. The first is that cost sharing will be kept limited, geared to the ability to pay of the lowest-paid employees. If cost sharing is limited under laissez-faire, even with tax neutrality, then inefficiency and inflation will continue.[3]

The second possibility is that the tax change would induce significant and uniform cost sharing. Inefficiency and inflation might thereby be contained, but only at the expense of what many would regard as serious inequity. Under such uniform cost sharing, low-income households would experience severe financial hardship, and might be unable to afford necessary medical care.

For example, suppose the typical private policy requires a deductible of $1,000, a coinsurance rate of 20 percent, and an out-of-pocket ceiling of $2,000, or 10 percent of the income of a $20,000 household. Such a burden may be bearable for the $20,000 household, especially if the company does not require immediate payment of cost

---

[3] As Mark Pauly explains in his paper in this volume, a household's choice of insurance with limited or no cost sharing can be optimal under certain conditions. A household must balance the benefit of additional risk reduction against the "welfare cost" of the additional "third-party inefficiency" (demand inflation) that results. In the absence of externalities, a household purchasing *individual* insurance would face a premium that reflects expected demand inflation. A highly risk-adverse household might choose an insurance policy with little cost sharing; yet its coverage would optimally balance risk reduction and demand inflation. In the collective choice of a single group insurance policy at the workplace, however, the majority of employees may agree to less cost sharing and a higher premium than they would prefer for themselves, because of concern for equity for low-paid, unhealthy employees. The inefficiency and inflation that results would be above-optimal—it would outweigh the benefits of additional risk reduction for the majority of employees.

sharing (in effect, extends a loan). But it may not be bearable for the $10,000 employee at the same workplace.

In my view, the failure of the private sector to achieve income-related cost sharing is a decisive weakness of the laissez-faire approach under tax neutrality. Medical care differs from other goods and services. Although many have little interest in whether person X obtains a TV, auto, or stereo, most do care whether X can afford the medical care his family needs. Economists call this a consumption externality. A state of affairs in which at least a minority cannot afford necessary medical care provides disutility for many in the society. Moreover, in contrast to food, clothing, and shelter, necessary medical care cannot be assured by providing a minimum cash income. The expenditure required to provide needed medical care varies greatly across households, in contrast to other necessities. Thus, significant uniform cost sharing under laissez-faire would achieve efficiency at the expense of equity.

An amendment to the laissez-faire approach could be offered. Private companies might be legally required to vary cost sharing, and be empowered to obtain the necessary data from households. Thus, households would be required to provide the same information to private companies that they already provide to IRS. But this raises the question: Why not let IRS relate cost sharing to income, so that households need not duplicate income reporting or worry about confidentiality? This is exactly the approach I shall set out shortly as the consumer cost-sharing strategy. The strategy envisions private insurance policies with significant, uniform patient cost sharing, supplemented by an income-related medical tax credit that assists households when their out-of-pocket burden is large relative to their income.

Thus far, the focus has been on group insurance at the workplace. Another fundamental weakness of laissez-faire is that employees of small firms, and persons between jobs, may well remain inadequately covered, as they are today. One philosophical view holds that these persons should be responsible for getting their own insurance. It is important, however, to recognize the obstacles to individual private insurance.

Individual insurance policies are much more expensive than group policies because the economies of scale in enrollment are lost. Private companies will only find it profitable to enroll individual households if they can vary the premium according to the expected medical cost, usually estimated from past experience. Of course, they will not find it profitable to vary the premium according to household income. Thus, a low-income household with poor health experience will be charged a premium that is very large relative to its income, or may even be refused insurance.

Laissez-faire could be modified to subsidize the purchase of in-surance by low-income, unhealthy households not covered at their workplace. It is still doubtful that universal, adequate coverage would be achieved. A minority would undoubtedly continue to be underinsured when catastrophic illness strikes. Although some would conclude that this is not society's problem, many would prefer a public policy that assures universal catastrophic protection. The issue is closely related to whether social security should be voluntary or mandatory.

In sum, a laissez-faire strategy, even with tax neutrality, may not succeed in containing inefficiency and inflation because concern for equity may limit uniform cost sharing under private policies. On the other hand, if the strategy succeeds in causing significant cost sharing, then low-income, unhealthy households may face significant financial barriers to medical care, and be vulnerable to severe financial hardship. Finally, universal catastrophic protection will almost certainly not prevail.

The Regulatory Strategy

At the opposite pole is the view that comprehensive regulation is the best way to manage the health sector. This approach rejects consumer cost sharing as inequitable and impractical. Instead, governmental regu-lation would be relied upon to limit excessive supply and cost.

Advocates of the regulatory strategy sometimes cite public utility regulation as evidence that their approach can work reasonably well. However, there is a fundamental difference between traditional public utility regulation and proposed health-sector regulation—a difference that makes health-sector regulation far more difficult. Consumers pay for their utility services, such as telephone, water, electricity, and natu-ral gas, according to their own use. Each consumer therefore has an incentive to limit his own demand. The task of traditional utility regu-lation is to prevent monopoly pricing, not to cope with inflated demand due to the absence of consumer cost sharing. In the health sector, the regulatory strategy must try to control the consequences of a zero effec-tive price to each consumer.

The difference can be grasped by imagining the challenge facing telephone regulators if all long-distance calls were "free" to the caller. Suppose each household received a fixed monthly bill ("premium"), and could then make unlimited long distance calls. Obviously, the volume of such calls would escalate rapidly, straining the capacity of the current phone system. The phone company, delighted to meet the accelerating demand, would seek a rapid expansion in its capacity. If supply were allowed to match demand, rapid "phone-sector inflation"

311

would ensue. The fixed monthly bill would rise sharply to cover the soaring cost per household. The expansion would be wasteful and inefficient because most households would be unwilling to pay the genuine cost of many of the calls they make.

How could the phone regulators respond? First, they might impose a ceiling on total phone company revenues. This method of "cost containment" would succeed in reducing the national telephone cost, because the phone company would be compelled to limit its capacity and service so that its total cost did not exceed its revenue limit. If limiting total cost were the sole objective, "cost containment" regulation would solve the problem.

The consequence of the revenue ceiling, however, would be chronic excess demand. Because long-distance calls would remain "free" to each caller, households would still seek an excessive number of calls. But they would be unable to complete a large fraction of attempted calls, because phone capacity would be limited by the revenue ceiling. If the regulation were not further refined to limit demand, widespread frustration would ensue. Calls would be free, but "getting a line" would involve long delays. Persons with urgent calls, who would have been willing to pay the genuine cost for prompt service, would often be unable to get through. Some persons would continue to enjoy "frivolous" calls—calls they would never have made were they charged full cost—others would be unable to reach a dying friend, or to complete a productive business transaction.

The next step, obviously, would be to extend the regulation from the supply side to the demand side. One approach might be to place households and business firms in various categories and allocate a quota of calls to each. Of course, it would be necessary to allow exceptions. A family with a dying relative on the opposite coast would need additional calls.

Because charging for additional calls is not permitted under the regulatory strategy, an appeals procedure might be required to decide exceptions. But consider how costly it would be to try to process appeals fairly. Persons would have an incentive to exaggerate need. The regulators would be unable to verify more than a small sample. What penalty would be imposed for "exaggeration"? Would such a penalty deter distortion?

The difficulty is of course analogous to hospital "utilization review," also regulation aimed at limiting demand to available supply in the absence of consumer cost sharing. Physicians, on behalf of their fully insured patients, are inclined to describe any request as necessary, even urgent. For example, should the patient stay the tenth day? If the day is "free," physician and patient might prefer it to home care, even if another hospital day is not essential. Yet the physician would not be a faithful advocate for his patient if he conceded to the hospital, or utilization board, that the tenth day was not essential but merely beneficial.

It is impossible for a utilization review board to determine the particular circumstances of each individual case. If a "hard line" is taken on appeals, inequities will result. The system will be insensitive to differences in individual circumstances and preferences. If the system is too "flexible," it will be abused, because the most aggressive and self-interested will take advantage by exaggerating urgency.

Thus, the reasonable success of today's phone regulation, when each consumer pays for his own long-distance calls, should not be cited as evidence supporting comprehensive health-sector regulation. The relevant analogy would be phone regulation when long-distance calls are free. Of course, such experience is rare, because few question the use of consumer cost sharing in public utilities, as well as virtually every sector of the economy.

It should be clear from the phone analogy that the important issue is not whether the regulatory strategy can limit total national cost. It can, through strict cost-containment methods. The important issue is the sensitivity of the system to the urgency of individual preferences. Resources should not be supplied to those with little urgency; they should be swiftly available to those with an urgent preference. A key question is: Who is to decide whether a particular service for a particular patient is urgent? The patient and his physician, constrained by cost sharing? Or a regulatory board?

Some critics of the regulatory strategy have argued that "the market" will always achieve less cost than government regulation. This mistaken assertion has enabled advocates of regulation to take the offensive. They have correctly argued that total cost can be reduced by strict limits on supply—through revenue or cost ceilings on providers, or specific limits on expansion of capacity and technology. They have correctly noted that Britain has allocated a smaller fraction of its GNP to the health sector under the National Health Service than does the United States. At a time of rapid cost inflation, it has seemed natural to make cost reduction the overriding goal, and to judge alternative strategies by this criterion.

The aim of health-sector policy, however, should be to obtain the right level of cost—neither too high nor too low—both in the aggregate and for each individual. Too little can be just as inefficient as too much, because efficiency means the allocation of resources in response to people's preferences.

For example, consider the supply of hospital beds. Without consumer cost sharing, patients and physicians have no reasons to weigh the cost of additional hospital days. Not surprisingly, observers believe stays are often excessive. Suppose the supply of beds is limited by regulation. It is hoped that only "excessive" days will be eliminated, and that truly necessary admissions will not be delayed, nor necessary stays shortened.

But with hospital days still free to patients, there is no reason to expect each physician to minimize length of stay when a longer stay might be beneficial and convenient though not absolutely essential. Under the fee-for-service system, patients expect their physician to be their advocate, and to guard their interest. Many patients would be alarmed if they thought their physician's loyalty was divided. Thus, most doctors will not assist hospitals and regulators in shortening stays.

A limit on bed supply, therefore, may lead to a shortage. Patients seeking admission may be required to wait, as often occurs in Britain. Regulators and hospital administrators would then decide who to admit first. Waiting lists are just as inefficient as excess beds. If people value quick admissions more than the cost of achieving such promptness, it is inefficient to prevent it in the name of cost reduction.

The outcome of the regulatory approach is ironic. In most other sectors of the economy, consumers are free to go beyond what is absolutely essential. Without regulatory approval, a consumer can seek a higher quality or style, however unnecessary, as long as he is willing to pay the cost. Under the regulatory strategy, consumers would not be free to seek what is merely beneficial. Because the absence of cost sharing invites wasteful use, regulators must counter with strict limits. Because consumers, guided by physicians, have an incentive to exaggerate urgency and demand, it is difficult for regulators to distinguish genuine from feigned urgency. The result is likely to be a "hard line," with supply curtailments that limit choice. Thus, the consumer who seeks an "excessive" refrigerator will meet no obstacle, as long as he is willing to pay for it. But if he finds a speedy admission for semi-elective surgery highly beneficial, he may be unable to obtain it. Consumer choice will be limited most where it matters most: in medical care.

Thus, the fundamental weakness of the regulatory strategy is that it has no effective method for allocating resources in response to the genuine preferences of individual consumers. It is unable to ascertain the degree of urgency of demand of individual consumers, because, in the absence of cost sharing, consumers guided by their physicians have an incentive to exaggerate urgency. In response to exaggerated demand, unable to measure the intensity of genuine preference, regulators must limit supply, and prescribe rules for its allocation with the aim of satisfying the most urgent needs while avoiding wasteful use. How sensitive can a regulatory board be to differences in individual preferences when the medical condition falls under a particular classification? Will simplifying rules prevent responsiveness to particular differences? It is insensitivity to genuine individual preference and urgency, not inflation of total cost, that is the central shortcoming of the regulatory strategy.

The Consumer Cost-Sharing Strategy

Advocates of regulation generally believe that consumer cost sharing in the health sector would be impractical, inequitable, and ineffective. In the past, consumer cost sharing has rarely been income related, and it is difficult to see how private companies would be able to vary cost sharing with ability to pay, as explained earlier. Without such variation, I fully agree that cost sharing is inequitable.

The key to fair, practical cost sharing is to use a modern instrument of public policy: a tax credit on the federal personal income tax. This instrument enables universal coverage, variation of cost sharing with income, and complete confidentiality. The medical tax credit must be supplemented by guaranteed medical loans to handle households' cash flow problems. The tax credit is envisioned as a complement to private health insurance policies with significant uniform cost sharing, and as an adequate insurance policy for every household not covered by private insurance. The tax credit therefore constitutes "insurance of last resort."

An example will illustrate. First, consider a household without private insurance. Suppose it has an income of $20,000. Under the medical tax credit, it might have to bear the first $1,000 (its deductible) of its annual medical bill out of pocket. It would be entitled to file for a tax credit equal to perhaps 80 percent of its additional medical bill (a coinsurance rate of 20 percent), until its total out-of-pocket burden ($1,000 plus 20 percent of the additional bill) reaches $2,000 or 10 percent of its income (its ceiling). This would occur when its annual bill reached $6,000. It could then file for a tax credit equal to 100 percent of the bill in excess of $6,000. Thus, its out-of-pocket ceiling would be $2,000. If the physician charges $1,200, and the hospital charges $300 per day, the patient must spend sixteen days in the hospital before reaching the "free-care" range. Because the average hospital stay is eight days, only a minority of patients would reach the free-care range—in sharp contrast to the current situation, in which virtually all patients are always in the free-care range.

It is possible to increase the percentage of inpatients for whom cost remains relevant without altering the out-of-pocket ceiling of 10 percent. If the tax credit were 85 percent instead of 80 percent, a patient would have to stay 22 days before cost became irrelevant; yet the maximum burden would remain $2,000, or 10 percent of income. Thus, it is indisputable that the tax credit rates can be set so that most hospital patients will not reach the free-care range, yet all patients would be protected by an adequate out-of-pocket ceiling.

The tax credit would replace the current medical deduction on the Form 1040 federal income tax return. The current deduction fails to provide an out-of-pocket ceiling; moreover, it actually provides a greater subsidy rate above the 3 percent threshold for high-income households than for low-income households. (This is a feature of any deduction, as opposed to credit.) The medical tax credit table would vary the household's deductible, coinsurance rate, and ceiling directly with its income. The rate structure could be graduated, so that the ceiling for a $10,000 household might be 9 percent of its income, while the ceiling for a $30,000 household might be 11 percent. In the example that follows, it is assumed that the ceiling is 10 percent for all households.

Now suppose the household has private insurance. If its cost-sharing burden under its private policy were less than its burden would have been without insurance (after receiving a tax credit), then it would not be entitled to any credit. On the other hand, if its cost-sharing burden under its private policy were greater, it would be entitled to a tax credit equal to the difference between the two burdens. Thus, private insurance coverage would never raise the burden on a household.

For example, suppose a private insurance policy has no deductible, and 20 percent coinsurance. Then a $6,000 medical bill would impose a $1,200 burden on a household. If the household's income is $20,000, then under the tax credit schedule given earlier (80 percent credit, 10 percent ceiling), it would not be entitled to any credit, because its burden would have been $2,000 without private insurance. If the household's income were $10,000, it would be entitled to a credit of $200, because its burden would have been only $1,000 without private insurance (assuming the ceiling is 10 percent of income).[4]

---

4 The taxpayer with private insurance would compute his tax credit as follows: The insurance company would be required to provide the taxpayer with his total annual medical bill and total cost sharing under the private policy. Using the medical tax credit table, the taxpayer would find the tax credit to which he would have been entitled without insurance for the same medical bill. He would then subtract that hypothetical credit from his annual medical bill to obtain his out-of-pocket burden without insurance. If his cost sharing under the private policy exceeds his burden without insurance, he would be entitled to a tax credit equal

It should be emphasized that if the household buys private insurance, the private policy would "go first," and the tax credit would "go last." The tax credit would be computed only after the insurance company's contribution towards the household's medical bill was determined. Thus, it would be impossible for a household to seek private insurance to cover its cost sharing under the tax credit. Such a strategy would only be possible if the tax credit "went first," and the private policy "last." The interaction of private insurance and the tax credit is explored further in the appendix.

The tax credit would apply equally to all medical care (inpatient, outpatient, office, and home care), avoiding the bias of many private plans that cover only inpatient care. Low-income households would now file a tax return solely to obtain medical tax credit. The credit would be "refundable," so that IRS would pay the household if its credit exceeded its tax liability. Eligibility for the tax credit would not depend on whether the taxpayer itemizes. A medical tax credit bill has been introduced in Congress by James Martin of the Health Subcommittee of the House Ways and Means Committee.[5]

A guaranteed medical loan program is an essential complement. The tax credit is designed to assure that each household, if given a reasonable period in which to pay, can afford its out-of-pocket burden. Many households, however, will be unable to pay immediately. Moreover, it will take up to a year for the tax return and credit to be filed and processed. To handle the cash flow problem, each household must be guaranteed convenient access to a medical loan at reasonable terms.

As I have described in detail elsewhere,[6] the government should contract with private health insurance companies and loan institutions to operate the loan program. Each household would receive annually a health credit card from IRS. The household would simply send its credit card, loan application, and medical bill to the designated lender. The lender would process the bill, and promptly pay the hospital and physician, just as private insurance companies do today. When the credit has been filed and processed, IRS would use the tax credit to pay the lender. (IRS would have no role other than processing the tax credit; it would not monitor providers.)[7] The lender would then bill the patient for the remainder.

---

to the difference. If cost sharing under the private policy is less than the burden without insurance, he would not be entitled to any tax credit. The taxpayer would be guided through this calculation by standard tax return instructions.

[5] "Medical Expense Tax Credit Act," H.R. 3974, a bill presented by Rep. James Martin and Rep. James Jones in the House of Representatives, May 7, 1979.

[6] Seidman, "Medical Loans."

[7] Hospitals and physicians would be eager to assist persons with little education in applying for a loan because full, prompt payment would depend on it. These

Thus, most patients would pay little or nothing out of pocket for perhaps a year after incurring a large medical bill. Because private health insurance companies are experienced in monitoring and processing medical bills, it is hoped they will participate fully in the loan program (just as they helped administer Medicare).

The income-related tax credit plus guaranteed loan program is the key to resolving the impasse over cost sharing under private insurance policies. Without the supplementary credit (and loan), uniform cost sharing under a private policy might overburden a household with a medical bill that is large relative to its income. This concern has been a central reason for the opposition to such cost sharing. The tax credit, however, would provide "insurance of last resort" that is income related. It guarantees that private-policy cost sharing will not overburden any household. It therefore provides the setting in which to introduce the final element of the strategy: a new tax incentive to encourage significant cost sharing under private policies.

There are several ways to encourage private-policy cost sharing. The first, favored by many health and public finance economists, is simply to end the current tax subsidies to private insurance. This would be achieved by including any employer contribution to insurance in the taxable income of the employee. Virtually all economists agree that a proper definition of household income includes such contributions. The partial deductibility of household premium expenses under the personal income tax should also be eliminated. The termination of tax subsidies to insurance should induce many employees to prefer policies with lower premiums (and therefore, greater cost sharing).

Given the "insurance-of-last-resort" tax credit, however, elimination of all tax subsidy to private insurance might induce many households to end private coverage. To prevent this, a substantial tax incentive for private insurance with significant cost sharing should be retained. Only tax subsidy for insurance with little or no cost sharing would be ended. The aim would be to induce covered households to retain restructured private insurance, and to induce uncovered households to obtain such insurance.

Several designs of the new tax incentives are possible. One design would include the employer's contribution in the employee's taxable

---

providers would surely help such patients complete the necessary form (as they do today under Medicaid). Similarly, the designated lender would be eager to help such patients in filing a tax return, because reimbursement of the lender by IRS would depend on it. The lender would inform the patient that if he would otherwise not file a tax return, the lender—with his permission—would complete a streamlined return on his behalf, solely to claim tax credit. Thus, it should be possible to provide full assistance to persons who might have difficulty filing a return on their own.

income, but provide a tax credit for the employee if the policy provides catastrophic protection. The credit should be no greater than the estimated cost of an adequate policy, so that the employee must bear the full cost of more extensive insurance (in fact, the credit can be less than the estimated cost, because the employee may be expected to bear part of the premium cost). A low-income employee must be able to buy a policy with a lower ceiling, and therefore, a higher premium, than a high-income employee. Thus, the credit must vary inversely with income to assure that each can afford an adequate policy. Other designs are also possible.[8]

Whichever design is adopted, households would of course be free to obtain insurance with little or no cost sharing. But they would now have to pay the full cost of such insurance without the benefit of tax subsidy. Relative to the current situation where tax subsidies encourage insurance without limit, any of these designs would introduce a new tax incentive that encourages significant cost sharing in private policies.

The tax credit, loan, and tax incentive for cost sharing would provide the framework for a healthy competition between fee-for-service providers and health maintenance organizations (HMOs). In the past, the unlimited tax subsidy for fee-for-service insurance has reduced the attractiveness of delivery systems that provide care at moderate cost. Once households must bear the cost of an expensive policy, they will weigh efficiency more carefully.

Health policy should not promote one delivery system over another, but rather should promote a fair competition. Some households prefer provider prepayment (an HMO), so that the provider does not have an incentive to perform additional services as under fee for service. On the other hand, some prefer fee for service, so that the provider does not hesitate to perform additional service, as it might under prepayment. There are pros and cons to each arrangement. What matters is not which arrangement reduces cost per se, but which provides the cost-quality-risk package most attractive to each individual household. The cost-sharing strategy is designed to increase the freedom of choice of each household.

---

[8] The basic idea for the tax credit for private catastrophic insurance was suggested by Mark Pauly in correspondence with the author. Another design would retain tax deductibility for an employer contribution only for insurance that contains a minimum of perhaps 20 percent coinsurance for perhaps the first $6,000 of annual medical bill. Premium expense for a prepaid health maintenance organization, however, would be tax deductible even without cost sharing, because prepayment to providers in itself promotes cost containment. Still another design would place a cap on the size of the employer contribution that can be excluded from employee taxable income, so that each employee must bear the full cost of insurance above the cap. Bills with each of these designs have recently been introduced in Congress.

It must be recognized that the tax credit is a modern policy instrument. It is only in the past two decades that the personal income tax has extended its coverage to nearly the entire population. Earlier, it would have been impossible to relate cost sharing to income in a practical, confidential manner. It is understandable that many who were concerned with equity historically supported "free" medical care, and opposed any patient cost sharing.

The tax credit implies that such opposition to cost sharing should be reconsidered. A sophisticated income tax system has for the first time enabled a balance to be struck between equity and efficiency. Cost sharing can now be geared to each household's ability to pay. It is possible to guarantee that every household can afford whatever care it needs, yet at the same time to provide most households with an incentive to weigh cost.

Would Consumer Cost Sharing Work?

Although the tax credit makes cost sharing practical, the question remains: Will it be effective? Critics of cost sharing like to depict the following scenario. The patient, barely conscious, survival in doubt, is about to be wheeled into the operating room on a stretcher. As his stretcher approaches the operating room, he manages to whisper: "Where's my *Consumer Reports*, and what's the other hospital charging?"

Advocates of cost sharing fully agree that it is unrealistic to expect a patient to shop around for a hospital, or question each service ordered by his physician. Patients rely on their physician to make choices, and such reliance will be unaffected by cost sharing. Yet cost sharing should still be effective. It is through the physician, the key decision maker in the health sector, that advocates expect cost sharing to work.

Today, physicians rarely receive feedback from patients concerning the cost of hospitalization. The reason is that few patients pay even a fraction of their own cost. In fact, many never even know the cost, or see a hospital bill. Physicians know that the average patient wants cost ignored by his physician because the bill is fully paid by a third party.

Under the medical tax credit, and the introduction of significant cost sharing in private insurance policies, the situation of the average patient would change radically. The average patient would pay a fraction of his own hospital bill. At the time of admission, most patients would continue to ignore cost, and remain preoccupied with their medical problem. Two months later, however, having recuperated, the average patient would take interest in his hospital bill. Although a medical loan might defer the burden, he would be able to estimate his ultimate out-of-pocket expense.

At this point, at least an important minority of patients would review their physician's behavior. Was the tenth day, the last, necessary? Was every test essential? Was my hospital X more expensive than hospital Y; if so, was its quality sufficiently greater? In contrast to the current situation, physicians would soon anticipate feedback, and the expectation would begin influencing their behavior.

Some physicians take seriously the trust relationship. When care is free to their own patient, they correctly reflect their patient's preference by ignoring cost. When their patient must pay a fraction of the cost, however, the physician knows his patient would want him to eliminate unnecessary cost. Suppose the doctor knows that for medical condition A, costly hospital X is superior to hospital Y; but for condition B, they provide equal quality. Under complete insurance, the physician might place all patients in hospital X for convenience. Under cost sharing, the ethical physician would still place a patient with condition A in costly X, but would place a patient with condition B in Y.

Other physicians, concerned primarily about their own self-interest, might nevertheless do the same. They would recognize that patients may later resent their lack of concern for cost. Eventually, a reputation for ignoring the financial burden on patients may affect their inflow of patients, and their income.

Is it realistic to expect at least a minority of physicians to weigh the financial impact on the patient? A current example is suggestive. Today, many insurance policies cover inpatient care more fully than outpatient care or home care; some exclude home care completely. It is common for a doctor to note the insurance aspect with his patient, and explain that he will treat him as an inpatient rather than outpatient, and extend the length of hospital stay, rather than secure a nurse for home care, because this will reduce the cost to the patient. Some physicians may do this because they feel the trust relationship requires it; others may regard such behavior as an investment in a good reputation. Patients, of course, appreciate such behavior. Under our reforms, it seems reasonable to expect many physicians to alter their current disregard for cost, and inform their patients of their new approach.

Once at least an important minority of physicians change the criteria by which they select hospitals, the incentives for hospital managers will alter radically. Today, most hospitals compete vigorously for physicians, who in turn bring patients. Because cost is irrelevant for their patients, physicians enjoy the luxury of choosing the most technologically advanced hospital, and the convenience of excess

321

capacity, regardless of cost or inefficiency. Naturally, hospital managers respond to physician demand by escalating cost.

Suppose patient cost sharing causes a fraction of physicians to prefer the hospital that achieves a given quality at minimum cost. Consider the case where area hospitals initially have a total bed capacity that just satisfies area demand (allowing for appropriate reserve capacity for unusual inflow). Consider what happens if hospital X greatly expands its bed capacity. Area demand is divided among area hospitals, so that all have excess capacity, raising the bed cost per patient. Today, with nearly complete insurance, area hospitals simply raise their bill per patient to the insurers to cover the cost of excess capacity. The regulatory strategy tries to contain this tendency by requiring "certificate of need," by which hospitals must obtain approval for expansion.

Under cost sharing, however, the tendency toward excess capacity would be automatically checked, as it is throughout most sectors of the economy. If hospital X contemplates an expansion that would cause excess capacity, it would now expect each area hospital to try to restore full utilization by reducing its price. Because quality is unchanged, the lower price would now attract a fraction of physicians, with their patients, because the latter would now benefit from a lower price. X would find it could not simply raise price to cover the cost of excess capacity, because the price increase would deter physicians, choosing on behalf of their patients. Anticipating a loss on its bed expansion, X would generally decide not to proceed.

The same process would work to limit the current competition for new technology that sometimes leads to "wasteful duplication." If a particular technology is useful for only a specific class of patients whose needs can be clearly identified before hospitalization, then it is socially optimal for only a subset of area hospitals to acquire the technology if this would be sufficient to handle area demand. It would be wasteful for all hospitals to obtain the technology, so that each hospital under-utilizes it. The regulatory strategy tries, through planning and "certificate of need," to secure such specialization of hospitals, and to avoid duplication.

Under cost sharing, suppose hospitals X and Y already possess technology Q, and their capacity is adequate for area demand. If hospital Z contemplates acquiring Q, it would recognize that X and Y would attempt to retain full utilization by reducing price, which would now attract physicians, who would bring patients. Thus, Z would be unable to set its price high enough to cover the cost of excess capacity. It would conclude that acquisition of Q would not be financially worthwhile. Z might instead decide to specialize in treatment of illness H, which requires technology R, for which area capacity is not yet satisfactory. Thus, we might expect some specialization by area hospitals. The tendency to wasteful duplication would be automatically curtailed.

Is this simply theory? The automatic checking of excess capacity and wasteful duplication is evident throughout most of the economy. It is not simply physicians who have a "technological imperative." Consider the stereo industry. Electronics engineers also love costly, technologically sophisticated stereos. Most would naturally prefer to design and construct the finest sound systems scientifically possible, even if the cost might be $3,000 per stereo. But management vetoes mass production of such stereos. Because consumers pay the cost of each stereo they buy, each company must make stereos that people are willing to buy. Thus, the "technological imperative" of electronics engineers is held in check.

Suppose stereos were paid fully by a third party. Then management would be glad to indulge the "technological imperative" of the engineers. In fact, because consumers would all prefer the finest stereo, companies would be forced to make only the most advanced stereos, regardless of cost. A mistaken observer might conclude that the fault lies with the training of engineers that indoctrinates them with a love of technology. In fact, the fault would lie with the absence of consumer cost sharing.

In responding to the current incentives for excess capacity and duplication, it is important not to swing the pendulum to the other extreme, and stifle innovation and healthy competition. The regulatory strategy encounters great difficulty distinguishing between the two. With complete third-party payment, hospitals have an incentive to expand capacity and technology, whether excessive or not. Each has an incentive to claim that its expansion introduces an important innovation. The regulatory board is confronted with proposals that are difficult to evaluate. Each hospital can bring scientific and technical testimony to support its case. If the board takes a "hard line," valuable innovation and competition may be limited. If it takes a "soft line," wasteful duplication will continue.

Consider how cost sharing helps distinguish automatically between the two. If hospital X genuinely believes technology R is a useful innovation that does not simply duplicate what is already adequately available, it will expect to attract enough physicians and patients to fully utilize the new technology. Other hospitals will find older, less advanced technology for treating the same medical condition becoming underutilized, as patients switch to X. These hospitals will either be forced to concede patients to X, counter with a better innovation, or, if area demand is sufficient, also acquire R. The pressure of competition benefits patients. On the other hand, if technology R is really no better than what other hospitals already have, then X will not expect to attract enough patients to fully utilize it. X will therefore avoid acquiring R, recognizing that it would merely duplicate existing technology.

Once again, this process is at work throughout the economy, where consumers pay for what they buy. Of course, the process does not work perfectly. Management makes mistakes; miscalculations occur. The same would be true in the health sector. Nevertheless, the issue is whether the automatic mechanism works better than full reliance on regulation and planning. It is possible that cost sharing, supplemented by selective community planning, would achieve the best result. It would seem unwise, however, once the automatic mechanism is understood, to refuse to use it in a sector as important as health.

Consider another example of the impact of cost sharing. Today, a physician may order a battery of tests, although it may be true that if the first test shows result A, then the other tests would be unnecessary. Assume time is not pressing. With full third-party payment, it may be more convenient for the patient to do all tests at once. Under cost sharing, however, it seems likely that many physicians would order the tests sequentially. If the first shows result A, the cost of subsequent tests would be avoided. Few physicians would be eager to respond to the complaint of a patient who later recognized he had incurred a substantial cost unnecessarily.

Cost sharing should help tailor resource allocation to individual circumstances. Consider the length of stay. Suppose patient A has a spouse who can stay at home full time. Because an additional day in the hospital now costs the patient out of pocket, he may prefer to go home. Patient B, however, lives alone, and needs someone's assistance full time. B may prefer to stay in the hospital, despite its cost. It must be emphasized that the out-of-pocket burden will be income related. Thus, if A and B earn low incomes, their share might be $20 per day; if they have high incomes, their share would be perhaps $120 per day. Resources will go to those with the most urgent preference, given their options. Under the regulatory approach, both A and B might request an additional day, both claiming their request was urgent. It would be impossible for a regulatory board to investigate each person's circumstance and options. It is possible that both might be permitted to stay, thereby increasing the wait of someone urgently seeking admission; or neither allowed to stay, imposing a hardship on B. The likelihood that A would not be permitted, while B would, is surely low.

If physicians weigh cost on behalf of their patients so that demand reflects genuine urgency, then supply can be allowed to respond freely to demand. In contrast, in the absence of cost sharing, demand exaggerates urgency, and regulators must prevent supply from wastefully matching inflated demand. Limiting supply below demand, however, has harmful consequences. Chronic excess demand for particular services—such as hospital admissions—reduces the freedom of choice of a minority of consumers, who find they are unable to promptly obtain services they value highly. Regulators will try to ration the limited supply according to genuine urgency, but they will be unable to avoid imposing inequities, because they cannot know the genuine urgency of each individual patient. Control over the use of medical facilities will be partly transferred from individual patients, guided by their physicians, to the regulators who ration the limited supply.

In contrast, when supply is allowed to match demand under cost sharing, each patient, guided by his physician, will be able to obtain promptly whatever service he values highly (for which he is willing to pay an income-related fraction of the cost). Each patient and physician will decide urgency, without requiring approval from regulators. In my view, the retention of freedom and choice by individual patients and physicians is a crucial advantage of cost sharing over regulation.

It is sometimes feared that cost sharing will cause patients to skimp on medical care. Once again, this fear is a natural response to cost sharing that is unrelated to income. When cost sharing is geared to ability to pay, every patient will be able to afford the care he needs, however costly. It is true that physicians, on behalf of patients, will now reduce unnecessary services; this is the purpose of cost sharing. But why should it be feared that patients will now prefer the lowest quality? Throughout the rest of the economy, consumers must always pay the higher cost of higher quality. This fact does not deter many from going beyond the minimum quality available. Most people regard medical care as extremely important. Under cost sharing, they would continue to prefer high-quality care, and the medical credit and guaranteed loan would ensure that such care could always be afforded, regardless of the patient's income.

There is a philosophical view that holds that some people will be shortsighted; although they can afford to pay a fraction of the cost, they will avoid necessary care until it is too late. Society should try to prevent the consequence of such myopia by eliminating cost sharing. Some people will no doubt behave this way. The cost-sharing strategy assumes that society's central responsibility is to ensure that every household can afford the medical care it needs. It is then up to each household to decide between medical care and other goods and services. Under cost sharing, households will generally pay less than the full cost of their own medical care, while they must pay 100 percent of the cost of other goods and services. Thus cost sharing does provide a substantial inducement to medical care. It does not, however, go to the extreme of a zero price.

The view that any out-of-pocket burden will discourage the short-sighted, and that therefore the system must be designed to prevent such persons from harming themselves, is clearly strongly paternalistic. At the other extreme is the laissez-faire advocate, who believes persons not covered by workplace insurance should be expected to obtain their own, even if its cost is high relative to household income. Income-related cost sharing takes an intermediate position. It is paternalistic to the extent that it guarantees universal catastrophic protection, so that a shortsighted household cannot leave itself inadequately covered. But it is not so paternalistic that it tries to protect individuals unwilling to pay even a fraction of the cost of their own medical care, when that fraction is geared to the household's ability to pay.

Conclusion

The consumer cost-sharing strategy, implemented by a tax incentive to induce significant cost sharing under private policies along with a medical tax credit and guaranteed loans, should achieve a better combination of equity and efficiency than the two major alternatives—the laissez-faire strategy and the regulatory strategy.

The central weakness of the laissez-faire approach is the inability of the private health insurance companies to vary consumer cost sharing with household income because of data and verification requirements. Even if the current tax subsidy to private health insurance is removed, concern for low-income employees may limit uniform cost sharing under private policies, so that "third-party" inflation and inefficiency continue. On the other hand, if significant uniform cost sharing does result from removal of the tax subsidy, low-income employees will be unable to afford necessary care. Moreover, persons uninsured at the workplace may be unable to afford adequate individual insurance, so that universal income-related catastrophic protection will not result, and financial hardships due to illness will continue.

The main shortcoming of the regulatory strategy is its inability to ascertain the degree of genuine urgency of individual preferences for particular services, because physicians, on behalf of patients, have an incentive to insist all demands are urgent, in the absence of cost sharing. Unable to distinguish genuine from feigned urgency, the regulators will have difficulty avoiding inequities and inefficiencies, as some patients obtain costly resources they value little while others must wait for services they urgently desire. The regulatory strategy may lower total national medical cost. Its weakness is not that it must be more costly, but that in limiting total cost by limiting supply, it will make the health-care system less sensitive to the varying needs and preferences of individual patients.

Under the cost-sharing strategy, implemented by private-policy cost sharing and the medical tax credit, society will continue to provide generous assistance to households in need of medical care. The assistance will be confidentially linked to each household's ability to pay. Unlike private health insurance companies, IRS possesses the data to vary cost sharing with household income. In contrast to the laissez-faire result, universal income-related catastrophic coverage will be assured. Every household will be able to ·afford whatever medical care it needs. Loans will be guaranteed to every household, so most will not have to pay out of pocket for perhaps a year (until the tax credit is filed and processed) after incurring a medical bill that is large relative to its income. Although most households will continue to be covered by private insurance policies, these policies will now have significant patient cost sharing. The medical tax credit plus guaranteed loan will provide "insurance of last resort," helping with out-of-pocket payments under private policies, and providing adequate insurance for households without private insurance.

In contrast to the regulatory strategy and the current situation, most households will ultimately bear a share of the cost of their own medical care, including hospital care. Most physicians, on behalf of their patients, will therefore conserve wherever this would not sacrifice desired quality. In response to the new orientation of physicians, hospitals will compete to provide a given quality at minimum cost. Automatically, as in other sectors of the economy where consumers care about cost and price, excess capacity and wasteful duplication will be discouraged; at the same time, innovation will be encouraged. Choice will be retained by each physician and patient who will be free to order the services they want, constrained only by cost sharing. Choice will not be limited due to supply restrictions by regulators, except in very special cases.

The consumer cost-sharing strategy therefore strikes a balance between equity and efficiency that should make it a desirable public policy for the health sector.

Appendix: The Interaction of Private Insurance and the Tax Credit

Figure 1 shows the relationship between the household's out-of-pocket burden and its annual medical bill. The three-part segment N shows the burden of each medical bill in the absence of private insurance, when

FIGURE 1
THE INTERACTION OF PRIVATE POLICY COST-SHARING
AND THE TAX CREDIT

Out-of-Pocket Burden (B)

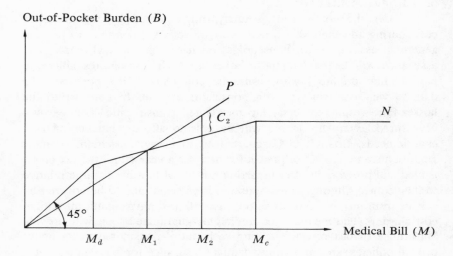

the household relies fully on the tax credit. M_d is the deductible under the credit. M_c is the medical bill at which the household reaches its out-of-pocket ceiling.

Segment P shows the burden at each medical bill under a particular private insurance policy, in the absence of the tax credit. Policy P has a constant coinsurance rate from medical bill 0.

Now consider the interaction of private insurance and the tax credit. As long as P is less than N, the household is not entitled to any tax credit, so its burden is given by P. Beyond M_1, however, P exceeds N, so that the household is entitled to a tax credit equal to the difference between P and N, thereby reducing its burden to N (at M_2, a credit of C_2).

The ratio of the increase in the burden to the increase in the medical bill ($\Delta B/\Delta M$) is given either by the coinsurance rate of the private policy, or the coinsurance rate of the tax credit, at each M.

Prospects for Competition under Health Planning-cum-Regulation

Clark C. Havighurst

This paper addresses some aspects of the important question whether competition and regulation can coexist in the health-services industry. Devotees of competition, being chronically critical of regulation, will find many reasons to doubt that coexistence is possible, but there should be no illusion among these market advocates that a negative conclusion on this question will speed the repeal of regulation so that market forces can take over. Indeed, because regulation has deeper roots than competition in this industry, any judgment that competition cannot survive in a regulated climate is likely to cause policy makers to give up on promising competitive strategies rather than to deregulate the industry. For these reasons, and because health-sector regulation, by itself, will probably do more to legitimize poor economic performance than to prevent it, it is important that we seek ways to assure that competition can indeed grow and flourish in a regulated environment.

I believe that regulation in this industry need not stifle desirable competition. This paper attempts to provide a basis for hopefulness. I discuss first the emerging awareness in Congress of competition's possibilities and, second, some specific legislative developments in the design of certificate-of-need regulation. On the basis of these glimmers of hope, I can visualize a scenario in which command-and-control regulation is progressively relaxed as private incentives and competition take over more and more of the resource allocation job in the health care sector. There is no denying that many obstacles could frustrate this scenario of phased deregulation, and only a little cynicism grounded in regulation's track record in this and other industries will be enough to convince many observers to discount my optimism. But I will argue that the phased deregulation strategy is tenable and deserves support. In any event, because immediate deregulation is not an option, phased deregulation is the only alternative we have to further regulatory encroachment.

NOTE: Work on this paper was supported by Grant No. HS01539 from the National Center for Health Services Research, Department of Health and Human Services. Portions have been adapted from work originally supported by the Federal Trade Commission.

329

Congress's Recent Discovery of the Competitive Option

The first session of the 96th Congress has been marked by a significant increase in interest in procompetitive strategies in health policy. Ideas for removing distortions in private incentives and permitting such incentives to guide the private financing system's future development are suddenly much in evidence, and many policy makers are beginning to appreciate competition's potential value in bringing pressure to bear on costs. Because they occurred so quickly, these recent developments might be viewed as a fad, but the basic idea of relying on consumer choice and market forces has enough substance and is reinforced by enough evidence and enough logic to be taken seriously. As a long-time advocate of market forces in this industry, I can confess to feeling not only some satisfaction at the turn events have taken but also some pressure now to deliver on promises that were easy to make when the trend was running the other way.

There are many reasons for the new viability of competitive strategies. The able advocacy of Alain Enthoven is a crucial factor, but would probably not have been sufficient in the absence of new evidence of the cost-effectiveness and competitiveness of HMOs. Credit for these developments goes in large measure to Paul Ellwood and Walter McClure, whose labors on behalf of HMOs are well known and whose ability to publicize the developments they have nurtured has also been valuable. At the same time, the Federal Trade Commission (FTC), which launched a substantial antitrust and consumer protection effort in the health-care sector in 1975, has given the market strategy a visible advocate—and thus increased credibility—within the federal government. Moreover, the FTC's antitrust enforcement campaign has revealed and dealt with important causes of the private financing system's poor service to the public in the past. In doing so, the FTC has provided a firmer basis for expecting competitively induced innovation to occur in the future. Similarly, increased understanding of how the tax laws have distorted consumers' incentives in buying health insurance (contributing to the destruction of cost-consciousness in buying medical care) has strengthened the perception that the private sector has not yet had a real opportunity to show what it can do to bring costs under control.

While the market strategy was becoming increasingly credible, the regulatory attack on the cost problem was in disarray. Existing regulation has been able to demonstrate no more than minimal achievements, as costs have continued to escalate in real terms. Indeed, the administration's hospital cost-containment bill, by far the most heavy-handed regulatory proposal to date, can be interpreted as a confession of the failure of previous efforts. Moreover, by giving the Congress a glimpse of the future under regulation and of the necessity for extremely arbitrary controls, the administration's bill has intensified congressional interest in nonregulatory alternatives. The recent defeat of the cost-containment legislation in the House of Representatives appears to reflect doubts concerning regulation's fairness and efficacy and may increase the sense of urgency about implementing alternative approaches. In the background of all these developments is, of course, a national mood reflecting distrust of government in general and of governmental regulation in particular.

Evidence that competition has emerged as a promising strategy appears in a variety of recent legislative proposals, each embodying in some form the principle of consumer choice under appropriate incentives. First, proposals to require employers to offer their employees several health plans, rather than only one, have been offered by Congressman Ullman, Senator Schweiker, Senator Durenberger, and others. The employer's dollar contribution would have to be the same whichever plan the employee chooses, so that employees will be aware of cost differences at the margin. The goal is to give employees the final choice with an opportunity to economize. By the same token, these plans would reduce the role of employers and labor unions, who have interests and agendas of their own and consequently may have been less inclined to economize and to experiment with less comprehensive benefits than many individuals would be. The "multiple-choice" idea, which is capturing many imaginations despite possible questions concerning its actuarial and practical feasibility, differs fundamentally from the "dual-choice" provisions in the HMO act, which were designed to help federally subsidized HMOs, not to foster competition as such.

Closely related to the multiple-choice idea is the new awareness of the tax laws' contribution to cost inflation through the inducement of overinsurance. Several proposals have set forth ways to avoid the dilution of cost-consciousness that occurs when a saving in health insurance premiums, paid out as increased wages, is subject to income and payroll taxes. Most of these proposals create substantial political problems because they threaten to increase taxes on those usually influential groups who have earned or negotiated liberal benefits.[1] Nevertheless, the new willingness to consider tax law changes, as revealed in recent hearings, confounds those who have long said that such changes, while

---

[1] Most of the existing proposals would establish a dollar limit on the amount of employer-paid insurance premiums that may be excluded from the employee's taxable income. Other more politically appealing approaches may be available, however. See statement of Clark C. Havighurst, in U.S. Congress, House of Representatives, Committee on Ways and Means, *Restructuring the Financing of Health Insurance, Hearings on H.R. 5740*, 96th Congress, 2nd session, February 25, 1980.

perhaps desirable to correct incentives, were politically infeasible and that regulation was therefore the only alternative available.

Competition and consumer choice are also prominently featured in the latest and most comprehensive proposals for national health insurance. Senator Kennedy touts his proposed Health Care for All Americans Act as featuring competition. Indeed it does provide a framework in which consumer choice, undistorted by tax considerations, could operate. However, its regulatory and collective bargaining features greatly narrow the range of matters on which competition could focus. The Carter administration's original blueprints for its National Health Plan (Phase I) also gave competition a significant place, indicating that consumers under the federal "Health Care" system would be allowed, at federal expense, to opt out of it into private-sector plans. Interestingly, competition's place in the administration's proposal was more fully spelled out in the summary documents—prepared, it would appear, in the White House—than in the more detailed specifications prepared by HEW or in the bill itself.

Another current legislative proposal would allow Medicare beneficiaries not only to enroll in HMOs but to benefit themselves—to the extent of the additional benefits that an HMO might be able to offer— by such an economizing choice. This procompetitive idea was first put forward by Paul Ellwood in the early 1970s and has been almost singlehandedly frustrated since then by a powerful member of the Senate Finance Committee staff. It would not only help HMOs but also break Medicare's strong commitment to retrospective cost reimbursement. Even more significantly, it would embody a "voucher" approach, giving federal beneficiaries an opportunity to choose for themselves with costs in view.

If the technical problems of calculating correct capitation payments and avoiding adverse selection can be solved, this experiment could grow into a system in which the federal government subsidizes its beneficiaries' purchasing power in ways that strengthen rather than impair the competitive market. A recent editorial in the AMA's *American Medical News* reveals the kind of double-think that is needed to oppose the principles underlying this procompetitive proposal: "If Medicare benefits can be furnished through an HMO (or whatever means) at reduced costs, the benefits should redound to all Medicare beneficiaries."[2] Obviously, the AMA would prefer that Medicare beneficiaries not have an incentive to choose a low-cost provider.

While the foregoing legislative proposals suggest that the idea of competition is alive and well on Capitol Hill, each of them presents

---

[2] "An HMO Double Standard," *American Medical News*, August 3/10, 1979, p. 4.

technical difficulties, and none of them is yet law or close to actual enactment. There are, however, two legislative developments that provide tangible, even dramatic, evidence that Congress has reexamined the fundamentals of health policy and has, for the first time, assigned competition a role to play. These two developments are both contained in the Health Planning and Resources Development Amendments of 1979.[3] One is the broad exemption from certificate-of-need requirements for HMOs. The other is new language endorsing competition as an allocator of some health resources that Congress has added to the planning law. Though less heralded than the HMO exemption, this latter legislative change may turn out, in the long run, to be more important in influencing the health-care system's future development. These two legislative changes provide the text for my substantive remarks on the compatibility of competition and health planning-cum-regulation.

Why Competition and Regulation Both May Seem Needed

Regulation exists in the health services industry for highly plausible reasons. Because prevailing systems for financing health services encourage inappropriate spending, it has been natural for policy makers to believe that central control is necessary to prevent abuses in pricing and utilization. There is indeed no denying that established private and public payment mechanisms do not well serve the consumer's or taxpayer's interest in cost containment. Nowhere in the system is there any mechanism for systematically comparing costs and benefits. As a result, providers and insured patients can spend money in the common funds with accountability only for the most egregious excesses.

Policy makers can hardly be blamed for perceiving that this state of affairs required a remedy in the form of public regulation of hospital rates, publicly sponsored utilization controls in public programs, and public certification of need for new facilities, new capital investments, and new services. Although conceived to deal with the cost problem, such measures have proved difficult to implement and have had only limited impact, if any. No doubt regulation's sponsors had few illusions that regulation, even at its best, could perfectly accommodate difficult tradeoffs between cost and other values or could do more than perhaps stabilize the share of GNP represented by health services. Certainly the most thoughtful advocates of regulation have embraced it not because they believe it is an ideal instrument but because they have seen no realistic alternative.

---

[3] Public Law No. 96-79.

The most plausible arguments against regulation have not challenged the view that resources are probably being badly misallocated in the health-care sector. Instead, the prescription of regulation has been seen as founded on an incomplete diagnosis of the problem and as inappropriately focused on suppressing symptoms rather than on addressing the underlying market failure. Regulation's critics argue that, if the financing and delivery system were organized differently, this system would provide necessary financial protection for consumers without generating an undue amount of inappropriate spending. This observation immediately calls attention to the reasons why third-party payment takes its present dysfunctional forms and does not feature cost containment—avoidance of the so-called moral hazard—as a major objective in benefit design, administration, and relationships with providers. If the present organization of the financing and delivery system is not inevitable, symptom-suppressing regulation may be an inappropriate response to the problem perceived.

A number of specific causes of the recognized market failure have been identified by market advocates. The tax law's inducement of overinsurance in the private sector is one of them. Another is the long-standing dominance of organized providers over private financing plans; provider organizations have used direct control of some "Blues" and similar plans, occasional boycotts of innovating plans they do not control and of providers cooperating with such plans, and effective collective bargaining with plans of all types to restrain the evolution of private health insurance in directions that would have triggered significant price competition among providers.[4] A third item that may be added to the list of factors distorting the design and operation of private financing mechanisms is the incentives of unions and employers as insurance-purchasing agents for employees; because employers and unions are locked into a quasipolitical relationship with the rank-and-file, they may define the workers' interests differently than the workers, acting as individual purchasers with the costs in view, would define them. It will be noted that each of these causes of the market's past failures is remediable by legislation and antitrust enforcement, and, after long being taken entirely for granted, is now being actively addressed.

As this diagnosis of the health care system's problems reveals, market advocates focus primarily on the private sector, its past failures,

---

[4] Clark Havighurst, "Antitrust Enforcement in the Medical Services Industry—What Does It All Mean?" *Milbank Memorial Fund Quarterly*, vol. 58 (Winter 1980), pp. 89–124; Clark Havighurst, "Professional Restraints on Innovation in Health Care Financing," *Duke Law Journal* (May 1978), pp. 303–387; Federal Trade Commission, *Staff Report on Medical Participation in Control of Blue Shield and Certain Other Open-Panel Medical Prepayment Plans* (Washington, D.C.: 1979), especially pp. 125–192 and 283–301.

and its potential strengths. Public financing programs, while large and important, are seen as simply mirroring insurance practices that developed in the private sector under conditions of market failure; the codification of these practices in public programs was inevitable in a political environment in which providers' preferences for the existing system had to be respected. By the same token, market advocates see the private sector as capable of leading public programs out of the wilderness by providing new options and approaches that public programs can either emulate or allow beneficiaries to purchase in the private sector with subsidized buying power. (The proposed HMO option under Medicare is an example.)

Market advocates have focused their attention on the private sector and have hoped for its reinvigoration through competition. By contrast, regulation advocates have been primarily concerned with public programs, and have generally envisioned a future involving an expansion of such programs and of direct public payment for health care. With this orientation, they have naturally perceived effective regulation as essential to make public programs, as currently designed, workable and to permit the desired expansion to occur. To HEW and the staff of the Senate Finance Committee, for example, the private sector must have long seemed an anachronism—a vestige of an earlier era and the domain of dominant private interests—and not as a mechanism whose faults could be corrected. It may thus be noted that where one comes out in the regulation-versus-competition debate has depended heavily in the past on where one was coming from and was headed. But, although regulation and competition advocates have had little common ground in the past, I believe there is a greater basis for accommodation today.

The most encouraging thing about the recent shift in the health policy debate is that it leaves behind, probably once and for all, the idea of a monolithic federal financing program. Thus, even Senator Kennedy has embraced in a limited way the idea of competition in the private sector, sponsoring a voucher-type system to encourage consumers to seek value in a health plan. Because it has been possible to shift attention to the private sector's competitive performance without giving up the goal of solving the underinsurance problem, the new focus of the policy debate offers an opportunity for bringing regulation advocates and market advocates closer together. Although HEW will not soon get over its fixation on its own programs or give up its pursuit of bigger and better ones to administer, the meaningful debate over policy development is now going off in other, more constructive directions. I expect that the next few years will see a mounting campaign to use regulation and competition in combination to achieve the ultimate goal of a system guided fundamentally by consumer preferences, yet responsive to concerns of social justice.

One reason for my thinking that regulation can keep the private sector's development as a major goal is that most economic regulation of the health care system has so far not been entrusted directly to HEW but has been left at the state and local level. Here, because the focus is not primarily on federal programs and on short-run budgetary concerns, attention can be given to the existing system in its entirety and to its evolution in the consumer's interest. Despite their accountability to HEW and its regulations, state and local planner-regulators have an overriding statutory mandate from both Congress and the state legislatures to make their local health care systems perform efficiently. I will argue that, although serious doubts about the planner-regulators' incentives and ideology still exist, there is a potential here for procompetitive development. Decentralization of regulatory and planning authority provides opportunities for experimentation in regulatory policy. Even if the regulators are profoundly anticompetitive in most health-service areas, the private sector's innovative capabilities and competition's allocational efficiencies may yet be demonstrated in some places. Once demonstrated, these lessons should spread.

Market advocates are surely right that, if we were so fortunate as to have a working competitive market—without tax subsidies for overinsurance, without trade restraints by organized providers, without employer paternalism and union leaders' demagoguery, and without federal programs founded on the principle of retrospective cost reimbursement—we could be proud of it. They are less certainly, but still probably, right in their belief that policies to remove, suppress, or modify the many distorting influences in the present system are desirable and would yield significant benefits in the long run.

They would be less clearly right, and very possibly wrong, if they should argue for adopting such policies and eliminating regulation at one stroke. I, for one, would vote for such a "let-'er-rip" approach, but I would do so with some trepidation because I have less than total confidence in the antitrust enforcers and the courts, in the health insurers' innovative capacity, in consumers' ability to detect their true interest, in providers' willingness to compete, and in our willingness to give the marketplace time to show what it can do before we introduce a new generation of controls. But, because revolution is not an option at the moment, I am reasonably content with the alternative of trying to design and administer regulation so that we can have both competition and regulation working side by side, each doing what it can do best.

In the short run, it is probable that regulation will be used to allocate resources in a larger sector of the health-care industry than will be entrusted to market forces. But, ultimately, if other policies such as tax-law changes, increased consumer choice, and antitrust enforcement take hold and if the planner-regulators act responsibly in the light of the innovations that begin to emerge, regulation will recede, leaving the market in command of most of the field. Simplistic as this scenario may be, it seems to me both reasonably hopeful and politically feasible. It requires present agreement only on allowing a mixture of means, and leaves the end result to be determined by evolution and by future decisions concerning competition's efficacy. It also promises to provide rich opportunities for experimenting with both market and nonmarket strategies, thus letting experience rather than theory guide us to the better outcome.

The most hopeful sign of all for the success of my scenario is that Congress, attuned to the problems of the entire health-care system and not just to the problems of Medicare and Medicaid, has now retreated from its previous inclination to entrust regulators with plenary authority, including the power to suppress desirable competitive developments. As the ensuing discussion shows, the regulators' efforts have lately been channeled by law toward those areas where they are most likely to serve a true public need and least likely to do significant harm. Moreover, the regulators have been reinstructed on their duties and explicitly told to foster competition where it is socially desirable. Regulatory policy has thus changed direction, opening possibilities for competition that did not previously exist. The remainder of the paper documents the changes in regulatory policy embodied in the Health Planning and Resources Development Amendments of 1979 and attempts to assess the new possibilities for blending regulation and competition in a constructive effort to put the health services industry on the right track. I hope I will be understood as preferring the right track to the wrong track, not the "left" one.

New Directions for the Planner-Regulators

Before 1979, there was little political or statutory support at the federal level for a procompetitive approach to health-sector regulation. The Health Planning and Resources Development Act of 1974 was strikingly devoid of language that could be construed as charging planner-regulators with a responsibility to consider competition in their deliberations. Even the Health Maintenance Organization Act of 1973, which actively supported HMO development, failed to provide any real indication that HMOs were valued as anything more than a desirable and cost-effective alternative. There was practically nothing in the law or its legislative history to indicate that Congress appreciated that HMOs' cost-effectiveness arose primarily because they had to compete in the marketplace on the basis of price or that HMOs might be valuable primarily because of the competitive stimulus that they might supply in the system as a whole. Anyone looking at federal health legislation as it existed before 1979 would have had to conclude that competition was not favored and that Congress had chosen to put all of its eggs in the regulation basket.

The Breakthrough in Utah. The first legislative event of 1979 that signaled a possible weakening in the singleminded commitment to regulation in the nation as a whole occurred in the state of Utah. Although no state certificate-of-need law prior to 1979 had given competition even an honorable mention, the Utah legislature enacted in March 1979 its Procompetitive Certificate of Need Act.[5] Though literally a contradiction in terms, that official title and the new law's substance put Utah on record in favor of maintaining a market-oriented health-care system under state regulatory oversight administered in compliance with federal law.

The unique features of the Utah law resulted from a combination of factors. Resistance in the state to pressures from the federal government to adopt a traditional certificate-of-need law led the legislature to commission a major investigation of health-care costs in Utah and of alternative methods of controlling them. As a consultant to Lewin & Associates, Inc., the contractor, I suggested introducing procompetitive principles into certification of need as a possible way of accommodating conflicts that existed in the state. A surprisingly broad consensus developed in support of the bill and of the basic idea of promoting competition at the same time that regulation was being imposed. That consensus has so far survived and may permit several other procompetitive steps to be taken. It remains to be seen whether the consensus will hold together as implementation of the new law begins and as the implications of the underlying idea become clearer.

Several provisions in the Utah law are relevant to competition. The lengthy statement of legislative purpose indicates that regulation is imposed only to deal with the perceived market failure traceable to "prevailing" methods of paying for services. The statement makes clear that, if the payment system should become more responsive to consumers' cost concerns in the future, the scope of regulation should be correspondingly reduced.[6] The legislature further declares that "need" for a health service or facility depends in part on "the efficacy of

---

[5] Utah Code Annotated, §26–34–1 et seq. (1953).

[6] Ibid., §26–34–2(1).

competition," and states its intention that the law serve "to promote the development of increased competition and improved market conditions to the extent possible in the state."[7]

The new law includes the value of competition among the criteria for decision making on certificates of need. It also requires decision makers to consider whether the demand side of the market is capable of allocating supply appropriately. It directs their attention to "the existence and capacity of public or private reimbursement and utilization review programs, and other public and private cost control measures to give effect to consumer preferences and establish appropriate incentives for capital allocation."[8]

The law also imposes some limitations on the regulators' power to protect existing providers against competition in order to protect revenues needed to cross-subsidize other services. Finally, the new law directs the certificate-of-need agencies "in their planning and review activities [to] foster competition and encourage innovations in the financing and delivery systems for health services that will promote economic behavior by the consumers and providers of health services and that lead to appropriate investment, supply and use of health services."[9]

Interest in Congress. Because the Utah law seemed a promising effort to blend concern about maintaining and strengthening desirable competitive impulses in the health care industry with regulatory control of excesses, it occasioned some notice and comment in Washington. The staff of the health subcommittee of the House Committee on Interstate and Foreign Commerce, which had already been exposed to the idea of making competition a consideration in federal law, was briefed on the Utah act, and its basic principles ultimately appeared in the House version of the health planning amendments of 1979.

In the Senate, the idea of introducing competition as a consideration in certificate-of-need decisions first emerged in testimony that I gave before Senator Kennedy's subcommittee on the hospital cost containment legislation. The idea that regulators should be accountable for what they do to competition and should not sacrifice it unnecessarily was expected to appeal to Senator Kennedy, who was sponsoring legislation to require federal regulatory agencies in nonhealth fields to issue "competition impact statements" in connection with major regulatory initiatives.[10] Ultimately, Senator Schweiker introduced language

---

[7] Ibid., §26–34–2(4).

[8] Ibid., §26–34–11(1)(m).

[9] Ibid., §26–33–8.

[10] S. 382, 96th Congress, 1st session (1979).

embodying the same basic principles without opposition from Senator Kennedy or his staff. The resulting version was significantly different from the House bill, but the general principles were essentially the same.

The 1979 Amendments' References to Competition. A combination of the Senate and House language emerged from the conference committee that met in August. The following paragraphs briefly discuss the specific changes in the 1974 health planning law made by the 1979 amendments. These amendments all appear in section 103 of Public Law 96–79 under the heading "The Role of Competition in the Allocation of Health Services." The committee reports are of particular interest and are referred to at several points. The House committee's extensive statement of congressional purpose is particularly instructive.

The key provision for ascertaining Congress's purpose is section 1502(b) of the amended Public Health Service Act, which provides extensive findings concerning competition's role in allocating health care resources. Each of the substantive provisions touching on competition, which are discussed below, has specific reference to section 1502(b). Adapted from language in the House bill, it provides as follows:

(b)(1) The Congress finds that the effect of competition on decisions of providers respecting the supply of health services and facilities is diminished. The primary source of the lessening of such effect is the prevailing methods of paying for health services by public and private health insurers, particularly for inpatient health services and other institutional health services. As a result, there is duplication and excess supply of certain health services and facilities, particularly in the case of inpatient health services.

(2) For health services, such as inpatient health services and other institutional health services, for which competition does not or will not appropriately allocate supply consistent with health systems plans and State health plans, health systems agencies and State health planning and development agencies should in the exercise of their functions under this title take actions (where appropriate to advance the purposes of quality assurance, cost effectiveness, and access and the other purposes of this title) to allocate the supply of such services.

(3) For the health services for which competition appropriately allocates supply consistent with health systems plans and State health plans, health systems agencies and State health planning and development agencies should in the performance of their functions under this title give priority (where appropriate to advance the purposes of quality assurance, cost

effectiveness, and access) to actions which would strengthen the effect of competition on the supply of such services.

Though not a ringing endorsement of competition under all circumstances, section 1502(b) substantially clarifies the concept of regulation embodied in the planning act and advances understanding of why competition has not been as effective in the past as it should have been. The reference to "prevailing methods of paying for health services by public and private health insurers" identifies the financing system as the source of the problem. The reference to "*prevailing* methods" implies the possibility that different methods might exist in the future, permitting competition a larger role. Similarly, the reference in paragraph 2 to services "for which competition does not *or will not* appropriately allocate supply" suggests that in the future competition's role might be enlarged.

These nuances should serve as a signal to the regulators that they should not assume that what needs regulation today will need regulation tomorrow. The House committee report was particularly explicit on this point, declaring that

> If . . . an innovative financing, reimbursement or service delivery arrangement affecting institutional health services were designed so that the method of payment by patients (1) created incentives for patients to respond to prices charged and (2) placed the providers at financial risk for unnecessary or excessive services, the committee would expect that planning agencies would, in awarding certificates of need, consider whether the effect of that new arrangement will be to properly allocate the supply of those services.[11]

Paragraph 2 of section 1502(b) appears to identify "inpatient health services and other institutional health services" (the latter a defined term including significant outpatient services provided by institutional providers) as being among those "for which competition does not or will not allocate supply" and which therefore must be allocated by regulatory means. The previously quoted sentence from the House report makes it clear, however, that paragraph 2 was not intended to declare such services subject to command-and-control regulation for all time and under all circumstances. Instead, the committee was simply stating its presumption that, because of the current extent and character of third-party coverage of such services, regulation is probably required. Because the House report contains no

---

[11] U.S. Congress, House of Representatives, *Health Planning and Resources Development Amendments of 1979*, H. Rept. 96-190 to accompany H.R. 3917, 96th Congress, 1st session, 1979, pp. 53–54.

analysis of the various services and ignores possibly relevant distinctions among them—between acute care hospitals and nursing homes, for example—this presumption should probably not be taken too seriously. In any event, it is certainly rebuttable in specific instances. Moreover, if one were to attach great weight to the special emphasis given the need to regulate inpatient and other institutional services, one would also have to infer the existence of an opposite presumption—against regulation—with respect to all other services, such as office-based diagnostic and therapeutic equipment.

Section 1502(b) apparently was not intended to give more than general guidance as to the particular services likely to require command-and-control regulation in the future. What comes through clearly is simply that Congress wants the regulators to regulate where it is necessary and not to do so where it is not. Congress has called attention in at least a general way to the kind of market failures that warrant intervention.

The Senate committee report on the planning amendments demonstrates that Congress has indeed arrived at a new perception concerning the permanence of the need for regulation. The 1979 report restates some crucial language from its 1974 report on the original planning law almost in the same words, but with a seemingly small amendment that reveals an altogether different conclusion about competition's future place. In its earlier report, in a much-quoted statement, the committee stated its view that "the health care industry does not respond to classic marketplace forces."[12] It has now restated that proposition as follows: "In the view of the committee the health care industry *has not responded* to classic marketplace forces [emphasis added]."[13] Underscoring its new perception, the committee repeats and amplifies the thought and goes on as follows:

> Despite the fact that the health care industry has not *to date* responded to classic marketplace forces, the committee believes that the planning process—at the Federal, State, and local level—should encourage competitive forces in the health services industry wherever competition and consumer choice can constructively serve to advance the purposes of quality assurance and cost effectiveness [emphasis added].[14]

---

[12] U.S. Congress, Senate, *National Health Planning and Resources Development Act of 1974*, S. Rept. 93-1285 to accompany S. 2994, 93rd Congress, 2nd session, 1974, reprinted in *U.S. Code Congressional and Administrative News*, vol. 1974, p. 7878.

[13] U.S. Congress, Senate, *Health Planning Amendments of 1979*, S. Rept. 96-96 to accompany S. 544, 96th Congress, 1st session, 1979, p. 52.

[14] Ibid., p. 53.

At another point, the Senate committee states its view that past policies in health sector regulation have been unduly neglectful of competition and declares its desire that the regulators avoid the vices of which regulators in other industries have been guilty:

> The Committee realizes that since initiation of the Act, the orientation of the planning process has become increasingly centralized, threatening to leave out competition altogether. With these provisions, the Committee introduces into the health planning law the recognition that planning agencies at all levels have as important a responsibility to promote competition among health care providers as the obligation to encourage cost containment, facility closure or shared services. The experience with other public regulatory authorities has been one of creating industry cartels which emphasize market stability rather than innovation and consumer preference. The Committee intends to protect against such tendencies in health sector regulation.[15]

Another amendment of the nonsubstantive portions of the planning law serves even more clearly to reveal congressional expectations about competition's potential place. To the act's already long list of "national health priorities," previously notable for the absence of even an oblique reference to competition, the amendments add a new priority as follows: "The strengthening of competitive forces in the health services industry wherever competition and consumer choice can constructively serve, in accordance with [section 1502(b)], to advance the purposes of quality assurance, cost effectiveness, and access."[16]

In keeping with this theme but on a more substantive level, the amendments set forth a new assigned function for health systems agencies, namely "preserving and improving, in accordance with section 1502(b), competition in the health service area."[17] This new affirmative duty to strengthen competition could serve as a mandate to HSAs to participate actively in the reform of the financing system, which would in turn permit command-and-control regulation to encompass a progressively reduced portion of the field.

The amendments' other substantive provisions bearing on competition take the form of two additional criteria that certificate-of-need agencies are to employ in their decision making. The first new criterion would have them weigh, "in accordance with section 1502(b), the factors which affect the effect of competition on the supply of health

---

[15] Ibid., p. 85.

[16] Public Health Service Act, §1502(a)(17).

[17] Ibid., §1513(a)(5).

services being reviewed."[18] Here the message is that the ability of the market to allocate resources of the type in question must be considered with care. The clear implication is that, if competition works reasonably well, the market should be left the allocative task.

The other new criterion would have the regulators consider "improvements or innovations in the financing and delivery of health services which foster competition, in accordance with section 1502(b), and serve to advance the purposes of quality assurance and cost effectiveness."[19] Again, the possibility of changes in the financing and delivery system, allowing the demand side of the market more effectively to discipline the supply side, must be a factor in deciding whether regulatory allocation is necessary.

The Significance of the New Regulatory Mandate. Taken together, the 1979 procompetition amendments to the Health Planning and Resources Development Act fundamentally alter the character of the health planning and certificate-of-need enterprise. Previously, the command-and-control mentality and the idea of allocating resources through central planning supplied the act's sole foundation. Now, the law embraces a mix of strategies and gives clear instructions to the planners and regulators that allocation by market forces is to be preferred if it can reasonably be expected to serve the public interest.

The significance of the new regulatory mandate can only be appreciated if one is aware that no other federal regulatory statute has ever been equally explicit and compelling in its mandate to promote competition. Only the Airline Deregulation Act of 1978[20] stands as a comparable effort to restore competition in a regulated industry. Surprising as it may seem, Congress has taken just about the longest step it could possibly take, at this time and under all the circumstances, toward deregulation of the health sector. Later discussion shows why this is true.

The procompetition language in the health planning amendments bears a close similarity both to President Carter's 1978 executive order directing executive-branch agencies to weigh the economic impact of regulatory initiatives,[21] and to several pending legislative proposals to extend similar requirements to independent regulatory agencies.[22] Al-

---

[18] Ibid., §1513(a)(11).

[19] Ibid., §1513(a)(12).

[20] Public Law 95-504, 92 Stat. 1705.

[21] Executive Order 12044 (March 23, 1978), 3 C.F.R., 1978 Comp., pp. 152–156.

[22] For example, the Carter administration's S. 755, Senator Abraham Ribicoff's S. 262, and Congressman Clarence Brown's H.R. 77, all introduced in the 96th Congress, 1st session, 1979.

though the similarity to these initiatives is substantial, the health planning amendments are much better calculated, and much more likely, to make a real difference in regulatory outcomes.

Because those other measures were triggered in large part by concern over the high compliance costs occasioned by some "social" regulation, they less clearly establish the restoration of competition as a paramount regulatory objective. Moreover, because the mandates in those measures are not aimed at any one industry, the regulators will find it easy to conclude that the message was intended for someone else. Finally, there has been considerable hesitancy to allow the courts to review specific regulatory actions in the light of these new instructions. Thus the message is largely hortatory, depending for its effectiveness solely on what it may convey to the agencies about the attitudes of their political overseers.

The health planning amendments, on the other hand, are specific to one industry, are enforceable in court, and reflect an emerging seriousness in Congress about competition in the health sector. Thus these amendments seem to be of a different order. Indeed, Congress appears to have departed from its customary practice of leaving the regulators' mandate vague and inconsistent, thus passing to them the burden of making the fundamental choices.

Though it seems incredible to state it, the only tenable reading of the language set forth above is that Congress has opted for competition, where it works, in health care. Congress, being Congress, will undoubtedly waffle on that choice in future legislation, but I believe that a real and salutary change of policy has occurred. That such a major policy change could occur without huge controversy is, I think, a tribute to the wisdom of the new policy and to its susceptibility to both market and regulation advocates. Other explanations of how this procompetitive language slipped through are harder to assess. Either the special interests failed to appreciate its implications or they believe a procompetition policy can forestall regulation and is the lesser of two evils.

The Regulators' New Mission. The aim of the procompetition language in the 1979 health planning amendments is that planner-regulators, before exercising their jurisdiction to limit entry and restrict competition in a particular category of health services, should assess the affected market's actual and potential ability to allocate resources of the particular type involved. If competition appears to be a reasonably reliable social control mechanism under all the circumstances, then regulation should foster it rather than supplant it by command-and-control intervention. Wholehearted acceptance of this simple conceptualization of the regulators' task would greatly affect the regulatory agenda, the nature of health planning, the substance of many regulatory decisions, and, in the long run, the nature of the health-care system as a whole.

Unfortunately, many agencies, faced with this radical restatement of their regulatory function, will probably continue business as usual, claiming that they have always had due regard for competition's potential but have found it minimal in most instances. Nevertheless, the new instructions will not be so easy to evade. Applicants will learn to frame their proposals in terms that require the agency to make reasoned findings on competitive impact. Moreover, courts can be expected to force the agencies to be explicit on such matters and to have substantial evidence to support their views.

Although the courts may insist that the regulators give competition a fair hearing, it would be unfortunate if the regulators accepted no more responsibility for competition than the courts require them to accept. Ideally, the agencies will make explicit their judgments on the market's efficacy, either in their health plans or in their recommendations and decisions on certificates of need, and will develop some sophistication in assessing the arguments on either side. There is no question that better understanding of the competitive process and its functioning under the peculiar incentives of this industry is required, but conscientious regulators, aided by new research, should be able to make progress in dealing with this new set of issues.

It would appear that the immediate issue in every certificate-of-need proceeding should be whether market forces sufficiently discourage, or do not unduly encourage, inappropriate investments in unneeded services of the type in question. But the step of assessing the workability of competition has usually been omitted. Presumably this has occurred because regulators assume that the competitive market is universally incapable of determining "need" for any of the facilities or services covered by a certificate-of-need law. The 1979 amendments invalidate this assumption. They require competition's efficacy to be assessed in every case. Indeed, the congressional committee reports make clear that subjecting a new facility or service to a certificate-of-need requirement creates nothing stronger than a presumption, rebuttable in specific circumstances, that the market has not been generally capable of allocating that category of resources efficiently. Moreover, although "need" has usually been thought of as a function of medical, demographic, and geographic factors, a new facility or service might also be "needed" as a competitive force without regard to other circumstances. Nothing in the state laws precludes interpreting the mandate of the agencies to include an assessment of the need for *competition*, and the recent amendments explicitly require such an assessment.

The crucial question that the planner-regulators must face is, of course, whether competition is desirable or not in particular circumstances. It is part of the genius of the 1979 amendments that they largely beg this difficult and controversial question, leaving it to be resolved in specific cases by the planner-regulators themselves. But the amendments undeniably reopen the previously closed question of competition's potential. The planner-regulators likewise have a responsibility to reopen their minds on the same question, even though it is a matter on which many of them have strong preconceptions. Unfortunately, as later discussion notes, it may take more than an act of Congress to make the health-care system's planner-regulators consider competition's possible efficacy in the industry solely on the merits.

Congress has provided some guidance for assessing when the market can responsibly be entrusted with allocative functions. The 1979 amendments state a preference for strengthening market forces "wherever competition and consumer choice can constructively serve . . . to advance the purposes of quality assurance, cost effectiveness, and access." Judged by customary drafting practice in regulatory legislation, this language, together with other signs of congressional intent, gives the planner-regulators a relatively concrete standard for deciding in specific cases whether or not to assert their command-and-control authority over market-entry and investment decisions by private actors. The regulators are to consider with particular attentiveness those conditions on the demand side of the market that determine whether price considerations are sufficiently reflected, either directly or indirectly, in consumer choices that the market can be counted on to balance all of the competing values reasonably well.

Thus actual or potential changes in health-care financing must be evaluated for their possible effect on the broader market's ability to discourage inappropriate investments.[23] These changes include not only the growth of HMOs but innovations in health insurers' benefit packages, their reimbursement and administrative practices, their relationships with providers, and their premium-setting techniques. The relevance of these factors is underscored by one of the 1979 amendments' new criteria for decision making, which directs attention to "improvements in the financing and delivery of health services which foster competition . . . and serve to promote quality assurance and

---

[23] For a discussion of how insurers might seek to control costs in a more competitive market, see Clark Havighurst and Glenn Hackbarth, "Private Cost Containment," *New England Journal of Medicine*, vol. 300 (June 7, 1979), pp. 1298–1305.

cost effectiveness." Because these new procompetitive directives to the planner-regulators appeared in the same legislation that created a broad exemption for HMOs, it is clear that Congress was not using competition simply as a code word for HMO development. Congress must have contemplated competition's specific relevance to services rendered under more traditional methods of payment.

The other new criterion introduced by the procompetition amendments requires the planner-regulators also to weigh "the factors which affect the effect of competition on the supply of the health services being reviewed. " This criterion calls attention to the specific characteristics of the service in question and its financing insofar as they bear on competition's impact and the need for command-and-control intervention. Among the factors that would influence the ultimate judgment are the scope and character of third-party payment for the given service, the service's discretionary or nondiscretionary character, opportunities for providers to inflate the cost of the basic service, the nature of the substitutes for the service in question (whether higher- or lower-cost), the value of nonprice competition as a stimulus to desirable improvements in quality and accessibility, and the presence or absence of a capital investment.

Another important factor for regulators to judge in deciding whether to interpose their own judgment in place of the competitive market is the amenability of the service in question to other forms of cost control. If the threat of higher costs could reasonably be expected to stimulate private health insurers to take protective action against the proliferation of expensive overutilized services, that threat could be viewed as a desirable stimulus to innovation and the emergence of market forces. Thus the planner-regulators might construe their new procompetitive mandate as a charge not only to let such pressures build but also to undertake educational and other efforts to assure that the private sector will respond to them in appropriate ways. The private cost-containment actions thus stimulated would strengthen the market pressures bearing both on the providers of the service in question and on other insurers, who would also have to take steps to address the cost problem. Even public programs could be regarded as capable of protecting themselves against abuses by various means.

I am currently working on a book that argues, among other things, that planner-regulators should regard stimulation of reforms in the financing system as an important responsibility and that the foregoing strategy of challenging financing plans to take over the cost-containment job is an appropriate one. Although it is controversial, this redefinition of the regulators' role opens up a path to measured introduction of market forces and to deregulation of local markets for health services.

Regulation has usually inhibited change, but the regulatory strategy recommended here would stimulate it. The Civil Aeronautics Board's aggressive deregulation of the airlines, prior to a legislative direction to deregulate, provides an example for health-sector regulators to follow.

Obviously, if one adopts an ideal view of regulation, it is easy to see it as inevitably superior to the competitive marketplace. But regulators' supposed strengths are often illusory. It is difficult to implement an ideal model of regulatory responsibility in a political world, to obtain the data necessary to make the model work, and to make sound judgments on the myriad factual issues and value choices presented. Indeed, the regulatory ideal is as irrelevant for practical purposes as is the textbook model of the free market.

For these reasons, the regulators must learn to limit their interventions on pragmatic grounds. They must sometimes defer to market forces on the basis of a realistic assessment of the comparative advantages of an imperfect market and imperfect regulation. Moreover, an agency might also sometimes decline to assume a command-and-control role simply because it has better things to do with the resources at its disposal. Even believing that it had something to contribute, the agency might still conclude that its limited resources would be better spent in other activities. The agency might, for example, seek to encourage local employers, insurers, and providers to participate in restructuring the financing and delivery system to reduce the need for regulatory controls.

Can Regulators Face Competition Questions on Their Merits? These proposals carry the assumption that regulators are not only wise and sophisticated but also free to pursue the public interest singlemindedly. The history of regulation, of course, suggests that this is far from the case. Therefore we must be concerned that regulators, who will still possess considerable discretion to suppress useful competition rather than encourage it, will not serve as a force for change in the direction of restoring the competitive marketplace.

Successful regulation of entry in the health care sector requires a mixture of toughness and liberality. Toughness is required in saying "no" to proposals for desirable facilities and services that, even though they would survive and be heavily used in an unreliably competitive marketplace, seem unlikely to add more than a little to the quality or benefits of medical care—not enough to be worth their cost. On the other hand, liberality is required where, even though duplication of services seems a danger and apparent needs are already being met, a satisfactorily competitive market exists and incentives are not too badly distorted.

Although the need for these regulatory postures is clear, there is good reason to fear that politically exposed regulators in the health care sector will adopt precisely the opposite stance. They will be liberal toward new investments in unreliably competitive circumstances and tough in excluding promising competitive developments.

It should be clear why, in a political world, regulation is more likely to restrain competition where it is helpful than where it is dysfunctional: Prestigious institutions and established provider interests can be appeased by such policies and would be offended by any other. Unless competition threatens provider interests, political support for its suppression will be weak. Moreover, where existing providers' natural impulse to grow can be gratified without harming their competitors, the claims of "quality," "need," and "fairness" will be difficult for a few cost-conscious voices to contest. Unable to resist these claims and protectionist pressures in many cases, planner-regulators will seek to demonstrate their backbone by stamping out "duplication" where competition is most threatening to providers. Even if some successes are achieved in curbing investments by existing institutions, the hardships thus imposed can be compensated for by curbing competition from outsiders.

Experience in other regulated industries underscores these fears. Such experience reveals the fundamental truth that protection from competition is the regulator's stock in trade, the currency with which he purchases cooperation and peace from the regulated interests. In the cooperative enterprise that is health planning—which in many places originated as a hospital cartel—the likelihood that history will repeat itself seems great.

Obviously, this is not the place to examine in depth the political economy of certificate-of-need regulation. There are substantial reasons to doubt that competition will always receive a fair hearing or be generally viewed by health planner-regulators as a constructive instrument. Nevertheless, there is also a significant possibility that the regulatory agencies in this industry have been structured in such a way as to ameliorate some of the problems that have been encountered elsewhere. For example, some steps have been, or can be, taken to address such common causes of regulatory abuse of the public trust as the excessively political climate of decision making, the regulators' special responsiveness to and protectiveness toward their regulated constituency, the lack of consumer representation in the regulatory process, and the weakness of the planning component in the agencies. In particular, the usual lack of precision in statutory mandates has been partly overcome in the 1979 amendments, and the political climate may increasingly support procompetitive regulation.

For these reasons and some others, I am inclined to take regulation at its face value in this industry and to urge upon the planner-regulators their responsibility for responding to the mandate that they have now been given. I expect a positive response by at least some of the regulators because I do not believe in predestination—we still cannot predict how specific regulators will perform their tasks. I also sense that many planners and regulators will recognize a good idea when they see it.

The key point is that only a minority of planner-regulators need embrace market forces as the vehicle for stimulating rapid and meaningful change in their health service areas. Out of this minority's creative efforts could come new ways of organizing and paying for health services that will then be available for use in other markets and in public programs. This is the way a few competitive HMOs found the loopholes in a provider-controlled system and paved the way for other private developments and major policy change. Because the planners and regulators are here to stay, it seems desirable that we appeal to their reason and open up their minds to new possibilities. I cannot help but believe that, in more than 200 HSAs, there are at least a few Alfred Kahns waiting to be unleashed on the task of responsibly deregulating this industry.

Confining Regulation's Scope by Legislation—
Coverage and Exemptions

Legislative decisions concerning the types of health-care providers, facilities, and services that are to be covered by regulation focus attention directly on the ability of market forces and competition to benefit consumers. Coverage of a regulatory law should ideally be determined on the basis of which mechanism—regulation or competition—has the comparative advantage in allocating resources efficiently. But coverage issues in health-sector regulation have not always been defined in this way. Until recently, it appeared that a strong presumption ran in favor of collective decisions on all aspects of the health-care delivery system. Apparently only the political power of particular interests stood in the way of comprehensive regulation of the system as a whole. Fortunately for competition, recent developments in federal legislation show that coverage issues are henceforth more apt to be faced with an eye to the utility of market forces. To the extent that particular providers are left out from under the regulatory umbrella, competition will have a surer opportunity to show what it can do.

It might be supposed that, because the planner-regulators have now been given a clear statutory mandate to foster competition, the coverage of a state certificate-of-need law would be largely inconsequential for competition. As we have seen, however, giving regulators a statutory directive to weigh competitive values is alone not enough to guarantee that competition will be given its due. Moreover, the administrative costs of regulation—to both government and private actors—are far from negligible. These costs should be avoided by imposing jurisdictional limits wherever regulation's benefits are less than certain.

McClure's Exemption Strategy. Walter McClure has recently presented a lengthy and well reasoned argument for employing explicit statutory exemptions as the crucial element in a mixed market and regulatory strategy.[24] Apparently despairing of ever overcoming the perversities of politically exposed regulators, he argues for a system in which statutory exemptions sharply distinguish those health-care providers who are subject to effective market control from those who are not. McClure specifies at length the conditions that would have to be met in order to qualify for such an exemption.[25] In general, he has sought to define and exempt those nonmonopolistic "health-care plans" that integrate the delivery and financing of care to a degree that is sufficient, in his judgment, to warrant a conclusive presumption that they not only face, but are organized to respond to, market pressures to contain costs. Thus, in other words, McClure seeks to generalize from the lessons of the HMO movement, expanding the definition of market-sensitive health-care plans to encompass more than the term HMO has traditionally included.

McClure's approach to promoting competition is attractive, but it may be too categorical to have much hope of success. A strong legislative bias exists, as McClure observes, in favor of treating all competitors uniformly, even if they differ in ways that would justify subjecting them to different regulatory regimes. Even if legislators could be persuaded to grant seemingly preferred status to certain providers, they would be inclined to delineate the exempt category by an extensive technical definition, thereby imposing new regulatory requirements such as appeared in the original federal HMO legislation. Thus, new regulation may be the price one pays for an exemption.

Another reason why legislators might not grant broad exemptions is that an unregulated competitive sector can be expected to erode the revenues of the regulated sector by "cream-skimming" tactics. Moreover, most of McClure's unregulated health plans would necessarily

---

[24] Walter McClure, "On Broadening the Definition of and Removing the Regulatory Barriers to a Competitive Health Care System," *Journal of Health Politics, Policy, and Law*, vol. 3 (Fall 1978), pp. 303–327.

[25] Ibid., pp. 307–322.

have many dealings with regulated providers. This contact would make it difficult both to maintain a clear line between the exempt and non-exempt sectors and to give exempt providers the freedom in acquiring inputs that their exposure to effective market forces would seem to justify.

In short, the legislature, in considering an exemption proposal, would face all of the same pressures, temptations, and technical arguments that regulators face when they are asked to tolerate competition and its implications. For these reasons, McClure's exemption strategy, while appealing, will be difficult to realize fully through explicit legislation.

McClure is certainly correct in advocating a broad exemption from regulation for those health-care plans whose market environment and internal organization warrant the conclusion that market forces can control their performance. One can insist, however, upon the parallel importance of those provisions in the 1979 health planning amendments that charge the regulators to have due regard for competition and its values. McClure's exclusive emphasis on the exemption strategy probably reflects a belief that, in a political debate on these issues, one should not concede that regulators ever could be trusted. His fear would be, of course, that the more radical exemption approach might be bypassed in favor of a change in the regulators' mandate that, as we have seen, could prove to be merely cosmetic, leaving the regulators in a position to frustrate desirable competitive change.

But, putting aside the interesting matter of how best to advocate the exemption strategy, the ideal legislative approach—assuming total deregulation is not an option—is obviously to write a certificate-of-need law embodying both the principles under discussion. Thus, a certificate-of-need law should have coverage provisions no broader than are needed to deal with documented market malfunctions *and* should include a strong mandate to the planner-regulators to intervene in a command-and-control mode only when necessary to suppress the symptoms of a true market failure and to pay at least equal attention to possibilities for correcting the market's remediable shortcomings. These two approaches to enhancing competition deal with somewhat different problems and should not be seen as mutually exclusive. It is reassuring to discover that Congress, in the 1979 health planning amendments, approached coverage issues in precisely this spirit. Congress accepted in a substantial way the McClure exemption approach while at the same time changing the criteria for regulatory decision making.

The HMO Exemption in the 1979 Amendments. Disregarding warnings in the literature that subjecting HMOs to certificate-of-need requirements would invite protectionist regulation and destroy competition,[26] Congress, in the 1974 legislation, required the states to enact certificate-of-need laws covering the creation of HMOs, their construction of new inpatient and outpatient facilities, and their introduction of new services. Even though reform-minded planners and regulators might have been expected to encourage HMO development, numerous HMOs encountered significant difficulties in obtaining needed certificates of need.[27] Even where the planners and regulators were not unfriendly, long delays and uncertainty added to HMOs' already considerable management problems. Moreover, the regulatory machinery allowed existing institutions and competing providers, actively represented in the HSAs and politically powerful, to delay approvals and often to impose burdensome requirements.

As it became clear that the predictions of the early critics were being realized, Congress began to give attention to amending the law to improve HMOs' ability to become established and grow under regulation. The 1979 amendments are a triumph for HMOs in their battle against overregulation. Where Congress had previously mandated that HMOs be covered, it now has moved to prohibit their coverage.

The Senate bill would have prohibited the states from imposing certificate-of-need requirements on the organization of new HMOs and on HMOs' introduction of many new services and construction of new outpatient facilities. As to HMO inpatient facilities and therapeutic and diagnostic equipment, the Senate bill would have provided special and highly favorable criteria for reviews in the case of applications by HMOs qualified under the federal HMO legislation.

The House bill went considerably further. It would have prohibited the states from imposing any significant certificate-of-need requirements on HMOs. Moreover, the House bill made no distinction between federally qualified HMOs and other ones. Indeed, it would have extended the exemption to any prepaid health plan whether or not included within any formal definition of HMO.

The House bill would also have extended the exemption to a non-HMO provider of health services if an HMO or other prepaid provider agreed to use the proposed new facility or service and provide at least 75 percent of the revenues from its use. The basic idea here was that, because the prepaid plans were forced by competition to be responsive to consumer needs and cost concerns, their judgments of

---

[26] For example, Clark Havighurst, "Regulation of Health Facilities and Services by 'Certificate of Need'," *Virginia Law Review*, vol. 59 (October 1973), pp. 1204–1215.

[27] Clark Havighurst, "Health Maintenance Organizations and the Health Planners," *Utah Law Review*, vol. 1978, no. 1, pp. 140–151.

need as reflected in their contracts with providers could be accepted as an adequate demonstration that a true need existed.

The language in the House bill first appeared in what was called the "Gramm amendment," named after Rep. Phil Gramm of Texas, a leading advocate of deregulation and of the introduction of market forces in the health-care sector. The Gramm amendment took a firm position, consistent with the McClure exemption strategy, of extending exemptions to any new investment validated by the demand side of the market. The amendment would have eliminated regulatory oversight with respect to any explicit and prospective purchasing decision made by a financing entity that served a defined group of cost-conscious consumers who had chosen the plan in a competitive environment.

The far-reaching Gramm amendment did not survive the House-Senate conference. The resulting legislation still retains, however, a broad exemption for HMOs of all kinds. A total exemption from certificate-of-need requirements is provided for all HMOs having at least 50,000 subscribers, thus permitting such HMOs to construct hospital and other institutional facilities and to acquire diagnostic and therapeutic equipment without restraint. An HMO qualifying for this exemption need not be federally qualified, and the applicable definition of HMO is an extremely broad one. The exemption also extends to a provider who has entered into a fifteen-year lease for the use of the proposed facility with a 50,000-subscriber HMO.

As to HMOs to whom the foregoing exemption does not apply, states are permitted to regulate only their institutional health services, major medical equipment, and certain capital expenditures. Special criteria are supplied for use in such regulation. These special criteria, drawn largely from the Senate bill, require the agencies to consult only the needs of the HMO subscribers, not to consider the effects of the HMO on incumbent providers. They also require regulators to approve the proposal unless existing providers are willing to provide the HMO with the needed services and facilities on reasonable terms.

The terms of the new law are complex, but their aim is to grant a total exemption for the creation of HMOs, for HMOs' construction of outpatient facilities, and for many other capital investments. Such regulation as is retained over smaller HMOs' construction of inpatient facilities and acquisition of diagnostic and therapeutic equipment (such as CAT scanners) is to be exercised in such a way that the HMO cannot be denied facilities that its members need.

Although this new exemption is broad, it might be assumed that the rejection of the Gramm amendment indicates a less than total willingness on the part of Congress to embrace the idea of unregulated competition under sweeping exemptions for market-sensitive health plans, along the lines of the McClure exemption strategy. However, the Gramm exemption was not curtailed because of doubt that market forces would discipline such plans and therefore adequately assure that unneeded facilities would not be constructed. Instead, the concern that prompted the conference revision appears to have been the possibility that the Gramm amendment could be used as a loophole. A sham HMO, by entering into a contract with a party wishing to build a hospital, could confer an exemption on that party even though the HMO would not in fact be able to follow through on its contract and actually use the hospital to the extent contemplated.

The concern was a valid one, for, once a hospital was built under the exemption and turned out to serve few HMO subscribers, it would be available for use by the rest of the community. Such a development might contribute to an excess of hospital beds and further cost escalation. The draftsmen's solution was to add the requirement that an HMO qualifying for the exemption have at least 50,000 subscribers, thus assuring that it is bona fide and could be relied upon to use the facility in question. As Senator Kennedy noted, Congress was concerned that "if you're going to call it a duck, it really is a duck."[28]

The HMO exemption in the 1979 amendments reveals in part the difficulty of carving out exemptions for unregulated health plans when those plans must have dealings with regulated providers. The amendments thus underscore both the value of the exemption strategy and its limitations. They also reveal, however, Congress's willingness to accept the argument that in many instances competing providers are sufficiently subject to market forces to obviate regulation. Indeed, the House committee report states that the exemption for HMOs was based "on the committee's belief that the supply of those services would not be excessive if they were not regulated and that market forces of supply and demand may appropriately allocate them."[29]

Thus, as innovation in financing plans and increasing competition among them increasingly permit the demand side of the market effectively to discipline the supply side and to discourage inappropriate investments, the appropriateness of regulation will diminish. Both through exploitation of statutory exemptions and through regulatory decisions to withdraw regulation in the light of new market conditions, competition should eventually be able to demonstrate that it deserves a major role in allocating health resources.

---

[28] "Health Planning Bill Awaits Final Congressional Action," *Congressional Quarterly*, vol. 37 (September 8, 1979), p. 1920.

[29] U.S. Congress, House of Representatives, *Health Planning and Resources Development Amendments of 1979*, H. Rept. 96-190 to accompany H.R. 3917, 96th Congress, 1st session, 1979, p. 53.

Other Coverage Issues in the 1979 Amendments. The health planning amendments dealt with other coverage questions besides the HMO exemption. The issue was not whether to drop a provision for mandatory coverage and to replace it with an outright federal exemption from state regulation for the previously covered service. Rather, the issue was whether to extend the mandatory coverage of state laws to encompass home health services and clinical laboratories. Both extensions had been vigorously urged by established providers of those services, whose desire to suppress competition was obvious, and by the planner-regulators themselves, who contended that wider power would improve their ability to rationalize the system. Congress rejected both proposals.

Although Congress's action leaves it open to the states to regulate market entry by home health agencies and clinical labs, the House committee report indicates substantial doubt that such regulation is appropriate. In its discussion of competition's role, the committee cites both services as being among those that would not be oversupplied in the absence of regulation and that the market could appropriately allocate.[30] The evidence would seem to support these views. Home health care is widely thought to be in short supply practically everywhere. Because it substitutes for inpatient care, suppression of its availability probably would raise costs rather than lower them. Clinical labs are also potential sources of economies that could be lost if regulation impairs growth or the appearance of new providers. Both services could benefit from quality improvements and innovation, which competition is likely to stimulate. Because home health care involves no appreciable capital investment and clinical lab equipment is highly mobile, both services are likely to disappear when demand is not forthcoming. In short, none of the plausible arguments for regulation are present, and it would seem wise for the states to decline to regulate. Although twenty or more states already regulate home health care, the new procompetition mandate to the regulators in the 1979 amendments would seem to compel them to adopt a laissez-faire attitude toward entry by competent providers.

What is striking here, as in the case of the HMO exemption, is that Congress now strongly rejects the idea, previously implicit in the health planning legislation, that planning and regulation are their own excuse for being. Congress has been consistent in using an exemption to preserve an unregulated sector where the incentives are clearly reliable. Moreover, it has issued an explicit procompetition directive to the regulators who must decide, in more complex circumstances, whether the

---

[30] Ibid., pp. 75–76.

market can do the allocative job. In every case, Congress is concerned with discovering whether a market failure exists and with confining the scope of command-and-control regulation to those specific circumstances where it does.

Conclusion: A Scenario for Deregulation

The 1979 amendments to the National Health Planning and Resources Development Act of 1974 may be viewed either as a symbolic gesture toward an idea—competition—that was in fashion for a short time in the spring and summer of 1979 or as a sign of a major shift in national health policy. It is too soon to tell which view is correct. But the substance of the change made in the regulators' mandate and in Congress's own stated view of the industry's problems can be neither denied nor ignored.

Because I think the idea of competition is a good one that will succeed if given a fair chance, I am inclined to be sanguine about the future. But predictions are precarious, and only perseverance will produce the long-run changes in the financing system that are essential before the market can assume a major allocative role. All that can be said conclusively at this point is that Congress has done a surprising and potentially significant thing and done it rather well. The burden of giving effect to the new policy now falls largely on the health-care system's planners and regulators. No one should have unbounded faith in them, but their mission, though changed in midcourse, is now fairly clear.

A final point has to do with deregulatory strategy. It would not be wrong to question whether regulation and competition, like oil and water, can ever really mix, even in a transitional period during which explicit deregulation strategies are employed. McClure's exclusive attachment to an exemption strategy may be based on a perception that one may have either regulation or competition but not both. Similarly, Alfred Kahn, our leading practitioner of deregulation, has reported how, as chairman of the CAB, he underwent "a conversion from a belief that gradualism is desirable to advocacy of something . . . close to total deregulation."[31]

What needs to be clarified is that the deregulation scenario that is envisioned in this paper, and for which Congress has set the stage, does not involve gradual relaxation of regulatory controls. Instead, it contemplates instant deregulation of particular health services as soon as market conditions make such action wise in particular markets.

---

[31] Alfred Kahn, "Applying Economics to an Imperfect World," *Regulation*, vol. 2 (November/December 1978), p. 20.

Unlike the airlines industry, health care involves many discrete services offered by local and largely immobile providers and facilities. Each service in each market area is a separate candidate for regulation or deregulation, with local circumstances most often being decisive. Where a broad statutory exemption is not appropriate in Congress's eyes, as it was for HMOs, the states may make their own judgments to cover or not to cover particular facilities and services. But, whatever a state does with respect to coverage, the planners and regulators are accountable under federal as well as state law. They are now bound to assess on a continuing basis the specific need for command-and-control regulation for each service in the light of both then-prevailing market conditions and potential market performance. A number of conditions remain to be fulfilled, but evolution toward the installation of the competitive marketplace as the chosen allocator of health-care resources is an increasingly realistic possibility.

Commentaries

Linda A. Burns

With the possible exception of cost containment per se, no single issue in the health care field seems to generate as much controversy among health providers and payers as the role of health maintenance organizations (HMOs) in both the financing and delivery of health services. Proponents believe that HMOs are the solution to much that ails our health care delivery system—rising costs, inappropriate utilization, uncoordinated care, and lack of consumer choice, to name but a few of the problems. Detractors believe that HMOs compromise the high-quality care that is rendered to individual patients as well as the primacy of physician-patient relationships.

It is clear that the real impact of HMOs lies somewhere between the extremes. The HMO movement is neither the panacea nor the culprit in our health care delivery system. It is equally clear that the HMO movement will have a major impact on hospitals, physicians, and insurers. Within the hospital industry, HMOs will not necessarily have an identical impact for each hospital. The same may hold true for insurers or physicians.

Within the context of this debate, Dr. Harold Luft contributes a solid piece of work that enables health policy makers to focus on the important issues of the role of HMOs in cost containment, competition, and national health insurance (NHI). In general, Dr. Luft provides an excellent review of the literature and summary of what we know and what we do not know about HMOs. He is appropriately guarded in his advice to health policy makers about extrapolating the results of selected HMO studies to the nation as a whole.

My purpose in commenting on Dr. Luft's paper is to share with you my perspective as a hospital administrator on how HMOs may be expected to influence the way in which health services are organized. I'll address the following points: the role of HMOs, the definition of HMOs, their performance, and the quality of their care. Additionally, I will offer observations on how behavior of individual hospitals may be expected to change in response to the introduction and expansion of HMOs within an individual community as a way of illustrating the role of HMOs in stimulating competition in the health industry. Finally, the current findings with respect to HMOs will be discussed in light of their implications for NHI.

Role of HMOs in Health Industry

Dr. Luft prefaces his findings by saying that the current interest in HMOs stems from their potential role in cost containment for the health industry. Much of the current interest in HMOs on a national level among health policy makers centers on the potential role of HMOs for cost containment, but HMOs play other important roles in the industry as well.

First, HMOs extend financing for a full range of ambulatory services—including primary care, ambulatory surgery, and subspecialty care that can be provided on an ambulatory basis. Because inadequate financing of ambulatory care remains an obstacle to expansion of ambulatory services, the way in which HMOs finance health care removes the financial barriers to the provision of additional ambulatory services to HMO enrollees.

Second, with respect to the opportunities to substitute ambulatory care for inpatient care, HMOs could be expected to hasten the acceptance of ambulatory programs such as ambulatory surgery. Because HMO plans extend financing for a full range of ambulatory services, physicians need not resort to hospitalizing patients to assure that the charges for the surgical services will be paid by the insurer rather than the patients through their out-of-pocket expenditures. Under many other third-party health insurance contracts, surgical operations that could be performed on an ambulatory basis are, instead, performed on an inpatient basis because the insurer will reimburse inpatient service charges and will not reimburse charges for an ambulatory surgical procedure. Patients and physicians will act to minimize the patients' out-of-pocket costs which results in hospitalizing many patients for surgery that technically could be performed on an ambulatory basis. HMO plans, by removing the financing obstacles to extension of ambulatory services, could be expected to hasten innovation and acceptance of new ways of organizing and delivering services in the health industry as a whole.

Third, health-care administrators are interested in HMOs for the ways in which HMOs have introduced an improved operating or management discipline to the health-care industry. Managing a successful HMO requires administrators to closely monitor utilization of

361

services, productivity, and clinical practice patterns. HMO plans must revoke or reduce medical staff privileges of physicians who do not practice cost-effective medicine or who practice sloppy medicine from a quality-of-care perspective.

Finally, consumers may look to HMOs for a variety of reasons. They may seek continuity of care as well as information about local health services. Should they enroll in an HMO, consumers can assure themselves that they will gain access to a variety of consultants or specialists. Consumers, then, may avoid the high search costs for medical services.

Certainly, some of these features are not exclusive to HMOs; nonetheless, HMOs do play a role in the health-care system other than cost containment.

Definition of HMO

Dr. Luft identifies the critical features of an HMO. The definition he uses allows considerable latitude as to what type of organization would be considered an HMO. In reviewing the critical features, several observations are offered.

1. "The HMO assumes a contractual responsibility to provide or assure the delivery of a stated range of health services, including at least physician and hospital services." In a broad sense, this feature is similar to service benefit contracts that are the basis of Blue Cross plans. Unlike indemnity contracts, which pay a dollar benefit, Blue Cross plans are service benefit plans. Although Blue Cross plans, as corporate entities, are not the providers of health services, Blue Cross plans do have contractual arrangements with hospitals (which are legally obligated as Blue Cross participating hospitals) to provide services to Blue Cross subscribers. An HMO plan, similarly, may assure the delivery of services through contractual arrangements with providers who are organizationally and legally distinct from the HMO corporate entity. This is not to say that the contractual responsibilities of Blue Cross plans and HMO plans are identical, but neither are they as dissimilar as one might first suppose. Other critical features of the HMO definition might also apply to service benefit plans.

2. "The HMO serves an enrolled, defined population." Blue Cross service benefit plans also serve a defined set of subscribers or patient population.

3. "The HMO has voluntary enrollment of subscribers." Regarding Blue Cross plans, participation is voluntary in the sense that an employee whose employer provides insurance coverage through Blue

362

Cross may choose not to participate. One suspects that Dr. Luft meant to emphasize instead the notion of dual choice; that is, prospective patients are able to choose between an HMO plan or other insurance plan, provided they are made available through the employer.

4. "The HMO requires a fixed periodic payment to the organization that is independent of use of services." Blue Cross plans require a fixed periodic payment independent of use of services. What Dr. Luft seems to have overlooked is that an overwhelming portion of the population has already chosen to prepay their health insurance premiums. The important question now is how providers (hospitals and physicians) will be paid; this is the feature which should be stressed in the definition.

5. "The HMO assumes at least part of the financial risk and/or gain in the provision of services." To understand the concept of HMOs, it is essential to recognize that what primarily distinguishes HMOs or more broadly defined alternative delivery systems is that the HMO plan, as a corporate entity, has contractual arrangements for not only the financing of health care but also the delivery of services. In one sense, both Blue Cross plans and HMO plans as corporate entities are at financial risk in the provision of services, because in either case excessive provision of services can lead to financial losses. However, the critical element for understanding HMOs is that the financial risk or gain is placed not so much on the corporate entity as a whole, as Dr. Luft states, but is passed through to the providers of the services (such as hospitals and physicians) whether they are organizationally and legally part of the HMO plan or are distinct and separate corporate entities. In other words, incentives are constructed for providers to efficiently produce health. Although there are some exceptions, Blue Cross plans have not typically passed the financial risk back to providers.

The way Dr. Luft describes the nature of the financial risk clouds the issue of how the financial risk of an HMO corporate entity is different from the financial risk assumed by a Blue Cross plan. It is more helpful to define the notion of risk in more detail so that one realizes that providers are at risk, not just the insuring or financing arm of the HMO corporate entity.

Finally, Dr. Luft's definition does not explicitly acknowledge the emphasis that HMOs have traditionally placed on providing and financing a comprehensive package of health services including critical care, acute inpatient care, primary care, health education, and preventive health services. Theoretically, HMO plans could be organized to finance and provide only a subset of the total range of health services, such as subspecialty services. But historically, HMOs have offered a comprehensive package of health services.

363

HMO Performance

Regarding the review of HMO performance, it is important to remember Dr. Luft's admonition: "There have been no randomized, controlled experiments that involve the assignment of a representative group of people to a wide range of health insurance plans and health maintenance organizations." But Dr. Luft adds additional evidence that health policy makers should be concerned about generalizing HMO experiences to the nation as a whole. His findings are as follows:

- HMOs report lower total costs.
- Costs are lower because of fewer hospital admissions.
- Costs are *not* lower because of efficiencies in production of hospital services in HMO hospitals and/or reduction in so-called discretionary or unnecessary surgery.

The significance of his findings is great and adds emphasis to the possibility that the cost savings attributed to HMOs may result from a predisposition of HMO physicians or HMO enrollees or both to use less medical care. In other words, the cost savings may *not* result from the financial incentives in HMO plans. All the allegations of lower hospitalization, which are the principal source for cost savings in HMOs, may not be reproducible if other providers or patients are shifted from the fee-for-service sector to HMOs.

Let me offer a hospital administrator's perspective on what changes one might expect in the mix of cases in HMO hospitals, production technology within HMO hospitals, and surgical utilization rates, if financial incentives were working.

Dr. Luft observes that available data show no differences in cost-per-patient day between hospitals controlled by Kaiser plans or Group Health Cooperative of Puget Sound and non-HMO hospitals. Regarding case mix, as a hospital administrator, on one hand I would expect that HMO hospitals might have a higher per-diem cost than non-HMO hospitals because an HMO hospital would be expected to have a higher proportion of sicker patients requiring a more intensive mix of services than would a non-HMO hospital. Theoretically, fewer ill or injured patients would be treated on an ambulatory basis as physicians attempt to substitute modes of ambulatory care for inpatient care.

On the other hand, if financial incentives were working, I would expect HMO hospitals to have lower per-diem costs for a number of reasons. An administrator of an HMO-controlled hospital would seem to be able to exercise greater prerogatives than in a non-HMO hospital in the management and scheduling of patient care activities because of the common interests hospital administrators hold with physicians in containing costs.

Under cost-based reimbursement systems for hospitals, there is little effective direct link between physicians and hospital administrators and few communal financial ties. Administrators are working to maximize revenues and minimize expenses of the institution as a whole, while physicians individually are attempting to minimize their own personal costs; this clash of objectives becomes evident in the daily operating decisions of the hospital administrator.

For example, one of the biggest operating problems of an administrator is implementing admissions scheduling to provide an even distribution of demand for ancillary services such as laboratory and radiology. Also, the levels and configurations of nurse staffing can be improved through an even distribution of demand for nursing services. In non-HMO hospitals, physicians wish to be assured that the hospital maintains a capacity—an empty bed that is appropriately staffed along with readily available ancillary services—to accommodate their practice patterns, which vary depending on office practices, teaching responsibilities, and research schedules. Physicians balk at modifying their own admitting practices—for example, shifting their admissions from Monday to Sunday and more evenly distributing their elective admissions throughout the week—even though these actions could result in lower operating expenses for the hospital as a whole.

In an HMO hospital, the financial incentives of the HMO plan would seem to bind the hospital administrator and physicians in a common objective of containing overall costs. Improvements in operating efficiency of the hospital might be more easily achieved under such a plan where the physicians' and hospital's financial gains/losses are more closely linked.

Besides the scheduling of admissions, other efficiencies in the production technology of HMO hospitals might be expected in the scheduling policies of surgical suites as well as the size of the pharmacy formulary.

Also, in comparing HMO hospitals and non-HMO hospitals, researchers should recognize that patient services are not the only output of hospitals; there are also education and research activities. Comparisons should correct for participation in teaching and research activities.

On balance, higher per-diem costs imposed by case mix may wash out any efficiencies gained from other management practices. However, it is important to know if there is evidence of this; future research is required in these areas.

Dr. Luft also observes that the figures for discretionary procedures do not appear to be disproportionately lower in HMO hospitals than the figures for all surgery. One would think that if physicians in HMOs were under incentives to reduce utilization, the physicians would act to first reduce discretionary or elective procedures before making across-the-board revisions in all surgery. This does not appear to be the case. This again leads one to question the self-selection of providers in HMO plans.

As an administrator, I would expect that HMOs would have much higher rates of ambulatory surgical procedures than conventional insurers or providers. Also, I would expect that some procedures that would be performed in an ambulatory surgical suite might be transferred to a lower-cost physician's office or examination or treatment room.

Again, the significance of Dr. Luft's findings cannot be overstated: Cost savings in HMOs may be the result of self-selection of providers or patients or both. If financial incentives were working, we should look for and find evidence of the factors listed above.

Another important observation Dr. Luft made is that there is little evidence that costs in HMOs are growing less rapidly than in the overall medical-care sector. This suggests that HMOs may not decrease or stop the escalating rate of medical-care costs.

The same pressures brought to bear on hospitals in the production of inpatient services—price of market basket of inputs, pressures to acquire new technology, increasing intensity of care—would also appear to affect HMOs. Thus the cost savings from HMOs are most likely to represent a one-time savings.

Quality of Care

Regarding quality, Dr. Luft states that the average HMO appears to offer care comparable to or somewhat superior to the average fee-for-service practitioner, but not superior to that of the better conventional settings. This conclusion overlooks the most recent review of the literature, which found more significant indications of improved quality in an HMO setting.

John W. Williamson, Frances C. Cunningham, and David L. Ward of the Health Services Research and Development Center of Johns Hopkins Medical Institutions reported that nineteen of the twenty-five qualifying studies found that overall, the general quality of HMO health care was superior to that in the fee-for-service or other setting to which it was compared. Six studies found HMO care to be of similar quality as that in the comparison setting, and none reported HMO care to be inferior overall.[1]

Competitive Impact of HMOs

Dr. Luft surmises that the most important potential role for HMOs under NHI is as a catalyst for cost-containment by conventional providers responding to competition for enrollees.

If there is any disappointment in Dr. Luft's paper, this is the section I would have liked to see expanded. I agree with Dr. Luft regarding the potential role of HMOs in sparking competition. I would go further and suggest that the competition will take place not only between HMOs and other providers—whether other HMOs, fee-for-service physician practices, or hospital sponsored ambulatory care programs—but also between conventional insurers and new alternative delivery systems. Before I elaborate on examples of expected behavioral changes among providers, specifically hospitals, I wish to draw attention to the nature of the competition I envision.

The competition will *not* be on a service-by-service basis as decided by an individual patient at the time of his or her illness or by the physician acting on the patient's behalf. Rather, the competition will take place between financing systems and between provider organizations and combinations of organizations for a defined population over a specified period of time. In other words, competition will be evident as insurers compete with other insurers as well as HMOs for enrollees. Providers (such as hospitals) will compete with each other to secure an HMO contract to provide patient services to an HMO plan's enrolled population.

Competition can be defined as a state of events in which many purchasers, though not necessarily all, exercise a real choice in the selection of alternatives offered by sellers. In the health industry, one may presume that competition has always existed; however, the form of competition has generally been a "nonprice" competition. Examples of this include the competition that hospitals engage in by the acquisition of new technology in efforts to attract and retain physicians for the hospitals' medical staffs. Hospitals thereby establish, maintain, and enlarge the patient base and patient days upon which they depend for revenues.

Now, however, with the expansion of HMOs, there exists interest

---

[1] John W. Williamson, et al., "Quality of Health Care in HMOs as Compared to Other Settings, A Literature Review and Policy Analysis," Johns Hopkins Medical Institutions, Health Services Research and Development Center (unpublished), April 1979.

in expanding the degree of price competition in the health industry. I should emphasize "expanding" because examples of price competition in the hospital industry already exist. For example, providers price competitively for contact lens services, plastic and reconstructive surgery, abortions, laboratory services, ambulatory surgery and other ambulatory services, and most recently "free-standing emergency rooms."

As a hospital administrator, I will predict some of the ways hospitals might respond to the introduction and expansion of HMOs in a community. First, however, it is important to differentiate the degree of hospital involvement with HMOs. One can view hospital involvement with HMOs as a spectrum. On one end, the hospital has the highest degree of involvement: The hospital invests its capital to develop an HMO, guarantees an operating subsidy, and structures the organization and governance of the HMO as a subsidiary corporation of the hospital. At the other end, the hospital may have a contractual arrangement to provide services to an HMO. These services could include inpatient services, ambulatory services, management services, purchasing services, laundry services and many more.

A hospital may or may not accept financial risk when contracting with an HMO to provide inpatient services. The HMO might pay the hospital billed charges, not a discounted rate. Also, every HMO needs a hospital, not the other way around, so many hospitals might forgo involvement with an HMO. Therefore, when discussing the role of HMOs in a competitive hospital industry, one should recognize the degree and type of HMO involvement with hospitals.

Before describing some of the behavior changes among hospitals that might be expected, I will describe why hospitals would want to become involved with an HMO. A hospital might view HMO involvement as:

- an opportunity to extend comprehensive health services to its community
- a way to offer consumers a choice in the way their health services are financed
- a way to demonstrate leadership in cost containment
- a means of attracting a greater market share of admissions or locking in its existing inpatient base
- a way to increase patient referrals to hospital-based physicians and fee-for-service subspecialists
- an opportunity to develop or upgrade existing ambulatory care programs
- a way to respond to pressure from organized businesses concerning rising expenditures

- a way to maintain a seat at the table in discussions about the future ways in which health services are to be financed and organized.

Before recent changes in the health planning legislation, some hospitals assumed that involvement with HMOs would yield more positive reactions from local health systems agencies in securing approval for other hospital projects. Now, with the special considerations for HMOs, some hospitals may be expected to pursue HMO involvement as a means to exploit the certificate-of-need exemption for HMOs. Here we are witnessing public policy makers going full steam ahead to encourage HMO growth. Meanwhile, Dr. Luft is saying, "proceed with caution." Things may not always be what they appear to be.

First, these developments say something about the inadequacy and ill-advisedness of selected regulation. Second, these developments underscore the recognition that hospitals, like other institutions, will act to further their own interests given the opportunity. Under the new health planning law, if a community wishes higher levels of hospital services, it will be much easier for HMOs or existing institutions with HMO affiliations to add capacity than existing institutional providers without HMO affiliation (everything else being equal).

Within the hospital industry, the major form of competition is expected to be among hospitals competing with other hospitals to secure HMO contracts for inpatient services. This will take time to develop and will parallel the growth of HMOs. As an HMO's enrollment increases and the HMO plan begins to account for a significant block of patient days for a specific hospital, the purchasing power for hospital services will be concentrated. Hospitals will engage in price competition by offering the HMO a discount on hospital charges—a contractual allowance similar to Blue Cross plans. Just as hospital administrators try to woo physicians with large patient practices, hospitals will seek HMO contracts. However, rate review activities in some states may inhibit price discounts for specific payers.

Many of the evils that are alleged to result from the market concentration of Blue Cross plans may be reproduced by HMOs, particularly in market areas where HMOs represent a significant market share.

Physicians also can be expected to be affected by HMO development. With the increasing supply of physicians, one would expect physicians to form competing HMOs. Discussion of these and other issues related to HMOs will be left to future forums of this sort.

In conclusion, Dr. Luft provides an excellent and useful summary, with caveats for caution in these areas. I think there are additional reasons to be concerned. I look forward to participating in continuing public policy discussions concerning HMOs, competition, cost containment, and national health insurance.

Joseph P. Newhouse

Economists, myself included, are toilet trained to believe in not only the efficacy, but also the desirability, of the price system. Most economists view health insurance as a subsidy that interferes with the price system and hence with economic efficiency; in the usual analysis, the social cost (welfare loss) of a subsidy increases as the square of its rate.[1] On the other hand, insurance serves to protect the consumer from the risk of unanticipated expense.

Cost sharing in a medical-care financing is thus seen as an attempt to compromise between the objectives of risk reduction and economic efficiency. Compared with full insurance, it reduces the rate of subsidy and its associated social cost, but it attempts to preserve most of the risk-sharing benefits of full insurance. Thus, it is not surprising to find Laurence Seidman advocating cost sharing and citing a number of other economists in his corner.[2]

Seidman takes up the issue of income distribution as well as that of economic efficiency. He assumes the desirability of low medical prices for low-income households, and therefore argues that cost sharing should be income related. His argument, in brief, is that uniform (nonincome related) cost sharing will either be so low as to be ineffective (and therefore economically inefficient) or so high as to be inequitable. He considers a regulatory strategy as an alternative to cost sharing, but dismisses it for several reasons, especially its inability to match quantities supplied to individuals with their demands. He advances income-related cost sharing as a way to enjoy both efficiency and equity.

Although sympathetic to Seidman's proposal, I believe he overlooks both theoretical and practical problems with income-related cost sharing. As a result, I believe that Seidman overstates his case, and that the desirability of income-related cost sharing is not nearly as obvious as Seidman's paper makes it appear.

Seidman treats the medical-care sector as an aggregate entity. Consequently, he misses the important problem that inpatient services pose for any cost-sharing strategy, whether income-related or not.

[1] This assumes a linear demand curve and the optimality of the initial (presubsidy) position.

[2] Martin S. Feldstein, "A New Approach to National Health Insurance," *The Public Interest*, no. 23 (Spring 1971), pp. 93–105. Martin Feldstein was probably the first economist to argue Seidman's general position to a policy audience.

Inpatient services, which include hospital and inpatient physician services, are the majority of medical-care expenditures, although they are incurred by only a small minority of consumers. They cause a difficult problem for a cost-sharing strategy because individuals' expenditures for inpatient services are frequently large with respect to their incomes; more formally, the expenditure distribution is very heavily tailed.[3] As a result, it becomes difficult to simultaneously keep the consumer from bearing substantial risk and still provide the consumer and the physician appropriate price incentives.

Consider first uniform cost sharing for inpatient services. A moderate deductible of, say, $200 per person per year will have minimal effect upon the demand for inpatient services. Practically everyone in the hospital will have expenditures in excess of such a deductible. Consequently, although the deductible may have some effect on admission decisions, it will have virtually none on decisions affecting cost per day—the most rapidly rising component of hospital expenditure—nor on those concerning length of stay. On the other hand, a deductible sufficiently large to preserve incentives (one of a size such that most hospitalized patients would not collect any insurance benefits) would impose a degree of risk that most consumers would probably pay a good deal to avoid.

Would the income-related cost sharing proposed by Seidman differ in these respects from uniform cost sharing? Seidman assumes it would, but does not back up his argument with any empirical analysis. Under Seidman's proposal some (probably nontrivial) fraction of hospitalized individuals will be fully insured for the last dollar they spend (that is, face a zero price at the margin). The number of such people will, of course, vary with the details of the insurance plan. The demand of these individuals, once admitted, will be similar to their demand if no cost sharing existed at all.

Most hospitalized individuals, however, will face a 20 percent coinsurance rate. Although such a rate would have some effect upon demand (relative to no cost sharing), the welfare loss from allocative inefficiency for those facing a 20 percent coinsurance rate would, on conventional assumptions, still be approximately two-thirds as much as with full insurance.[4] Adding in the additional allocative inefficiency

---

[3] For example, the coefficient of variation in the 1963 CHAS-NORC survey data for hospital expenditure is 3.3 and for surgeon in-hospital expenditure 4.3, but the corresponding values for physician office visits and prescription drugs are 1.6 and 1.7 respectively.

[4] This calculation assumes a linear demand curve and initial (preinsurance) optimality, and makes no allowance for the cost of the additional risk imposed by the 20 percent coinsurance. (Such risk would increase the two-thirds value.) It also assumes that hospitals' supply curves would not be altered substantially

from those facing a zero price at the margin, it becomes apparent that income-related cost sharing will leave most of the allocative inefficiency in the inpatient sector untouched.

Put another way, Seidman's view that his strategy would "automatically" check excess hospital capacity and "automatically" curtail wasteful duplication seems to overlook the great amount of insurance his proposal leaves in force. I doubt that the hospital sector would look much different with income-related cost sharing than it would with no cost sharing.

Consider now outpatient medical services. Here the distribution of expenditure is much less thick-tailed, and the argument for a cost-sharing strategy is correspondingly stronger. But for outpatient services, *uniform* cost sharing at relatively moderate levels (say $200 per person per year) may suffice to avert much of the allocative inefficiency without raising questions of equity that are overly troublesome.[5]

Although income-related cost sharing of the kind Seidman proposes should also avert much of the welfare loss, it appears to have significant practical problems that uniform cost sharing does not. For example, what is the ability of low-income families to use the income tax credit Seidman proposes? As I understand the proposal, low-income families with medical expenditures would have to file a tax return to obtain reimbursement. How many such families currently do not file? Might such families have trouble with the mechanics of this system?

Another potential practical problem that Seidman does not deal with is the definition of the filing unit. The IRS now allows the married taxpayer to define the taxable unit. Suppose a nonworking wife has considerable medical expenditure and files separately, claiming no income. Are her expenditures fully reimbursed? To avoid defeating the purpose of the plan in this way, could husbands and wives be required to file jointly? If so, how would separations and divorces be treated? Would partial-year accounting periods be defined? Could this be done and appropriate incentives preserved? What if a couple separates, gets back together, separates again, and so forth, all over a one-year period? Would the resulting administrative complexity be worth the expense? To avoid such problems, would husbands and wives be required to file as a unit for the entire year? Apart from any legal

---

by 20 percent coinsurance—that is, that the degree of competition would not be appreciably affected. I doubt that any increased competition resulting from 20 percent coinsurance would change supply curves by an amount sufficiently large to alter the overall conclusion.

[5] The Health Insurance Study is designed to estimate effects of cost sharing on demand and health status. See Joseph P. Newhouse, "A Design for Health Insurance Experiment," *Inquiry*, vol. 11, no. 1 (March 1974), pp. 5–27 for a description.

issues such a requirement might raise, it appears to cause potentially serious practical problems. What if a husband has deserted and cannot be located? What if the parties prefer not to speak to one another?

Although I think workable solutions can probably be found for such practical problems, the administrative issues raised by income-related cost sharing deserve serious attention. The costs of resolving these issues may seriously compromise any gains from an income-related system.[6]

Where does this analysis leave us? Although the issue deserves careful empirical study, I am skeptical that cost sharing, income-related or not, is a useful tool for the inpatient sector. By contrast, a moderate uniform deductible may be quite useful for outpatient services. Seidman's implicit argument that no nonincome-related deductible exists that both preserves economic efficiency and maintains equity is not at all obvious if one limits oneself to outpatient services.[7]

What kind of strategy seems desirable for inpatient services? I share Seidman's lack of enthusiasm for a regulatory approach, but the difficulties with all other strategies mean it cannot be ruled out of consideration a priori.[8] My own preference with respect to inpatient services is to experiment with schemes that vary premiums for insurance depending upon the inpatient provider selected.[9] Such schemes have

---

[6] An earnings-related system, as opposed to an income-related system, appears not to raise such practical problems. Seidman's desire to be equitable toward the low-income *employee* (my emphasis) could be met by an earnings-related system; clearly, however, distributional issues would remain for the population as a whole.

[7] Of course, equity, like beauty, lies in the eye of the beholder; some would find a $1 deductible inequitable. I doubt, however, that many families would find a $200-per-person annual deductible an impossibly onerous burden. To the degree such a problem is important, the appropriate remedy appears to lie in altered income maintenance programs of the type proposed to deal with the effects of the recent increases in petroleum prices.

Seidman also implies that cost sharing only for outpatient services could induce a nontrivial amount of additional hospital utilization—that is, that the cross-price elasticity is substantial. The evidence does not support this view. See Joseph P. Newhouse, "Insurance Benefits, Out-of-Pocket Payments, and the Demand for Medical Care: A Review of the Literature," *Health and Medical Care Services Review*, vol. 1, no. 4 (July/August 1978), pp. 1, 3–15.

[8] Incidentally, I think Seidman leans too heavily on the English analogy in his discussion of regulation. Seidman believes regulation inevitably becomes "hard line," but neither Canada nor Sweden can be so easily characterized as hard line, in that their expenditure per capita is not that different from ours (as compared with the United Kingdom). Seidman also exaggerates the consumer's inability to pay for more than the minimum under a regulatory strategy; he ignores, for example, the existence of private-sector medicine in the United Kingdom.

[9] Joseph P. Newhouse, "Medical Costs and Medical Markets: Another View," *New England Journal of Medicine*, vol. 300, no. 15 (April 12, 1979), pp. 855–856; National Commission on the Cost of Medical Care, *Report of the National Commission on the Cost of Medical Care, 1976–1977*, vol. 1 (Chicago: American Medical Association, 1978).

been proposed by Ellwood, as well as Taylor and myself.[10] An increased market share for HMOs is in this spirit, as are certain new insurance plans.[11]

These proposals all attempt to increase competition among hospitals, but raise important uncertainties that appear to require limited implementation to resolve. The key uncertainties relate to the magnitude of administrative costs and, in some proposals, the importance of incentives to discriminate against sickly patients.[12] If these problems are manageable, such a procompetitive strategy seems attractive.

John B. Reiss

Although he first suggests that competition and regulation might coexist in the health-services industry, Havighurst essentially decries the value of regulation, concentrating on advocating more competition. Havighurst does not explain the nature of the competition he espouses for the industry. Presumably he desires the outcomes derived from the economists' theoretical competitive market model.

The competitive model analyzes how people buy and sell goods and services (commodities); it generates a series of conclusions accepted as socially and individually desirable. Each consumer can buy a collection of commodities such that the last dollar spent on any one commodity gives equal satisfaction. A consumer cannot gain more satisfaction by purchasing something different nor by increasing saving. Sellers manufacture and sell commodities such that the last dollar spent on producing and selling another unit of any commodity cannot

---

[10] Paul M. Ellwood, "The Health Care Alliance," in *Report of the National Commission on the Cost of Medical Care, 1976–1977,* vol. 2 (Chicago: American Medical Association, 1978); Joseph P. Newhouse and Vincent Taylor, "How Shall We Pay for Hospital Care?" *The Public Interest,* no. 23 (Spring 1971), pp. 78–92.

[11] Seidman does not indicate how HMOs are to be handled in an income-related cost-sharing strategy. It seems best to allow those electing an HMO a tax credit equal to the actuarial value of the fee-for-service insurance plan. This preserves neutrality, but the credit would vary with income, which increases administrative complexity somewhat. For a description of a new insurance plan, see Stephen Moore, "Cost Containment Through Risk-Sharing by Primary-Care Physicians." *New England Journal of Medicine,* vol. 300, no. 24 (June 14, 1979), pp. 1359–1362.

[12] In the case of HMOs and Health Care Alliances, providers have an incentive to discriminate against individuals whose expected demands exceed their premiums. If such potential discrimination is an important practical problem, I doubt that it could be legislated out of existence. Although open enrollment could probably be successfully mandated, providers, if they wished, could be rude to sickly patients, keep them waiting, and so forth in a manner that seems prohibitively expensive to prevent.

produce more by being spent on another commodity. The result is that society's resources are used to produce and sell the maximum possible quantity of commodities and that set of commodities generates maximum consumer satisfaction. So all actors, making self-interested individual decisions, are as well off as can be.

Underlying the ideal results of the competitive model are some heroic assumptions. The income distribution resulting from all the transactions is taken as given, though the society could determine it inequitable for noneconomic reasons. There are sufficiently large numbers of independent buyers and sellers in the market that no person or group can affect any price. All the participants have perfect knowledge about the commodities and can communicate with everyone else about them. There is complete mobility of labor, geographically and among occupations. A buyer's satisfaction derived from any commodity is independent of anyone else's preferences or judgments. There is no uncertainty. When these assumptions are violated, varying degrees of market failure result.

In "real-world" economic activity, the assumptions of the competitive model are violated frequently. Havighurst identifies a number of reasons for market failure in this industry. For example, he writes that provider control of insurance has restrained the development of price competition and that can be remedied by antitrust enforcement. He states that union and employer negotiations concerning health insurance ". . . may define workers' interests differently than the workers" and that can be corrected by legislation. Havighurst uses these and similar examples to argue that market failure can be corrected by legislative action or antitrust enforcement. Rosoff[1] raises serious doubts about how far antitrust enforcement can go in balancing "fostering competition . . . (with) . . . promoting quality in health care through professional self-regulation."[2] Other causes of market failure, discussed below, suggest that legislative action also cannot be used to eliminate all market failure because the nature of the health-care market is quite different from that for other commodities.

One basic cause of market failure in this industry is the social policy decision that everyone shall have access to health care whether or not they can afford it. One function of a market is to ration; if people have insufficient income or wealth to purchase all the commodities desired, they must make choices. Making health care available without regard to ability to pay eliminates the need to choose between

[1] Arnold J. Rosoff, "Antitrust Laws and the Health Care Industry: New Warriors into an Old Battle," *St. Louis University Law Journal*, vol. 23, no. 3 (1979), pp. 479–80.
[2] Ibid., p. 478.

it and other commodities. Health care is given a zero effective price, so the demand-limiting function of the market is removed.

Seidman recognizes that "the regulatory strategy must try to control the consequences of a zero effective price to each consumer." As Seidman develops his model of consumer cost sharing for health care, he assumes that this social policy decision can be modified significantly. Because the political decision process reflects consumer and voter preference, the social policy decision arises from a market-like phenomenon and cannot be assumed readily changeable. Market failure resulting from zero consumer price leads to rising expenditures due to increased demand and due to cost effects, such as the expansion of hospital purchases discussed by Feldstein.[3] Consequently, if health-care expenditures as a percentage of gross national product are to be held relatively constant, a nonmarket control such as regulation will have to be exercised. This social policy decision clearly changes the availability of health care and consumer access to it compared with an unfettered market outcome.

Even if the social policy choice were reconsidered, it is unlikely that Havighurst's competitive market, an example being the Seidman cost-sharing model, would result. It is not clear that consumers voluntarily would choose to pay more than a zero price for their medical care at the time of delivery. Medical care is not like any other commodity. With the exception of certain elective procedures, patients do not choose medical care in the ordinary sense; it is a lesser of evils. Consumption of medical care usually involves pain, suffering, inconvenience, and personal risk. Generally the consumer has little knowledge of the problem to be solved, let alone the alternative solutions. Once the consumer has entered the medical system, most judgments about the consumption of the product are made by others.

Probably most important, a consumer is faced with high expenditure uncertainty and personal risk. While healthy, most consumers have no way of estimating whether or when a health emergency may arise, nor, if it should arise, what it might be. Most consumers anticipate an incident of medical care will be expensive. Consequently, consumers are likely to have a preference for somewhat higher insurance premiums to reduce uncertain but probably much higher reductions in future income. In addition, the consumer faces risk in the receipt of medical care, and any reduction of that risk through increased spending is likely to be seen as cost-effective by the patient and physician even if ex post it can be shown to have been ineffective.

---

[3] Martin Feldstein, "Hospital Cost Inflation: A Study of Nonprofit Price Dynamics," *American Economic Review*, December 1971, p. 855.

376

Frech notes "that where the Blues have more market power, they will induce consumers to hold more complete insurance." Perhaps the cause and effect are opposite; after certain income levels, full-coverage plans reflect consumer preference with respect to health care, uncertainty and risk. Pauly suggests that if: "an insurer could observe that state of a person's health, and pay a fixed indemnity based on the level of that state . . . the person would simply pay a fixed sum . . . (and) . . . would have no incentive to purchase medical care worth less than its cost." This suggestion ignores the fact that insuring against uncertainty and risk has a positive value seldom included in actuarial assessments of benefits. Many arguments discussing "overinsurance" and "moral hazard" that favor the development of competitive market approaches ignore the elements of market failure identified here.

Seidman follows a line of reasoning similar to that of Frech and Pauly by suggesting that consumers participate in health maintenance organizations (HMOs) because they are willing to take fewer services. An equally credible argument is they join so they can obtain all the services they may need for a fixed payment. Indeed, Luft indicates there is no clear evidence HMOs are cost reducing, and even the initial reduction in expenditures for enrollees compared with community performance may result from causes which do not reduce total system costs. In a recent news article,[4] a Washington, D.C., HMO indicated it substitutes queuing by time for other forms of rationing because consumers have comparatively unlimited demand for health care when the effective price is zero. That action of the HMO is a form of private regulation.

The discussion above has suggested that all the heroic assumptions mentioned earlier are violated in this industry: market failure is endemic. In circumstances of market failure, fostering competition does not necessarily generate desirable results. For example, it is agreed generally that hospitals compete to add physicians to their staffs. To facilitate this competition, hospitals add to their technological and bed capacity, and construct amenities. Those activities lead in many places to the creation of excess capacity, unnecessary duplication of high technology medical services, and higher costs.

Such nonprice competition may be aided by the coverage and cost reimbursement policy of Medicare and Medicaid and a lack of conventional market pressures created by the full insurance coverage provided in the free market. Some government policies that encourage these results might and should be eliminated; for example, cost reimburse-

---

[4] B. D. Colen, "Group Health Plan Uses Delays to Control Costs," *Washington Post*, October 3, 1979.

ment could be changed to a pricing policy. However, the full coverage and small cost sharing are argued above to result from consumer preference; hence they are unlikely to change. Consequently, "competition" may induce perverse results in this industry.

Promoting insurance premium competition, advocated as a substitute to the more usual price competition[5] does not help, given the hypotheses of this paper. The more likely result is competition in the form of more expansive insurance coverage. Although premium competition for a given scope of coverage is not opposed, it is unlikely to solve the rationing problem and lead to significant reductions in expenditure.

In other markets in the U.S. economy there is lack of information, sometimes interdependence of buyers and sellers, and other causes of market failure. In none is there such a complete breakdown of the conditions necessary for some form of competition to exist as in the health-care industry. Consequently, the only way to resolve the conflict between the expansive demand for the product of this industry and its finite resources is use of a nonmarket tool: regulation.

Regulations are but one part of a legal structure. Regulations are written to implement statutory requirements established by the legislature. The prescriptions and limitations of the statute set the general approach for the regulations. For example, the Social Security Act requires Medicare and Medicaid to pay reasonable, actual costs. This requirement has been interpreted to preclude recognition of efficient economic behavior by permitting profit margins or other economic incentives. Therefore, if regulation is to act in place of nonexistent market forces, the statutes have to be drawn carefully.

Havighurst presents various regulatory problems which arise "in a political world." Regulations of a command, control, and punish nature can lead to such problems. There is a notion at large that regulation only can be command, control, and punish. Heath-care regulations typically have taken this form, but it is not the only possible choice. Regulations could provide rewards for undertaking desired activities and establish incentives that generate competitive behavior leading to market-like results. Examples are given below.

There are problems with the present federal regulatory scheme. Statutes authorizing particular programs sometimes conflict in their implementation instructions. For example, there are inconsistent statutory requirements applied to HMOs by the Public Health Service Act

---

[5] For example, Walter McClure, "A Comprehensive Market and Regulatory Cost Containment Strategy for Health Care," a draft paper prepared for the U.S. Department of Health, Education, and Welfare, Bureau of Health Planning and Resources Development, p. II–9.

and the Social Security Act.[6] Agencies regulating the industry frequently do not concern themselves with each others' programs. For example, while the Department of Health, Education, and Welfare is making considerable strides in coordinating the activities of Medicare, Medicaid, quality control programs, health planning, and related regulatory activities, in the past those concerned with solving payment problems did not consider the effect of their regulation on quality and so forth. Indeed, I would describe current practices as ad hoc anecdotal regulation: each regulation, rational in itself, is designed to solve a particular problem but not part of any carefully designed policy for the health-care system as a whole.

A rational regulatory scheme should be based on a clear articulation of national health policy. Because there are many competing interests in this industry, establishing policies concerning the use of the resources the nation devotes to health care will set the stage for regulatory programs.

There are also many competing goals to be achieved within the health-care system. These include the desire to limit resource use on the one hand and, on the other, to improve access for all people needing care; the need for low-cost efficient production and, at the same time, the need for high-quality services; the need to reduce the rate of increase of health costs and the need to broaden the spectrum of care provided.

Without a market to implicitly make these decisions, the forum provided by the legislative and regulatory processes permits competing preferences to be heard. The conclusions drawn by policy makers from those public debates should form the basis for regulatory actions. Regulatory actions, being based on policy compromises made among competing interests and goals, would have more likelihood of being consistent across various agencies. Regulatory conflicts would be easier to resolve in the light of established policies. For example, a clear policy regarding cost versus quality could eliminate certain regulatory inconsistencies, such as limiting nursing home expenditures to a historic cost base and at the same time raising quality standards and hence future costs.

Discussion of the competitive market model provides an interesting pointer for regulatory activities. In the market, people act in their perceived best interest. The "invisible hand" of the market "weighs" the competing interests and goals, distributing income and allocating

---

[6] John B. Reiss, Fred Hellinger, Iris M. Croft, Susan Pettey, Paul Pryor and Lisa Potetz, "An Analysis of Regulations Affecting Health Maintenance Organizations," Office of Health Regulation, Health Care Financing Administration, U.S. Department of Health, Education, and Welfare, September 5, 1979.

resources without apparent conflict. A statutory-regulatory system weighs the interests and goals in public discussion. As that is accomplished, a regulatory scheme could return the decision process, where possible, to a market-like environment. Rather than instruct "regulatees," regulations could provide rewards for behaving in accordance with the public policy. There would have to be an element of command, control, and punishment to regulations; where relevant, this element should apply to the transgressor, not everyone. Three examples follow.

The state of New Jersey is about to implement a payment scheme for hospitals based on payment for the case.[7] That scheme establishes a reasonable price per case for providing patient care, identifies the product, and motivates hospitals to improve their efficiency by allowing them to retain savings resulting from such efforts. Because the care is defined in medical and financial terms, the program not only provides economic incentives for the efficient provision of needed services, but virtually requires communication among physicians, administrators, and financial managers to solve problems, giving them a language they all understand. The program permits linkage of payment and quality so professional standards review organizations can ensure economic efficiency does not reduce the quality of care. Eventually it should be possible to develop criteria useful for planning decisions related to the case data, thus linking all the regulatory activities.

For the first time, patients will have price information related to a comprehensible product. That would not solve the entire information problem, but it would provide an important missing piece. Even if that knowledge did not lead patients to the least expensive institution, public knowledge of significant differences in cost among hospitals for the care of similar cases would raise the level of inquiry and put pressure on hospitals to provide care more efficiently in the long run.

A second example involves regulations concerning survey and certification of providers for participation in Medicaid and Medicare. Present rules require surveys be done every year for nursing homes and many hospitals.[8] This not only adds expense to facilities' operations, but causes problems for state survey agencies. State agencies usually have limited resources and cannot both follow up effectively with poor-quality facilities and continue unnecessary inspections of those of high quality.

---

[7] See John B. Reiss, Michael J. Kalison, Robert A. Knauf, Russell P. Catterinichio and Leo K. Lichtig, *A Prospective Reimbursement System Based on Patient Case-Mix for New Jersey Hospitals*, 8 volumes, New Jersey State Department of Health under HEW/HCFA contract number 600-77-0022, 1976–78; John B. Reiss, "A Conceptual Model of the Case-Based Payment Scheme for New Jersey Hospitals," *Health Services Research*, forthcoming, Summer 1980.

[8] 42 CFR 405 Subpart S.

An agency should be able to establish a survey program having incentives for the provision of high-quality care to patients. As an example, if a nursing home had a track record of excellent care over a series of years, it could be permitted to enter into provider agreements annually without a requirement for resurveying every year. Resurveying might be done once every three years, with provision for spot surveys to ensure no falling away from previous high standards. However, for the home with a poor track record, surveying might be completed once a month or even more often. The poor homes would experience increased surveillance and aggravation with no concomitant increase in payments, so the incentive for them to provide better quality care and eliminate the cost and hassle would be significant.

A third example relates to the health planning and certificate-of-need process. If a pricing system were established, such as that based on the case, it would be possible to eliminate control of market entry, at least for primary- and secondary-care services. It might still be necessary to maintain market-entry controls for tertiary services, because their regional distribution greatly affects their accessibility and availability to various population groups. General market-entry controls are inconsistent with a regulatory scheme for promoting resource allocation using economic and market-type incentives. The removal of controls implies we must let providers leave the market if they cannot compete at the set price.

These proposals, and similar ones, require changes in the present regulatory scheme. Some also may require statutory change—for instance, providing for significant economic incentives in Medicare and Medicaid payments. If market advocates agree that market failure is as severe as I suggest, they would be better off devoting their energy to promoting a statutory base permitting use of economic incentives in a "procompetitive" regulatory scheme than tilting at the windmill of "free competition."

Selected AEI Publications

AEI Associates Program